Perspectives in Exercise Science
and Sports Medicine: Volume 7

Physiology and Nutrition for Competitive Sport

Edited by

David R. Lamb, Ph.D.
The Ohio State University

Howard G. Knuttgen, Ph.D.
Pennsylvania State University

Robert Murray, Ph.D.
The Gatorade Company

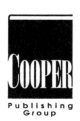

COOPER
Publishing
Group

33065665

Library of Congress Cataloging in Publication Data:
LAMB, DAVID R., 1939–
PERSPECTIVES IN EXERCISE SCIENCE AND SPORTS MEDICINE
VOLUME 7: PHYSIOLOGY AND NUTRITION FOR COMPETITIVE SPORT

Cover Design: Gary Schmitt

Library of Congress Catalog Card number: 88-70343

ISBN: 1-884125-09-3

Printed in the United States of America by Cooper Publishing Group, 1048 Summit Drive, Carmel, IN 46032
10 9 8 7 6 5 4 3 2 1

Contents

Contributors

Oded Bar-Or, M.D.
Chedoke Hospital
McMaster University
Hamilton, ON L8N 3Z5
CANADA

Ulf Bergh, Ph.D.
National Defence Research
Establishment
Department of Human Studies
Sundbyberg
S-172 90 SWEDEN

Edmund R. Burke, Ph.D.
3240 Wade Court
Colorado Springs, CO 80917

Priscilla M. Clarkson, Ph.D.
Department of Exercise Science
University of Massachusetts
Boyden Building
Amherst, MA 01003

Edward F. Coyle, Ph.D.
Human Performance Laboratory
Belmont Hall-Room 222
The University of Texas at Austin
Austin, TX 78712

J. Mark Davis, Ph.D.
Department of Exercise Science
School of Public Health
University of South Carolina
Columbia, SC 29208

E. Randy Eichner, M.D.
Section of Hematology
University of Oklahoma
Health Sciences Center
Oklahoma City, OK 73190

Björn Ekblom, Ph.D.
Karolinska Institute
Dept. of Physiology III
P.O. Box 5626
S-114 86 Stockholm
SWEDEN

Carl Foster, Ph.D.
Sinai Samaritan Medical Center
950 N. 12th Street
Milwaukee, WI 53233

George Gandy, M.Sc.
Department of Physical Education,
Sports Science, & Recreation
Management
Loughborough University
Loughborough, Leics., LE11 3TU
ENGLAND, UK

Carl V. Gisolfi, Ph.D.
Department of Exercise Science
N420 Field House
University of Iowa
Iowa City, IA 52242

Steven Gregg, Ph.D.
The Quaker Oats Company, Europe
Avenue des Pléiades 11
B-1200 Brussels
BELGIUM

Frederick Hagerman, Ph.D.
Dept. of Zoology & Biomedical Science
Ohio University
Athens, OH 45701

Craig A. Horswill, Ph.D.
Dept. of Endocrinology
Childrens Hospital
700 Children's Drive
Columbus, OH 43205

Mitchell Kanter, Ph.D.
Gatorade Exercise Physiology
Laboratory
The Quaker Oats Company
617 West Main Street
Barrington, IL 60010

Howard Knuttgen, Ph.D.
Center for Sports Medicine
117 Ann Building
Pennsylvania State University
University Park, PA 16802

L. Perry Koziris, M.A.
Center for Sports Medicine
117 Ann Building
Pennsylvania State University
University Park, PA 16802

William J. Kraemer, Ph.D.
Center for Sports Medicine
117 Ann Building
Pennsylvania State University
University Park, PA 16802

David R. Lamb, Ph.D.
School of Health, Physical Education, &
Recreation
The Ohio State University
129 Larkins Hall
337 West 17th Avenue
Columbus, OH 43210

Ronald J. Maughan, Ph.D.
University Medical School
Dept. Environmental/
Occupational Medicine
Foresterhill
University of Aberdeen
Aberdeen AB9 2ZD
SCOTLAND

Robert Murray, Ph.D.
Gatorade Exercise Physiology
Laboratory
The Quaker Oats Company
617 West Main Street
Barrington, IL 60010

Ethan R. Nadel, Ph.D.
John B. Pierce Foundation Laboratory
Yale University School of Medicine
290 Congress Avenue
New Haven, CT 06519

Ronald Rogowski, Ph.D.
Gatorade Exercise Physiology
Laboratory
The Quaker Oats Company
617 West Main Street
Barrington, IL 60010

Ann C. Snyder, Ph.D.
Dept. of Human Kinetics
423 Enderis Hall
Milwaukee, WI 53201

Lawrence Spriet, Ph.D.
School of Human Biology
University of Guelph
Guelph, Ontario N1G 2W1
CANADA

Dieter Strass, Ph.D.
Institute for Sports and Sport Science
University of Freiburg
Schwarzwaldstr. 175
7800 Freiburg i. Brsg.
GERMANY

John R. Sutton, M.D.
Dept. of Biological Sciences
Cumberland College of Health Sciences
University of Sydney
P.O. Box 170
Lidcombe, NSW
AUSTRALIA 2141

Ronald L. Terjung, Ph.D.
Department of Physiology
SUNY Health Science Center
766 Irving Avenue
Syracuse, NY 13210

Todd A. Trappe, M.S.
International Center for Aquatic
Research
1750 East Boulder Street
Colorado Springs, CO 80909

John P. Troup, Ph.D.
P.O. Box 1338
Groton, CT 06340

Clyde Williams, Ph.D.
Department of Physical Education,
Sports Science, & Recreation
Management
Loughborough University
Loughborough, Leics., LE11 3TU
ENGLAND, UK

Acknowledgement

The Gatorade Company is proud to support the continuing series of scientific texts published as *Perspectives in Exercise Science and Sports Medicine*. As with the preceding six volumes of *Perspectives*, this book resulted from the annual Gatorade Sports Science Institute Scientific Conference. The 1993 conference on *"Physiology and Nutrition for Competitive Sport"* involved top exercise scientists in a discussion of the scientific and practical aspects of sports physiology and nutrition. We hope that you find this text to be a valuable addition to your professional library.

Congratulations to the authors, reviewers, and editors for a job well done.

James F. Doyle
President
Gatorade—Worldwide

Foreword

Founded in 1954, the American College of Sports Medicine (ACSM) is the world's largest scientific society dedicated to exercise science and sports medicine. One of ACSM's key objectives is to promote dissemination of the current body of knowledge concerning safe and successful participation in competitive sport. Accordingly, as president of the College, I am very pleased and proud to welcome Volume 7 of *Perspectives in Exercise Science and Sports Medicine* to the scientific literature.

I commend Drs. Lamb, Knuttgen, and Murray, the editors of this important volume, for their excellent work in designing a book that addresses an important and timely issue. In addition, I congratulate them for assembling a team of authors who are the world's experts on their respective topics.

Finally, I wish to express my appreciation to the Gatorade Sports Science Institute (GSSI) for its longstanding and highly significant commitment to exercise science. GSSI's direct contributions to the field have been many and important. Furthermore, its support of numerous projects of the American College of Sports Medicine has advanced the College's development over the past decade. This volume is the latest in a long series of outstanding scientific products that have been generated through the sponsorship of the Gatorade Sports Science Institute.

Russell R. Pate, Ph.D.
President
American College of Sports Medicine

Preface

Since 1988, the various volumes in the **Perspectives in Exercise Science and Sports Medicine** series have addressed a wide range of topics related to the responses and adaptations of human beings to exercise. These volumes have been organized in terms of either a category of activity (prolonged exercise), a particular population group (youth), a physiological mechanism (fluid homeostasis, thermoregulation, energy metabolism), or a unique feature of physical performance (ergogenics). Each of the six previously published volumes has considered the human organism engaged in a combination of vocational tasks, conditioning activities, competitive sports, and laboratory experiments.

The Sports Medicine Review Board of the Gatorade Sports Science Institute organizes and sponsors the conferences that foster the series. Therefore, it was only fitting that a volume specifically focused on competitive sport be produced for the series. In this regard, the Institute decided not to consider sport as a general grouping of activities, but rather to address selected sports independently in the form of unique chapters.

Very few books and monographs exist in which the biological aspects of sport activity are examined and discussed in a comprehensive and extensive fashion. The aim of the author of each chapter in this volume was to complete an exhaustive review of the literature of a particular sport and to synthesize the important information into a manuscript that would be of great interest and use to scientists and coaches alike.

The sport activities of weightlifting, sprinting, swimming, wrestling, skating, rowing, road and track cycling, distance running, and cross-country skiing were selected and assigned to individual authors, each of whom had experience and expertise in conducting research in the respective activities. In most cases, the persons were not only qualified as respected scientists but they also had extensive practical experience as consultants to the governing bodies of the particular sports in their respective countries.

Successful performance in competitive sport is dependent upon the genetic potential of the athlete, individual strategy, group strategy in team events, physical conditioning, and nutrition. Conditioning can be further separated into exercises and activities designed to enhance strength, anaerobic power and capacity, and aerobic power and capacity. Genetic potential is considered in terms of the anatomical and physiological dimensions and capacities that each sport requires. Also discussed are the appropriate physiological preparation for competition and the optimal nutritional strategies for periods of training and for competitive events.

This volume is the final product of a conference entitled "Physiology and Nutrition for Competitive Sport" conducted in Rancho Bernardo, California, during the summer of 1993. The conference and the publication of the book are sponsored by the Gatorade Company with the proceeds from the sale of the book donated to the American College of Sports Medicine Foundation.

We are confident that the material presented in this volume represents the most accurate and comprehensive review of the available research on the many sport activities included. It is our hope that the presentation and discussion of this information will serve as a stimulus to the readers to play a part in the advancement of knowledge concerning the scientific basis of performance in competitive sport.

As usual, Kathryn Bowling and her associates at McCord Travel Management did a superb job of organizing the travel and many wonderful events in California. We are exceedingly grateful for their efforts. Our particularly heartfelt gratitude is extended to Joan Seye and Betty Dye for doing such great work in transcribing the discussions that appear at the end of each chapter. Finally, we acknowledge the contribution made by Ronald Terjung, who organized the manuscripts that became the introductory chapter.

David R. Lamb
Howard G. Knuttgen
Robert Murray

Introduction to Physiology and Nutrition for Competitive Sport

EDWARD F. COYLE, Ph.D.

LAWRENCE SPRIET, Ph.D.

STEVEN GREGG, Ph.D.

PRISCILLA CLARKSON, Ph.D.

FUNDAMENTAL PRINCIPLES

Among the principles common to each of the sports discussed in this book are those underlying the application of power against resistance or drag, the supply of energy by anaerobic mechanisms, and the development of optimal programs for training and nutrition. While some of these principles are discussed in each chapter in the context of each specific sport, it is possible to become justifiably so engrossed within the confines of the sport that the general physiological and nutritional principles are not always apparent. The purpose of this introduction is to briefly review some of these important principles in hopes that their applications in subsequent chapters may be more clear.

SPORT PERFORMANCE: SUSTAINABLE POWER OUTPUT VERSUS RESISTANCE OR DRAG

Success in running, swimming, bicycling, speed skating, rowing, and cross-country skiing involves propeling an athlete's body for a given distance. In the case of Olympic weightlifting and power lifting, success is determined by how much weight can be lifted in the appropriate movements, whereas a wrestler is judged by the degree of physical control over the opponent. These sports are quite different in terms of the patterns of muscle recruitment, the force and power produced, and the equipment used, e.g., bicycles, rowing shells, and barbells. Nevertheless, success in all of these seemingly diverse sports is a function of the rates of muscular energy production and the efficiency and skill with which that energy is directed against resistance or drag.

Resistance and Drag

As shown in Figure I-1, performance in sport is a function of the power output that can be sustained by the athlete throughout the competitive event relative to the resistance or drag that must be overcome. The nature of the resistance or drag (friction) that must be overcome by the athlete will, of course, vary according to the nature of the sport and the velocity at which the body moves through air or water. A weightlifter or power lifter must apply power to overcome the gravitational resistance offered by the barbell; the wrestler must apply power to overcome the

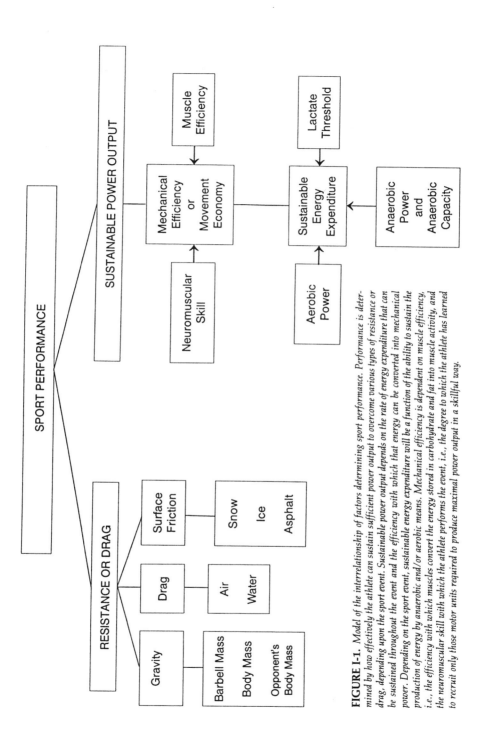

FIGURE I-1. Model of the interrelationship of factors determining sport performance. Performance is determined by how effectively the athlete can sustain sufficient power output to overcome various types of resistance or drag, depending upon the sport event. Sustainable power output depends on the rate of energy expenditure that can be sustained throughout the event and the efficiency with which that energy can be converted into mechanical power. Depending on the sport event, sustainable energy expenditure will be a function of the ability to sustain the production of energy by anaerobic and/or aerobic means. Mechanical efficiency is dependent on muscle efficiency, i.e., the efficiency with which muscles convert the energy stored in carbohydrate and fat into muscle activity, and the neuromuscular skill with which the athlete performs the event, i.e., the degree to which the athlete has learned to recruit only those motor units required to produce maximal power output in a skillful way.

resistance supplied both by gravity and by the muscular contractions of the opponent; neither lifters nor wrestlers are significantly affected by resistance offered by the air or water through which their bodies move. On the other hand, runners, swimmers, rowers, skaters, cyclists, and cross-country skiers must supply power to overcome the friction offered by air, water, ice, snow, and road or track surfaces.

Air and Water Drag

Resistance and drag forces are what the athlete must overcome, so it is sometimes appropriate to normalize power production according to the factor presenting most of the resistance. For example, bicycling power should often be normalized to cycling velocity because on a flat course when cycling at speeds greater than 13 km/h, most of the resistance to the power generated by a cyclist is created by the air that the cyclist's body moves through; relatively little bicycling power is lost to friction of the moving components of the bicycle or to the rolling resistance of the contact between the tire and road (Kyle, 1991). It is also important to realize that the air drag increases as the square of the velocity, i.e., if speed is doubled, the drag increases fourfold. Furthermore, the cycling power needed to achieve this doubled velocity increases eightfold (i.e., as the cube of the velocity) (Kyle, 1991).

Air drag offers great resistance in any sport requiring the athlete to move at relatively high velocities; such sports include speed skating (30–40 km/h at distances of 0.5 to 10 km) and sprint running (25–35 km/h at distances of 0.1 to 0.4 km). In fact, the air creates so much resistance in speed skating that the skaters must assume a tightly crouched posture to reduce the frontal area exposed to air. Although this posture reduces leg power, it reduces air drag to an even greater extent and thus produces higher skating velocities. Swimmers move at low velocities because they encounter large drag forces from the water as well as from the turbulence at the surface of the water. This drag encountered by a swimmer is not simply a function of body mass, but also of the body geometry as it moves in the prone or supine position through the interface between water and air.

It is obvious that in events such as bicycling, speed skating, and possibly sprint running, each of which requires the athlete to move through the air at high speeds, the ultimate race time will be determined by the power generated relative to the air resistance, which can be roughly estimated from the athlete's frontal surface area. The same analogy applies to swimming, but the drag against both water and air is much greater than air drag alone, and the physical factors causing the drag are quite complicated. The main point is that the race velocity in these sports is a function of power production relative to some index of the drag encountered at racing velocities. Therefore, velocity, i.e., performance, can be increased by improving power output and/or by reducing drag.

Sports such as distance running and cross-country skiing are carried out at velocities of 15–25 km/h; thus, air drag offers relatively minor resistance. Instead, these athletes must transport their body masses against the resistance offered by gravity. In these events, power production needed to generate a particular velocity is a function of body mass, and power should be related to body mass, e.g., $\dot{V}O_2max$ is usually expressed in $mL \cdot kg^{-1} \cdot min^{-1}$ (Martin & Morgan, 1992). However, it has also been suggested that running economy (Bergh et al., 1991) and cross–country skiing $\dot{V}O_2max$ (Ingjer, 1991) should be scaled to some exponent of body weight.

In weightlifting, power lifting, and some other sports, competitive performance is little affected by either drag forces or by having to support one's body mass. In such sports, it is the absolute power that can be sustained by the athlete that is critical to success; expressing that power per unit body mass is inappropriate. Of course, the governing bodies of these sports have long recognized the importance of raw power and have thus adopted body weight classifications to minimize the advantage of having a greater muscle mass to produce more power.

In rowing, the athletes assume a body posture that presents a low profile; this minimizes air drag, which is already quite low because the rowing shells move at relatively low velocities. Furthermore, water drag is reduced in rowing because the shells are smooth and streamlined. In this sport it is advantageous for athletes to be larger and more powerful because the racing velocity achieved is largely a function of the absolute power generated. Therefore, as in weightlifting, power production in rowing is typically not expressed in relation to body weight or in relation to some index of the drag encountered, but rather as watts or as oxygen consumption in liters per minute.

SUSTAINABLE POWER OUTPUT

Sustainable power output (W), i.e., work per unit time, is the power that the athlete can sustain for the duration of the competitive event. Bicyclists and rowers rely upon their equipment to transfer muscular energy to the environment; this equipment can be developed as stationary cycle and rowing ergometers so that the power used for propulsion can be easily determined. Sustainable power output for prolonged aerobic exercise is a function of the energy expenditure ($\dot{V}O_2$) that can be maintained during the event and the mechanical efficiency (i.e., the ratio of the mechanical power produced to the metabolic energy expended). The power production is directly measured by the ergometer, and the energy expenditure is calculated from measurements of the steady-state $\dot{V}O_2$ and the respiratory exchange ratio to determine the caloric equivalent for each liter of oxygen consumption.

Sustainable Energy Expenditure

Movement in sport is ultimately achieved by converting chemical energy from bodily stores of carbohydrate and fat into the mechanical energy of muscle action, with the majority of the chemical energy liberated in this process being lost as heat. The mean rate of energy expenditure that can be sustained for the duration of a competitive event is called the *sustainable energy expenditure*. When an athlete competes in an event for roughly 15 min or longer, all but a small fraction of the energy is provided from aerobic metabolism, and it is safe to assume that about 5 kcal of chemical energy are derived from carbohydrate and fat stores for each liter of oxygen consumed. Accordingly, the measurement of oxygen consumption ($\dot{V}O_2$) provides a direct estimate of the sustainable rate of energy expenditure.

Anaerobic Energy Production in Competitive Sports. Energy is required from anaerobic metabolism whenever the demand for energy, i.e., adenosine triphosphate (ATP), is greater than can be provided aerobically. The need for anaerobic energy during competitive sport can be categorized as follows:

1. Anaerobic energy is needed at the onset of exercise when the immediate supply of oxygen (O_2) is inadequate and the cardiovascular system requires a finite time to increase O_2 delivery to the exercising muscles and enable oxidative metabolism to match the new level of energy demand. The higher the intensity of the activity, the greater will be the demand for anaerobic energy through the transition. The need for some anaerobic energy must occur at the onset of every event in all the sports described in this volume. At one end of the spectrum, almost all the energy required for power lifting and weightlifting must immediately come from anaerobic sources at the onset of the lifts, given the short durations and high power outputs of these events. On the other end, the amount of anaerobic energy required at the onset of the very long events in endurance skating, cycling, running, and cross-country skiing would be very small when expressed as a percentage of the total energy required.

2. Anaerobic energy is also required during the transition when increasing the exercise intensity from one power output to a higher power output. This will not occur in all sports but will certainly be important in sports requiring explosive power on an intermittent basis, as in wrestling and ice hockey and during cross-country skiing, running, and road cycling when climbing hills or attempting to break away from other racers.

3. In events in which the continuous demand for energy is greater than aerobic metabolism can provide, anaerobic energy will be re-

quired to maintain high power outputs even when the maximal O_2 uptake has been reached, e.g., in any swimming, skating, rowing, cycling, or running races lasting about 1–6 min. The best example may be world-class rowers, who typically compete for 5–7 min over 2000 m and have very high values for maximal aerobic power and for anaerobic power and capacity. It must also be remembered in this context that given muscles or muscle groups may at times be functioning just below or just above their aerobic potential, thereby requiring different amounts of anaerobic energy, even though the whole body power output may be 90–110% $\dot{V}O_2$max. An example of this would be leg, back, and arm muscle groups of a rower during the 5–7 min, 2000-m race.

Sustainable Energy Expenditure in Brief, High-Power Events. Unfortunately, the sustainable energy expenditure is difficult to determine during brief, high-power activities such as weightlifting and sprinting that rely largely on the anaerobic breakdown of phosphocreatine and muscle glycogen for energy. As described in Chapter 2, anaerobic energy production can be estimated either 1) invasively from exercise-induced changes in the concentrations of intramuscular phosphocreatine and glycogen as determined with the aid of muscle biopsies obtained before and immediately after exercise, or 2) non-invasively from measurements of oxygen deficit. When such measurements of energy production from anaerobic sources are coupled with simultaneous measurements of aerobic energy production, the approximate relative contributions of these two energy sources during various phases of exercise lasting from 0–180s is as shown in Table I–1. It is clear from the table that the percentage of the anaerobic contribution to energy production falls off rapidly as the exercise duration increases. The averages over the entire 180 s of exercise were 45% anaerobic and 55% aerobic. The cumulative proportions reported here are similar to most of the reports of anaerobic involvement in the coming chapters that discuss various events in many different sports.

Both phosphocreatine (PCr) degradation and anaerobic glycolysis are activated instantaneously at the onset of high-intensity exercise. Measurements of PCr and lactate from muscle biopsies taken following as little as 1–10 s of electrical stimulation (Hultman & Sjoholm, 1983) and after sprint cycling (Boobis et al., 1982; Gaitanos et al., 1993; Jacobs et al., 1983) confirmed the rapid breakdown of PCr and rapid accumulation of lactate. At the onset of less intense exercise, a similar instantaneous activation of both PCr degradation and anaerobic glycolysis occurs, but at a much slower rate as the mismatch between energy demand and aerobic supply is reduced during submaximal exertion.

Rate of Anaerobic Energy Production During Exercise. The rate of anaerobic energy provision is critical to the success of sports that require the devel-

TABLE I-1. *Relative contributions of anaerobic and aerobic energy production during sequential phases and cumulative periods of exhausting exercise lasting 180 s.* Data from Bangsbo et al. (1990)

Contributions of Anaerobic and Aerobic Energy During Sequential Phases of Exercise

Phase	Time	Anaerobic	Aerobic
1	0 - 30 s	80%	20%
2	30 - 60 s	60%	40%
3	60 - 90 s	42%	58%
4	90 - 120 s	36%	64%
5	120 - ~180 s	30%	70%

Contributions of Anaerobic and Aerobic Energy During Cumulative Periods of Exercise

Period	Anaerobic	Aerobic
0 - 60 s	70%	30%
0 - 90 s	61%	39%
0 - 120 s	55%	45%
0 - 180 s	45%	55%

opment and short-term maintenance of high power outputs. World-class power and weightlifters can produce power outputs that are 10–20 times greater than outputs required to elicit $\dot{V}O_2$max, but can only maintain them for a fraction of a second. Sprinters can achieve power outputs that are 3–5 times the power outputs that elicit $\dot{V}O_2$max, but they can sustain those power outputs for only about 10 s. However, power output over a 30–40 s sprint can still be sustained at twice the power output at $\dot{V}O_2$max. Estimates of anaerobic ATP provision rates have been calculated from studies reporting intramuscular substrate and metabolite changes following intense exercise lasting from 1.3 to 200 s (Spriet, 1994). These studies used non-elite athletes who performed sprint cycling, sprint running, repeated knee extensions, or who underwent electrical stimulation of their muscles. The highest measured rates for ATP production from PCr and anaerobic glycolysis during various types of exercise lasting from 1.3–10 s were approximately 1.4–2.1 and 1.4–2.2 mmol ATP·kg wet muscle^{-1}·s^{-1}, respectively. This can be compared to maximal rates of ATP provision from aerobic metabolism of roughly 0.4–0.6 mmol ATP·kg wet muscle^{-1}·s^{-1}, assuming a $\dot{V}O_2$max of 3–4 L/min and 15–20 kg of active muscle mass. The two sources of anaerobic ATP combined to provide about 2.5–3.0 mmol ATP·kg^{-1}·s^{-1} during sprint cycling for 6–10 s (Boobis et al., 1982; Jacobs et al., 1983).

The anaerobic ATP provision rates decrease when averaged over longer periods of time. In studies that examined intense exercise for 30 s, the average ATP provision rates from PCr and glycolysis were approximately 0.4 and 1.0 mmol ATP·kg^{-1}·s^{-1}, respectively. If it is assumed that about 25% of the produced lactate escaped the active muscle during 30 s of exercise, then the estimate for glycolysis would increase accordingly.

The large decrease in energy produced from PCr when averaged over 30 s indicates that the PCr store becomes depleted between 10 and 30 s of intense exercise.

When high intensity exercise was maintained for 50–90 s, the average anaerobic ATP provision rates from PCr and glycolysis decreased further to approximately 0.2 and 0.4 mmol ATP·kg^{-1}·s^{-1}. This indicated that no further PCr breakdown occurred beyond 30 s and that the glycolytic average was actually less than one-half of the 0–30 s average. Since a glycolytic rate of less than zero from 30 to 50–90 s is not possible, it suggests that the average power output that can be sustained for 50–90 s is much lower than for 30 s and that the escape of lactate during exercise is considerable, leading to a larger underestimation of glycolytic ATP production than during 30 s of exercise.

In summary, the highest rates of anaerobic ATP provision from PCr and glycolysis during maximal or near maximal high-intensity exercise are attained in the initial 10 s of exercise. If demanding exercise is extended for 30 s, the PCr store will be depleted between 10 and 30 s and the glycolytic ATP production rate will be about 50% of the rate during the initial 10 s. The average glycolytic ATP provision rate during 30 s of high-intensity exercise will be about 3–4 times greater than the rate of ATP production provided by PCr. With high-intensity exercise extended to 50–90 s, estimates of glycolytic ATP provision are unreliable because considerable lactate escapes the muscle.

Anaerobic Energy Production During Intermittent High-Power Exercise. Many sports require the athlete to repeatedly engage in bursts of high-intensity exercise with varying amounts of recovery time between exercise bouts. Examples include repeated fast breaks in basketball and repeated sprints in football. Most of the energy for short bouts of high intensity-exercise is derived from anaerobic sources; therefore, the ability to recover during rest periods is essential for success in this type of activity. Many studies have examined the performance effects of intermittent high intensity-exercise, but few have examined the anaerobic metabolism associated with this type of metabolic stress. Examples of the exercise models that have been studied and provided some conclusions include: 10 bouts of sprint cycling, each lasting 6 s with rest periods of 30 s; 4 bouts of sprint cycling for 30 s with 4-min rest periods; and 2 bouts of knee extension exercise to exhaustion in 3 min with 10–60 min of recovery (Bangsbo et al., 1992; Gaitanos et al., 1993; McCartney et al., 1986). Muscle biopsy measurements demonstrated that PCr was decreased by approximately 50% after 6 s and by 75–80% during longer sprints. The PCr is quickly resynthesized during recovery, reaching 50% of rest values by 30–60 s and about 80% by 2–4 min. With repeated sprinting, energy production from anaerobic glycolysis is progressively more difficult to achieve. Presumably, the accumulation of muscle lactate and the associated release of H^+ plays a major role in the inability to reactivate anaerobic glycolysis. Therefore, after repeated sprinting, the ability to provide anaerobic ATP is severely reduced and becomes dependent on PCr degradation.

Role of Maximal Oxygen Uptake and the Blood Lactate Threshold in Determining the Sustainable Energy Expenditure During Prolonged Exercise. The maximal rate of aerobic energy expenditure possible is a function of the athlete's maximal rate of oxygen consumption ($\dot{V}O_2$max) or aerobic power, but exercise cannot be sustained at $\dot{V}O_2$max for more than a few minutes. For longer events, the greatest sustainable $\dot{V}O_2$, i.e., the sustainable energy expenditure, is not limited just by $\dot{V}O_2$max, but more importantly by the blood lactate threshold, i.e., the greatest $\dot{V}O_2$ that can sustained before lactic acid accumulates rapidly in the blood (Coyle et al., 1988). Essentially, the blood lactate threshold represents the highest $\dot{V}O_2$ that can be maintained during exercise without eliciting the sensation of muscle fatigue associated with the accumulation of lactic acid, first in muscle, and then in the blood (Holloszy & Coyle, 1984). The lactate threshold provides a better reflection than $\dot{V}O_2$max of the exercising muscle's ability to produce aerobic energy for periods lasting 30–240 min (Coyle et al., 1988, 1991).

Mechanical Efficiency

Mechanical efficiency for a sporting event is the ratio of the mechanical power output to the total energy expended to produce that power. Typically, both power output and energy expenditure are expressed in watts, and the ratio is expressed as a percentage. For example, if a cyclist expends energy at the rate equivalent to 5 L of oxygen per minute (1745 W) to produce 400 W of power on a bicycle ergometer, the mechanical efficiency would be (400/1745)·100 = 23%. Two of the principal factors that determine the mechanical efficiency of an athlete in a sport event are: 1) the efficiency with which the active muscles convert the chemical energy stored in carbohydrate and fat to the mechanical energy required to shorten the contractile elements in the muscles, and 2) the neuromuscular skill with which the athlete performs the event. Before discussing these factors, however, it is important to review how the economy of movement is frequently used as an analogue of mechanical efficiency.

Economy of Movement as an Analogue of Efficiency. Although athletes obviously expend energy while swimming, running, skating, or skiing on flat courses, estimation of power output is difficult in these activities because there is little or no measurable physical work accomplished when the body mass does not move in a vertical direction (Webb, 1988; Williams & Cavanagh, 1983). Because power output is hard to quantify in these activities, mechanical efficiency is not usually determined. Instead, it is customary to calculate the economy of movement, defined simply as the velocity achieved by the athlete at a given rate of energy expenditure ($\dot{V}O_2$). This provides an indirect estimate of efficiency in which movement velocity provides an index of power output.

Role of Muscle Efficiency in Determining Mechanical Efficiency. Muscle efficiency has two components, the first being the efficiency with which chemical energy from carbohydrate and fat is converted to adenosine triphosphate (ATP), the only form of chemical energy that can power muscle contraction. The process of ATP synthesis is about 40% efficient, i.e., 40% of the metabolic energy in carbohydrate and fat is transferred into ATP synthesis, whereas 60% of the energy is lost as heat (Kushmerick, 1983; Kushmerick & Davies, 1969). This efficiency of ATP synthesis is fairly constant.

The second component of muscle efficiency, i.e., the efficiency with which the energy released during ATP hydrolysis is converted to muscle fiber shortening, is more variable than is the efficiency of converting stored fuels to ATP. The efficiency of ATP hydrolysis is dependent on the velocities of muscle contraction (Goldspink, 1978; Kushmerick & Davies, 1969). A peak efficiency of approximately 60% or more can be elicited from myofilaments contracting at one-third of maximal velocity; i.e., the velocity of peak efficiency (Kushmerick, 1983; Kushmerick & Davies, 1969). Thus, slow-twitch muscle fibers obviously have slower velocities of peak efficiency than do fast-twitch fibers (Fitts et al., 1989).

Mechanical efficiency when cycling at 80 rpm is directly related to the percentage of slow-twitch muscle fibers in the vastus lateralis muscles (Coyle et al., 1992). It seems that when cycling at this cadence, the velocity of muscle fiber shortening in the vastus lateralis is close to one-third maximal velocity of the slow-twitch fibers (Coyle et al., 1992). This makes slow-twitch muscle fibers substantially more efficient than fast-twitch muscle fibers at converting ATP into muscular power when cycling at 80 rpm (Coyle et al., 1992; Goldspink, 1978).

Muscle fiber type had a large effect on mechanical efficiency, which in turn had a large influence on sustainable power output during a 1-h bout of cycling in a homogeneous group of cyclists (Horowitz et al., 1994). The cyclists were paired and divided into two groups based upon the percentages (i.e., above or below 56%) of slow-twitch muscle fibers in their vastus lateralis muscles. One group possessed a normal distribution of fiber types, with an average of 48% slow-twitch fibers. The other group had 72% slow-twitch fibers on average. These two groups were identical in $\dot{V}O_2$max as well as in the $\dot{V}O_2$ maintained during the ride. Therefore, they possessed the same aerobic energy expenditure potential for this type of task. However, the cyclists with a high percentage of slow-twitch fibers displayed significantly higher mechanical efficiencies and were therefore able to sustain a 9% greater power output (342 W vs. 315 W) during the 1-h ride. Clearly, endurance cycling performance is heavily influenced by mechanical efficiency, which in turn appears to be dependent on the rider's muscle fiber type profile and the efficiency of ATP hydrolysis by the muscle.

Role of Neuromuscular Skill in Determining Mechanical Efficiency. No matter how efficiently one can transform chemical energy into mechanical energy in a given muscle fiber, the overall mechanical efficiency in a sports event will be poor if the athlete is poorly skilled, i.e., if muscle fibers contract that either do not contribute to the desired movement or actually detract from it. A good example of this phenomenon is the contrast in the freestyle swimming performances of novice and elite swimmers. The novice thrashes about with great energy expenditure but little forward velocity, whereas the elite swimmer has learned to swim rapidly and gracefully, using only those motor units required to execute the stroke effectively. Neuromuscular skill obviously plays a greater role in determining the mechanical efficiency for some sports, e.g., swimming and wrestling, than it does for others, e.g., running and power lifting, but even small differences in skill can have a major impact on performance at the elite level.

TRAINING PRINCIPLES

Improvements in sports performance require an increase in the sustainable output of force or power, often by an improvement in the ability to produce energy aerobically and/or anaerobically. Endurance events such as the marathon or tour cycling events represent one end of the spectrum, whereas events such as the 100-m dash and power lifting represent the opposite end. In between these two extremes are an abundance of sporting events that last 1–10 min. Many training programs have been developed by coaches, athletes, and scientists in which athletes train for hours each day attempting to improve performance, sometimes by as little as a fraction of a second.

The most widely accepted general training principles include the principles of overload, specificity, reversibility, and individuality. While these components of training programs have been studied extensively, most investigations have not used elite athletes. Consequently, it is not possible to determine precisely whether these principles are applicable to elite athletes, whose superior performances may result more from superior genetic endowments than from any specific training programs.

Progressive Overload

Adaptations to training will occur only if the training program places unaccustomed physiological burdens on the athlete in a progressive manner, i.e., the athlete's body must be exposed to progressively more serious disturbances in homeostasis. This progressive overload can occur by increasing training volume or training intensity or by altering the exercise-rest cycle.

Training Volume. The volume of training refers to the number of times a load or training session is administered over a given time. Training volume can be increased by requiring the athlete to train more frequently or for longer durations in each training session. In resistance training, greater training duration in a session is achieved by increasing the number of repetitions in each set of the resistance exercises and/or the number of sets performed. The optimal training frequency, i.e., the number of training sessions performed weekly, appears to be a function of training duration and the incidence of overuse injuries. For example, swimmers typically train more frequently than do distance runners, presumably because swimmers train in a non-weight-bearing water environment and are thus subject to fewer overuse injuries. Over the past decade there has been a growing tendency in many sports toward more frequent training sessions of greater duration.

There is obviously some limit beyond which increasing training volume is counterproductive. To help answer the question of whether swimmers should train 3–4 h daily for events that last only a few minutes, Costill et al. (1991) evaluated the influence of training volume on swimming performance in collegiate swimmers. Swimmers were divided into two groups, those who trained for approximately 10,000 m/d and those who trained for approximately 5,000 m/d. After 6 wk of training, the results indicated that the group training 10,000 m/d did not improve in aerobic power or swim performance any more than the group training 5,000 m/d. These results suggest that training volume may not be the primary determinant of success in a training program. However, it is possible that increases in training volume over many months and years may be useful in specifically training slow-twitch muscle fibers, may improve capillary density in the muscles, or may increase mechanical efficiency; each of these adaptations could eventually lead to improved performance.

Intensity. Training intensity, i.e., the quality of the training session, is increased by requiring the athlete to exercise at a faster pace (e.g., swimming, running, cycling, rowing, skating, and skiing), up a steeper incline (e.g., running, cycling, and skiing), with a greater load (e.g., rowing, weightlifting, and power lifting), or against a stronger or more skillful opponent (e.g., wrestling). The greater the intensity of training, the greater the fatigue and the longer the period of recovery necessary to ensure that subsequent exercise bouts can be sustained at an adequate intensity. It is widely believed that exercise intensity is the critical component in improving or maintaining aerobic power (Hickson et al., 1977; 1985).

Increasing training intensity improves total work capacity, which is a function of maximal power output and time to exhaustion (Sharkey, 1970), and has been reported to enhance athletic performance (Hickson et al.,

1977; Holloszy & Booth, 1975; Pollock, 1973). Hickson et al. (1977) demonstrated that aerobic power and endurance increase linearly during training as long as the exercise intensity *relative to* $\dot{V}O_2max$ is maintained constant; in other words, the absolute intensity of exercise must be increased as $\dot{V}O_2max$ improves if further improvement in $\dot{V}O_2max$ and endurance is sought. However, the rate of increase in $\dot{V}O_2max$ approaches zero as the genetically determined upper limit to $\dot{V}O_2max$ is approached.

Maintenance of training-induced adaptations appears to be dependent upon exercise intensity. When both exercise intensity and training frequency are decreased, there is a progressive decline in aerobic power, mitochondrial enzyme activity, myoglobin concentration, and exercise endurance (Hickson et. al., 1985). However, it is possible to maintain exercise-induced increases in aerobic power when training volume is reduced as long as exercise intensity is increased or at least maintained above 85% $\dot{V}O_2max$ (Brynteson & Sinning, 1973; Hickson, 1981).

Altering the Exercise-Rest Cycle. The body can also be forced to adapt to intracellular homeostatic disturbances by changing the amount of time devoted to exercise and recovery during training sessions. By breaking up the training into intervals of exercise interspersed with intervals of recovery, an athlete can perform a greater total volume of high-intensity exercise during a given training session than when the athlete exercises continuously. Additional overload can be achieved by progressively reducing the time of recovery between exercise bouts in a training session or by progressively increasing the intensity of exercise required during the recovery intervals, e.g., by requiring an runner to jog rather than walk during the recovery intervals. Although intermittent exercise schemes are widely accepted as desirable for training athletes who compete in events lasting less than about 10 min, it appears that continuous and intermittent training are equally effective for training athletes to compete in more prolonged events (Ballor et al., 1989).

Training Specificity

Adaptations to training are specific to the type of training performed. Stated simply, one cannot expect to become a champion in one sport event by training for another event. It is obvious that only the motor units that are overloaded will adapt to the training, so the movements in training should be as similar as possible to the movements used in competition. Early investigations by Klausen et al. (1971) showed that training effects are specific to the exercising limb and are not transferable to the contralateral limb or from legs to arms. Also, Saltin et al. (1975) investigated the effect of training on the central and peripheral adaptations resulting from one-legged exercise training and found that training adaptations were apparent only when exercising with the trained limb.

A neural adaptation specific to training intensity has been suggested by Coyle and co-workers (1981), who investigated the changes in peak torque following isokinetic resistance training at various velocities. Subjects who trained at 60°/s produced increases in peak torque without changes in skeletal muscle structure, whereas subjects who trained at 180°/s improved peak torque as the result of hypertrophy of Type II fibers. Presumably, the group trained at 60°/s must have improved the ability to recruit more motor units simultaneously by virtue of neural adaptations. Similarly, Rosler et al. (1986) found that improvements in leg power output resulting from a cycling endurance training program were specific to the contraction velocities employed in the training. At least part of this adaptation was attributed to neural adaptations.

The desirability of simultaneous participation in strength and endurance training programs has been questioned. Hickson and Rosenkoetter (1981) reported that subjects participating in a strength-only program had a 20% greater improvement in strength development than did subjects who trained in a strength-endurance combination program. Other investigators (Dudley & Djamil, 1985; Sale et al., 1990) have confirmed that concurrent training for strength and endurance appears to reduce the ability to increase muscular strength. However, strength training does not appear to adversely affect improvements in aerobic power induced by endurance training. Additionally, observations by Hickson et al. (1980) confirmed an absence of any negative effect of adding strength training to an endurance exercise program and showed that after a strength-endurance training program, endurance performance was enhanced during exercise lasting 4–8 min and to some extent during exercise lasting 71–85 min.

Reversibility of Training-Induced Adaptations

Training produces a variety of physiological adaptations that collectively enhance sport performance. In contrast, long periods of detraining, i.e., a severe reduction in or a total cessation of training, can reverse these adaptations because of the reduction in physiological demands on the body (Coyle et al., 1984). Detraining diminishes aerobic power (Coyle et al., 1984; Hickson et al., 1985) as well as the activities of the enzymes of energy metabolism (Chi et al., 1983; Henrikson & Reitman, 1977). The rate of reversal of these adaptations may be partly dependent upon the intensity and duration of the training program, but VO2 max declines substantially in as little as 2–3 wk, mostly as a result of a diminished plasma volume (Coyle et al., 1984). Coyle et al. (1984) reported that sedentary individuals who had undergone a modest training program of only 2 to 4 months exhibited a greater decline in mitochondrial content during detraining than did highly trained athletes who had trained intensely for many years.

Individuality of Adaptations to Training

The principles of training are similar for all individuals, but the degree of adaptation achieved may vary considerably among individuals, presumably because of differences in genetic endowment. In addition, the extent of improvement in a given individual may vary as a function of age-related changes in adaptability. Thus, the training of athletes can never be done strictly on the basis of some scientifically derived recipe; coaches must always be aware of individual differences in the adaptations their athletes achieve in response to different training regimens.

SPORTS NUTRITION PRINCIPLES

Research in sports nutrition has largely focused on laboratory studies of substrate utilization and exercise performance after various forms of nutritional intervention. Based upon results from many of these well-controlled studies, general recommendations can be made regarding carbohydrate, protein, fat, fluid, and micronutrient ingestion. This section will briefly review these recommendations and address whether athletes are currently following the advice of nutrition scientists.

Dietary Carbohydrate

Carbohydrate in Training Diets. Based largely upon the results of experiments lasting less than a week, it has been recommended that athletes undergoing intense training ingest 60–70% of their total energy intake as carbohydrate, compared to the 45% that is more typically consumed in Western cultures (Costill & Hargreaves, 1992). This high-carbohydrate diet is considered necessary to maintain muscle glycogen stores and enable athletes to work at higher training loads (Williams, 1993). It is believed by many that athletes who consume diets containing less than 40% carbohydrate may experience chronic fatigue during periods of intense training, thereby compromising the effectiveness of the training regimen (Coyle, 1991). However, diets containing 70–80% carbohydrate have not consistently improved performance compared to diets containing 40–45% carbohydrate in studies of athletes training for 7–28 d (Sherman & Wimer, 1991), perhaps because the performance tests used in some of these experiments were inappropriate. Still, high-carbohydrate diets have never been shown to adversely affect performance and should be consumed by all people, not just athletes, to minimize the risk of cardiovascular disease.

Despite a clear consensus that high-carbohydrate diets should be consumed on a daily basis during periods of strenuous training, athletes are not following this advice. Williams (1993) provided a review of several studies that assessed the dietary intake of 14 groups of athletes. For males, the range of carbohydrate intake was 43–60%, and for females the range was 48–60%, with only two groups ingesting 60% carbohydrate. Grandjean (1989) reported that the range of carbohydrate intake for 11 groups of male athletes was 43–54%, whereas the range for three groups of female athletes was 49–52%. These groups consisted of professional athletes, NCAA Division I athletes, and athletes participating in competitions sponsored by the U.S. Olympic Committee. Other studies have also reported that the dietary carbohydrate intakes of athletes were less than the recommended 60–70% level (Chen et al., 1989; Faber et al., 1990; Heinemann & Zerbes, 1989).

Carbohydrate Ingestion Before, During, and After Endurance Exercise. In addition to promoting the idea that athletes in training should consume plenty of dietary carbohydrate on a daily basis, sports nutrition experts also are in considerable agreement concerning recommendations for carbohydrate ingestion shortly before, during, and after intense endurance exercise.

Carbohydrate Ingestion Before and During Exercise. A high-carbohydrate meal consumed within 6 h of endurance competition may complete the restoration of glycogen stores in liver and muscle (Coyle, 1991). For example, Coggan and Swanson (1992) recommended ingestion of about 50 g of carbohydrate immediately before endurance competition, or ingestion of 200–350 g of carbohydrate 3–6 h before the event.

As reviewed by Coggan and Swanson (1992) and Coyle (1991), research has shown that carbohydrate ingestion during prolonged intense exercise or intermittent fatiguing exercise (e.g., soccer) can delay fatigue, presumably by helping to maintain blood glucose levels to support muscle energy needs. Brouns (1993) recommended that for exercise lasting longer than 45 min, at least 20 g, but optimally 80 g, of carbohydrate be ingested for every hour of exercise. Coyle (1991) and Coggan and Swanson (1992) have recommended ingestion of carbohydrate at rates of 30–60 g/h and 40–75 g/h, respectively.

Because of the importance of fluid intake during prolonged exercise, carbohydrate is generally ingested as a liquid. Thus, recommendations for carbohydrate intake are often expressed as solution percentages. A 6–8% carbohydrate solution seems to produce optimal rates of gastric emptying and intestinal absorption (Gisolfi & Duchman, 1992). For providing both supplemental energy as well as fluid replacement, a solution containing 5–10% carbohydrate is recommended, depending upon the volume ingested (Coggan & Swanson, 1992). As an example, a solution containing 5%–7.5% would be recommended if the volume ingested were 900–1,000 mL/h, whereas if the volume ingested were only 500–600 mL/h, a 7.5%–10% solution would be warranted.

Carbohydrate Ingestion After Exercise. Coyle (1991) identified three important factors that determine optimal conditions for carbohydrate ingestion during recovery from prolonged strenuous exercise: time of ingestion, amount of carbohydrate ingested, and the type of carbohydrate. The rate of muscle glycogen resynthesis is most rapid within 3 h after exercise, so ingestion of as much carbohydrate as can be tolerated should be ingested during this time. Thereafter, ingestion of 50 g carbohydrate every 2 h will result in an optimal rate of glycogen synthesis. Lastly, muscle glycogen is resynthesized more slowly when fructose is ingested compared to glucose, sucrose, or starch (Coggan & Swanson, 1992; Coyle, 1991).

Dietary Protein

The U.S. Recommended Dietary Allowance (RDA) of protein for adults is 0.8 g·kg body weight^{-1}·d^{-1} (National Research Council, 1989). Thus, the diet for an average individual consuming the usual amount of energy should contain 10–15% of that energy in the form of protein. However, several studies have shown that the RDA does not meet the needs of athletes involved in high-intensity endurance or resistance training. The reason athletes require greater amounts of protein is that strenuous exercise causes an increase in protein breakdown during and immediately following exercise and a subsequent increase in protein synthesis during prolonged recovery from exercise (Lemon, 1992). Increases in protein synthesis after endurance exercise may reflect an increased synthesis of mitochondrial (enzymatic) proteins; after resistance exercise, dietary protein contributes to an increased synthesis of contractile proteins in skeletal muscle fibers (Chesley et al., 1992; Lemon, 1992).

For endurance athletes, experts have recommended daily protein consumption in amounts of 1.2 g/kg body weight (Evans, 1993), 1.2–1.4 g/kg (Lemon, 1992), 1.6 g/kg (Lemon, 1991), and 1.8 g/kg (Brouns, 1993). For strength-trained athletes, Tarnopolsky et al. (1992) found that a diet containing protein in quantities of 2.4 g·kg^{-1}·d^{-1} did not produce an increase in protein synthesis greater than a diet with 1.4 g·kg^{-1}·d^{-1}. They recommended a protein intake of 1.76 g·kg^{-1}·d^{-1} for athletes undergoing strength training, but this high protein intake may only be required during the initial stages of a resistance training program. Lemon et al. (1992) examined protein requirements for strength athletes in the early stages of an intensive weight training (bodybuilding) program. Based on nitrogen balance techniques, they recommended that protein ingestion be 1.6–1.7 g·kg^{-1}·d^{-1}. Higher protein intakes (2.62 g·kg^{-1}·d^{-1}) over the 1-month training did not result in greater muscle mass and strength development than did a lower protein intake of 1.35 g·kg^{-1}·d^{-1}. Lemon (1992) recommended that strength athletes should consume 1.2–1.7 g protein·kg^{-1}·d^{-1}, with beginning weight trainers ingesting the higher amounts and more experienced athletes the lower amounts.

Although there is a consensus that serious athletes should consume more protein than is recommended for normally active individuals, several studies have shown that many athletes routinely consume 1.2–2.0 g protein·kg^{-1}·d^{-1}, which may make extra protein intake unnecessary (Lemon & Proctor, 1991). The reason for this typically high protein intake among athletes is that most of them also ingest more food than the general population, and 15–20% of the food energy is usually protein. Lemon (1992) provided the example that a daily 5,000-kcal diet with only 10% protein would result in a protein intake of 125 g, which for a 70-kg athlete would amount to about 1.9 g protein·kg^{-1}·d^{-1}. Thus, although athletes require more protein than do non-athletes, their higher caloric intakes are generally sufficient to ensure protein needs, and protein supplements are not warranted.

Dietary Fat

The recommended dietary fat intake for athletes is 20–30% of total energy intake; included in this amount is the intake of saturated fats, which should account for less than 10% of total energy. Although fat is utilized as an important fuel during endurance exercise, there is an adequate supply of fat in body stores to easily accomplish its role in energy metabolism (Brouns, 1993). Unfortunately, athletes may be ingesting diets considerably higher in fat than is advisable. Williams (1993) reviewed several studies documenting mean fat intakes of 27–43% for various male athlete groups, with only 4 of the 14 groups ingesting less than 30% fat. Grandjean (1989) reported that athletes were ingesting about 37% and 34% of their energy from fat for the males and females, respectively. Studies of athletes from other countries also reported high fat intakes, with mean values ranging from 33–49% (Chen et al., 1989; Faber et al., 1990; Heinemann & Zerbes (1989).

The diet consumed by most individuals in the U.S. contains about 36% of the total caloric intake from fat (National Research Council, 1989). Thus, diets of many groups of athletes are as high or even higher in fat intake than those of the general population. Because this high fat intake is at the expense of the recommended amount of carbohydrate ingestion, training ability could be compromised. The long-term health risks for athletes ingesting high-fat diets have not been seriously studied, but they are presumably similar to the adverse risks for heart disease associated with high fat intake in the general population.

Replenishment of Body Fluids

Body temperature rises during exercise, and the primary means of body cooling is sweat evaporation. Athletes performing prolonged exercise, especially in a warm environment, face the challenge of maintaining body temperature at the expense of fluid loss by sweating. Therefore, an important consideration in these conditions is the prevention of serious dehydration.

Body size, training status, exercise intensity, and environmental conditions all affect sweating rate (Brouns et al. 1992). Maximal sweat rate for a 70-kg male athlete could reach 1.8 L/h (Brouns et al., 1992). As fluid is lost from the body, the ability to thermoregulate diminishes. Thus, it is important to limit fluid loss and replenish any loss by ingesting liquids during and after exercise. For example, the American College of Sports Medicine (1984) recommends that runners drink 100–200 mL of fluid after every 2–3 km.

High sweat rates accompanying prolonged physical work in the heat may also compromise the body's electrolyte balance, as electrolytes, especially sodium and chloride, are lost with sweat. Under these conditions, there are several reasons why it is important to replenish electrolytes with fluid ingestion (Murray, 1987). Addition of sodium (along with glucose) to a replacement beverage may enhance intestinal absorption of water, and optimal concentrations of sodium increase the palatability of the drink, which should increase the volume ingested. Another reason why an electrolyte beverage would be preferable to plain water is to maintain the body's sodium status. This is illustrated by the fact that during prolonged endurance exercise, consumption of plain water accompanied by profuse sweat loss can result in hypotonic hyponatremia ("water intoxication"), a life threatening dilution of sodium concentration in the body fluids (Armstrong et al., 1993).

There appears to be no "ideal" oral rehydration solution that can be recommended for all conditions (e.g., pre-event, exercise, and recovery) (Gisolfi & Duchman, 1992). While plain water may be suitable for brief exercise, carbohydrate-electrolyte beverages are recommended for more prolonged exercise. A moderate amount of carbohydrate in a sports drink can provide an exogenous source of energy and, in combination with sodium, can facilitate fluid absorption from the intestine. Using the available scientific literature as a guide, Gisoli and Duchman (1992) have proposed detailed plans for fluid consumption before, during, and after exercise of various types under different environmental circumstances. However, rather than first adopting a new eating or drinking scheme immediately before or during a major competition, athletes should always try such regimens during their routine training sessions to ascertain their individual responses to these dietary modifications.

During the initial 24 h of recovery from prolonged exhaustive exercise, athletes should be encouraged to drink back all of the weight they lost during exercise; even a small amount of fluid weight that is not regained may impair the performance of subsequent exercise (Brouns, 1991). During this same 24 h period, they should also consume about 8–10 g of carbohydrate per kilogram of body weight, either as solid food or as a component of the fluid used to replenish body water. Several high–carbohydrate drink mixtures are commercially available for this purpose. Finally, to help ensure that most of the fluid consumed will remain in the body and not be excreted by the kidneys, athletes should ingest about 2 g of sodium chloride every hour for the first several hours after exercise (Gisolfi & Duchman, 1992). This electrolyte replacement goal can be achieved by consuming carbohydrate–electrolyte drinks or by adding the appropriate amount of table salt to the athlete's solid food.

Micronutrients

Vitamins. The B vitamins function in energy metabolism and in the production of red blood cells; most athletes ingest at least the RDA amounts of these vitamins, and there is no systematic evidence to support supplementation of B vitamins in the athlete's diet (Clarkson, 1991a). Of recent concern is whether athletes ingest enough antioxidant vitamins— A (beta-carotene), C, and E. The reason for this concern is that exercise may increase the production of free radicals which, in turn, increase lipid peroxidation that damages cellular membranes. Antioxidants inactivate free radicals and prevent or reduce lipid peroxidation (Alessio, 1993; Goldfarb, 1993). The intake of vitamins A, C, and E among athletes equals or exceeds the RDA (Clarkson, 1991a), but use of the RDA as a guideline for athletes has been questioned because increased amounts of antioxidants may be necessary to reduce the negative effects of exercise-induced lipid peroxidation (Alessio, 1993; Goldfarb, 1993). However, training increases the body's natural antioxidant defense system, and there is little evidence that antioxidant supplements actually benefit athletic performance.

Minerals. The dietary intake by athletes of magnesium and phosphorus for the most part appears adequate (Clarkson, 1991b; Clarkson & Haymes, 1994). However, many female athletes do not consume the RDA for calcium. This is of concern because an adequate calcium intake is necessary to ensure peak bone mass during growth and maintenance of bone mass in older women. Poor calcium intake is associated with stress fractures in athletes.

There is insufficient evidence to support claims that trace mineral status of athletes is compromised (Clarkson, 1991a, Clarkson & Haymes, 1994). Exercise increases the excretion of chromium and zinc in the urine, but the athlete's dietary intake of these minerals is usually adequate to replenish the losses. Also, although zinc intake by women athletes seems to be below the RDA, it is not known if their bodily zinc status is negatively affected.

For selenium and copper, the few studies of athletes reported that ingestion of these trace minerals met or exceeded the recommended levels and the status of these minerals in the bodies of the athletes was adequate. Female athletes are often iron depleted, but the incidence of iron depletion for athletes is no greater than that found for the general population. Iron supplements can improve the iron status of athletes who are iron depleted, but such supplements generally improve performance only if the athletes have been anemic.

General Nutritional Recommendations

For general health purposes, female athletes should be careful to ingest adequate amounts of calcium, zinc, and iron, and all athletes should ingest foods rich in antioxidants. Although there is not sufficient evidence to justify vitamin and mineral supplementation by athletes, many regularly consume such supplements (Clarkson, 1991a; 1991b), which often include large doses of selected micronutrients that may be unnecessary. Taking indiscriminately large doses of selected vitamins and minerals could be harmful because large doses of certain micronutrients can interact with the absorption or function of others. For example, ingestion of zinc at levels of 50% above the RDA can inhibit copper absorption. However, some athletes, especially lightweight rowers, wrestlers, and women distance runners and figure skaters, may have inadequate amounts of one or more vitamins and minerals due to poor dietary practices. Ingestion of foods rich in micronutrients should provide the required amounts. Athletes who are concerned that their diets may not contain the necessary quantities of all micronutrients could be advised to take multi-vitamin/ mineral supplements containing no more than the RDA. This would be considered an "insurance safeguard" and should present no harm.

Eating Behavior and Knowledge of Nutrition

In spite of well-established principles of sport nutrition, many athletes do not follow those principles and engage in inappropriate eating behavior. For example, 48% of women figure skaters were reported to be within the anorexic range (Rucinski, 1989) and 15% of elite female skiers demonstrated anorexic behavior or suffered from anorexia (see chapter 9 in this volume). Some male athletes may also have eating disorders. Depalma et al. (1993) reported that of 131 lightweight college football players, 74% had been binge eaters, 17% had experienced self-induced vomiting, 66% had reported fasting, and about 4% had used laxatives. Wrestlers are notorious for the practice of losing large amounts of weight in the hours prior to competition by acute dehydration, food restriction, vomiting, and use of laxatives and diuretics (Steen & Brownell, 1990).

The reasons for poor nutritional behavior by athletes are not known but probably include poor nutritional habits developed over many years and a lack of sport nutrition education for both coaches and athletes. Coaches may more readily attribute poor performance to being out-of-shape than to the possibility of poor dietary practices. Many athletes may not be able to identify a proper diet, so even if they are made aware of the need for a high-carbohydrate diet, they may be unable to identify what constitutes such a diet. Clearly, there is a need for better education of athletes and coaches concerning proper nutritional practices and dietary habits. Efforts should be placed not only on offering sound recommendations, but also on providing ways to identify proper foods and practical means to achieve optimal diets.

BIBLIOGRAPHY

Alessio, H.M. (1993). Exercise-induced oxidative stress. *Med. Sci. Sports Exerc.* 25:218–224.

American College of Sports Medicine (1984). Position stand on prevention of thermal injuries during distance running. *Med. Sci. Sports Exerc.* 16:ix–xiv.

Armstrong, L.E., W.C. Curtis, R.W. Hubbard, R.P. Francesconi, R. Moore, and E.W. Askew (1993). Symptomatic hyponatremia during prolonged exercise in heat. *Med. Sci. Sports Exerc.* 25:543–549.

Ballor, D.L., M.D. Becque, C.R. Marks, K.L. Nau, and V.L. Katch (1989). Physiological responses to nine different exercise:rest protocols. *Med. Sci. Sports. Exerc.* 21:90–95.

Bangsbo, J., P.D. Gollnick, T.E. Graham, C. Juel, B. Kiens, M. Mizuno, and B. Saltin (1990). Anaerobic energy production and O_2 deficit-debt relationship during exhaustive exercise in humans. *J. Physiol. (London)* 422:539–559.

Bangsbo, J., T.E. Graham, B. Kiens, and B. Saltin (1992). Elevated muscle glycogen and anaerobic energy production during exhaustive exercise in man. *J. Physiol. (London)* 451:205–227.

Bergh, U., B. Sjodin, A. Forsberg, and J. Svedenhag (1991). The relationship between body mass and oxygen uptake during running in humans. *Med. Sci. Sports Exerc.* 23: 205–211.

Boobis, L.H., C. Williams, and S.A. Wooton (1982). Human muscle metabolism during brief maximal exercise (abstract). *J. Physiol. (London)* 338:21P–22P.

Brouns, F. (1991). Heat-sweat-dehydration-rehydration:a praxis oriented approach. *J. Sports Sci.* 9:143–152.

Brouns, F. (1993). *Nutritional Needs of Athletes.* West Sussex: John Wiley & Sons.

Brouns, F., W. Saris, and H. Schneider (1992). Rationale for upper limits of electrolyte replacement during exercise. *Int. J. Sport Nutr.* 2:229–238.

Brynteson, P., and W.E. Sinning (1973). The effects of training frequencies on the retention of cardiovascular fitness. *Med. Sci. Sports* 5:29–33.

Chen, J.D., J.F. Wang, K.J. Li, Y.W. Zhao, S.W. Wang, Y. Jiao, and X.Y. Hou (1989). Nutritional problems and measures in elite and amateur athletes. *Am. J. Clin. Nutr.* 49:1084–1089.

Chesley, A., J.D. MacDougall, M.A. Tarnopolsky, S.A. Atkinson, and K. Smith (1992). Changes in human muscle protein synthesis after resistance exercise. *J. Appl. Physiol.* 73:1383–1388.

Chi, M.M.-Y., C.S. Hintz, E.F. Coyle, W.H. Martin, J.L. Ivy, P.M. Nemeth, J.O. Holloszy, and O.H. Lowry (1983). Effects of detraining on enzymes of energy metabolism in individual human fibers. *Am. J. Physiol.* 244:C276–C287.

Clarkson, P.M. (1991a). Vitamins and trace minerals as ergogenic aids. In: D.R. Lamb and M.H. Williams (eds.) *Perspectives in Exercise Science and Sports Medicine, Vol. 4: Ergogenics—Enhancement of Performance in Exercise and Sport.* Indianapolis:Brown & Benchmark Press, pp. 123–176.

Clarkson, P.M. (1991b). Minerals: exercise performance and supplementation in athletes, *J. Sports Sci.* 9:91–116.

Clarkson, P.M., and E.M. Haymes (1994). Mineral requirements for athletes: Calcium, magnesium, phosphorus, and iron. *Med. Sci. Sports Exerc.* (In Press).

Clarkson, P.M., and E.M. Haymes (1994). Trace mineral requirements for athletes. *Int. J. Sports Nutr.* (In press).

Coggan, A.R., and S.C. Swanson (1992). Nutritional manipulation before and during endurance exercise: effects on performance. *Med. Sci. Sports Exerc.* 24:S331–S335.

Costill, D.L., and M. Hargreaves (1992). Carbohydrate nutrition and fatigue. *Sports Med.* 13:86–92.

Costill, D.L., R. Thomas, R.A. Roberts, D. Pascoe, C. Lambert, S. Barr, and W.J. Fink. (1991). Adaptations to swimming training:influence of training volume. *Med. Sci. Sports Exerc.* 23:371–377.

Coyle, E.F. (1991). Carbohydrate feedings:effects on metabolism, performance and recovery. In: F. Brouns (ed.) *Medicine and Sport Science, Vol. 32: Advances in Nutrition and Top Sport.* Basel: Karger, pp. 1–14.

Coyle, E.F., A.R. Coggan, M.K. Hopper, and T.J. Walters (1988). Determinants of endurance in well trained cyclists. *J. Appl. Physiol.* 64:2622–2630.

Coyle, E.F., M.E. Feltner, S.A. Kautz, M.T. Hamilton, S.J. Montain, A.M. Baylor, L.D. Abraham, and G.W. Petrek (1991). Physiological and biomechanical factors associated with elite endurance cycling performance. *Med. Sci. Sports Exerc.* 23:93–107.

Coyle, E.F., W.H. Martin, D.R. Sinacore, M.J. Joyner, J.M. Hagberg, and J.O. Holloszy (1984). Time course of loss adaptation after stopping prolonged intense endurance training. *J. Appl. Physiol.* 57:1857–1864.

Coyle, E.F., L.S. Sidossis, J.F. Horowitz, and J.D. Beltz (1992). Cycling efficiency is related to the percentage of Type I muscle fibers. *Med. Sci. Sports Exerc.* 24:782–788.

Depalma, M.T., W.M. Koszewski, J.G. Case, R.J. Barile, B.F. Depalma, and S.M. Oliaro (1993). Weight control practices of lightweight football players. *Med. Sci. Sports Exerc.* 25:694–701.

Dudley, G.A., and R. Djamil (1985). Incompatibility of endurance- and strength-training modes of exercise. *J. Appl. Physiol.* 59:1446–1451.

Evans, W.J. (1993). Exercise and protein metabolism. In: A.P. Simopoulos and K.N. Pavlou (eds.) *World Review of Nutrition and Dietetics, Vol. 71: Nutrition and Fitness for Athletes.* Basel:Karger, pp. 21–33.

Faber, M., S.-J. Spinnler-Benade, and A. Daubitzer (1990). Dietary intake, anthropometric measurements and plasma lipid levels in throwing field athletes. *Int. J. Sports Med.* 10:140–145.

Fitts, R.H., D.L. Costill, and P.R. Gardetto (1989). Effect of swim exercise training on human muscle fiber function. *J. Appl. Physiol.* 66:465–475.

Gaitanos, G.C., C. Williams, L.H. Boobis, and S. Brooks (1993). Human muscle metabolism during intermittent maximal exercise. *J. Appl. Physiol.* 75:712–719.

Gisolfi, C.V., and S.M. Duchman (1992). Guidelines for optimal replacement beverages for different athletic events. *Med. Sci. Sports Exerc.* 24:679–687.

Goldfarb, A.H. (1993). Antioxidants: role of supplementation to prevent exercise-induced oxidative stress. *Med. Sci. Sports Exerc.* 25:232–236.

Goldspink, G. (1978). Energy turnover during contraction of different types of muscle. In: E. Asmussen and K. Jorgensen (eds.) *Biomechanics VI-A.* Baltimore: University Park Press, pp. 27–39.

Grandjean, A.C. (1989). Macronutrient intake of the US athletes compared with the general population and recommendations made for athletes. *Am. J. Clin. Nutr.* 49:1070–1076.

Heinemann, L., and H. Zerbes (1989). Physical activity, fitness, and diet: behavior in the population compared with elite athletes in the GDR. *Am. J. Clin. Nutr.* 49:1007–1016.

Henrikson, J., and J.S. Reitman (1977). Time course changes in human skeletal muscle succinate dehydrogenase and cytochrome oxidase activities and maximal oxygen uptake with physical activity and inactivity. *Acta Physiol. Scand.* 99:91–97.

Hickson, R.C. (1981). Skeletal muscle cytochrome c and myoglobin, endurance, and frequency of training. *J. Appl. Physiol.* 51:746–749.

Hickson, R.C., H.A. Bomze, and J.O. Holloszy (1977). Linear increase in aerobic power induced by a strenuous program of endurance exercise. *J. Appl. Physiol.* 42:372–376.

Hickson, R.C., B.A. Dvorak, E.M. Gorostiaga, T.T. Kurowski, and C. Foster (1988). Potential for strength and endurance training to amplify endurance performance. *J. Appl. Physiol.* 65:2285–2290.

Hickson, R.C., C. Foster, M.L. Pollock, T.M. Galassi, and S. Rich (1985). Reduced training intensities and loss of aerobic power, endurance, and cardiac growth. *J. Appl. Physiol.* 58:492–499.

Hickson, R.C., and M.A. Rosenkoetter (1981). Reduced training frequencies and maintenance of increased aerobic power. *Med. Sci. Sports Exerc.* 13:13–16.

Hickson, R.C., M.A. Rosenkoetter, and M.M. Brown (1980). Strength training effects on aerobic power and short term endurance. *Med. Sci. Sports Exerc.* 12:336–339.

Holloszy, J.O., and F.W. Booth. (1975). Biochemical adaptations to endurance exercise in skeletal muscle. *Annu. Rev. Physiol.* 38:273–295.

Holloszy, J.O., and E.F. Coyle (1984). Adaptations of skeletal muscle to endurance exercise and their metabolic consequences. *J. Appl. Physiol.* 56:831–838.

Horowitz, J.F., L.S. Sidossis, and E.F. Coyle (1991). Muscle fiber type influences efficiency and performance. *Med. Sci. Sports Exerc.* 23:S92.

Hultman, E., and H. Sjoholm (1983). Substrate availability. In: H.G. Knuttgen, J.A. Vogel, and J. Foortmans (eds.) *Biochemistry of Exercise, Vol. 5.* Champaign, IL: Human Kinetics, pp. 63–75.

Klausen, K., J.P. Clausen, B. Rasmussen, and J. Trap-Jensen (1971). Effect of strenuous arm and leg training on pulmonary ventilation, metabolism, and blood pH during submaximal exercise (abstract). *Acta Physiol. Scand.* 82:8A.

Kushmerick, M.J. (1983). Energetics of muscle contraction. In: L.E. Peachey, R.H. Adrian, and S.R. Geiger (eds.) *Handbook of Physiology, Section 10: Skeletal Muscle.* Bethesda, MD: American Physiological Society, pp. 189–236.

Kushmerick, M.J., and R.E. Davies (1969). The chemical energetics of muscle contraction II. The chemistry, efficiency, and power of maximally working sartorius muscle. *Proc. R. Soc., Ser. B.* 1174:315–353.

Kyle, C.R. (1991). Ergogenics of bicycling. In: D.R. Lamb and M.H. Williams (eds.) *Perspectives in Exercise Science and Sports Medicine, Vol 4: Ergogenics—Enhancement of performance in exercise and sport.* Carmel, IN: Brown & Benchmark, pp. 373–413.

Jacobs, I., P. Tesch, O. Bar-Or, J. Karlsson, and R. Dotan (1983). Lactate in human skeletal muscle after 10 and 30 s of supramaximal exercise. *J. Appl. Physiol.* 55:365–367.

Lemon, P.W.R (1991). Does exercise alter dietary protein requirements? In: F. Brouns (ed.) *Medicine and Sport Science, Vol. 32: Advances in Nutrition and Top Sport.* Basel:Karger, pp. 15–37.

Lemon, P.W.R. (1992). Nutritional factors in strength and endurance training. In: J. Karvonen and P.W.R. Lemon (eds.) *Medicine and Sport Science, Vol. 35: Medicine in Sports Training and Coaching.* Basel:S. Karger, pp. 160–173.

Lemon, P.W.R., and D.N. Proctor (1991). Protein intake and athletic performance. *Sports Med.* 12:313–325.

Lemon, P.W.R., M.A. Tarnopolsky, J.D. MacDougall, and S.A. Atkinson (1992). Protein requirements and muscle mass/strength changes during intensive training in novice bodybuilders. *J. Appl. Physiol.* 73: 767–775.

Martin, P.E., and D.W. Morgan (1992). Biomechanical considerations for economical walking and running. *Med. Sci. Sports Exerc.* 24:467–474.

McCartney, N., L.L. Spriet, G.J.F. Heigenhauser, J.M. Kowalchuk, J.R. Sutton, and N.L. Jones (1986). Muscle power and metabolism in maximal intermittent exercise. *J. Appl. Physiol.* 60:1164–1169.

Murray, R. (1987). The effects of consuming carbohydrate-electrolyte beverages on gastric emptying and fluid absorption during and following exercise. *Sports Med.* 4:322–351.

National Research Council (1989). *Recommended Dietary Allowances, 60th Edition.* Washington: National Academy Press.

Pollock, M.L. (1973). The quantification of endurance training programs. In: J.H. Wilmore (ed.) *Exercise and Sport Sciences Reviews*, Vol 1. New York: Academic, pp.155–188.

Rosler, K., K.E. Conley, H. Howald, C. Gerber, and H. Hoppler (1986). Specificity of leg power changes to velocities used in bicycle endurance training. *J. Appl. Physiol.* 61:30–36.

Rucinski, A. (1989). Relationship of body image and dietary intake of competitive ice skaters. *J. Am. Dietetic Assoc.* 89:98–100.

Sale, D.G., I. Jacobs, J.D. Macdougall, and S. Garner (1990). Comparison of two regimens of concurrent strength and endurance training. *Med. Sci. Sports Exerc.* 22:348–356.

Saltin, B., K. Nazar, D.L. Costill, E. Stein, E. Jansson, B. Essén, and P.D. Gollnick (1975). The nature of the training response: peripheral and central adaptation to one-legged exercise. *Acta Physiol. Scand.* 96:289–305.

Sharkey, B.J. (1970). Intensity and duration of training and the development of cardiorespiratory endurance. *Med. Sci. Sports* 2:197–202.

Sherman, W.M., and G.S. Wimer (1991). Insufficient dietary carbohydrate during training: Does it impair athletic performance? *Int. J. Sport Nutr.* 1:28–44.

Spriet, L.L. (1994). Anaerobic metabolism during high-intensity exercise (Chapter 1). In: M. Hargreaves (ed.) *Exercise Metabolism.* Champaign, IL: Human Kinetics (In press).

Steen, S.N., and K.D. Brownell (1990). Patterns of weight loss and regain in wrestlers: Has the tradition changed? *Med. Sci. Sports Exerc.* 22:762–768.

Tarnopolsky, M.A., S.A. Atkinson, J.D. MacDougall, A. Chesley, S. Phillips, and H.P. Schwarcz (1992). Evaluation of protein requirements for trained strength athletes. *J. Appl. Physiol.* 73:1986–1995.

Webb, P. (1988). The work of walking: A calorimetric study. *Med. Sci. Sports Exerc.* 20:331–337.

Williams, C. (1993). Carbohydrate needs of elite athletes. In: A.P. Simopoulos and K.N. Pavlou (eds.) *World Review of Nutrition and Dietetics, Vol. 71: Nutrition and Fitness for Athletes.* Basel:Karger, pp. 34–60.

Williams, K.R., and P.R. Cavanagh (1983). A model for calculation of mechanical power during distance running. *J. Biomech.* 16:115–128.

1

Olympic Weightlifting and Power Lifting

WILLIAM J. KRAEMER, Ph.D.

L. PERRY KOZIRIS, M.A.

INTRODUCTION

Olympic weightlifting competition is made up of two lifts, the snatch and the clean and jerk. The objective in the snatch (Figure 1-1 a-d) is to lift the barbell from the floor in one continuous motion to an extended-arms position overhead. The clean and jerk (Figure 1-2 a-f) involves two separate movements. The first (clean) requires lifting the barbell in one continuous motion from the floor to a position on the shoulders and chest. The second (jerk) is then lifting the barbell overhead to an extended-arms position. Both lifts require the competitor to complete the lift in an erect standing posture and to have the barbell under control.

The three lifts in power lifting are the squat, the bench press, and the deadlift. The squat (Figure 1-3 a-b) is initiated from a standing position

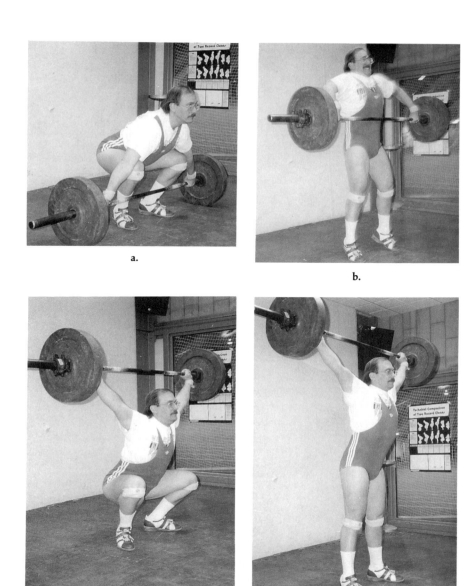

FIGURE 1-1 a-d. *The snatch lift.*

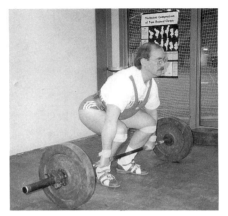

a.

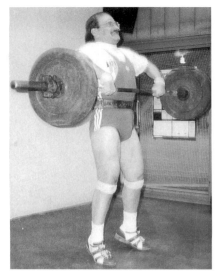

b.

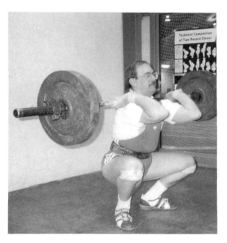

c.

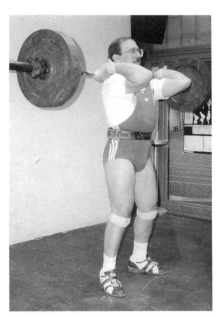

d.

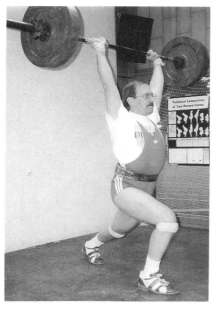

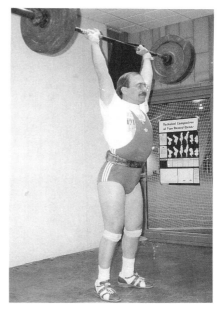

e.

f.

FIGURE 1-2 a-f. *The clean and jerk lift.*

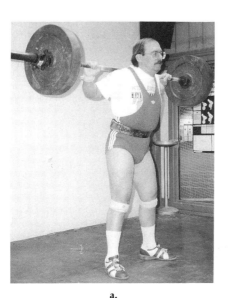

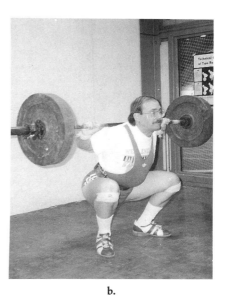

a.

b.

FIGURE 1-3 a-b. *The squat.*

OLYMPIC WEIGHTLIFTING AND POWER LIFTING   **5**

with a barbell across the competitor's shoulders. The objective is to flex the hips and knees to a position in which the thighs are parallel to the floor and to then return to the erect starting position. The objective in the bench press (Figure 1-4 a-c) is to lower a barbell from an extended-arms position to the chest while lying supine on a bench and to then push the barbell back to the starting position. The objective in the deadlift (Figure 1-5 a-b) is to lift a barbell from the floor to thigh level, ending in an erect standing position.

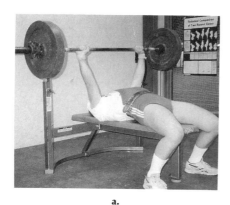
a.

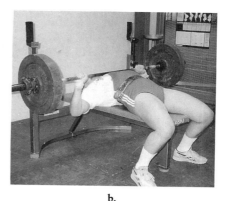
b.

c.

FIGURE 1-4 a-c. *The bench press.*

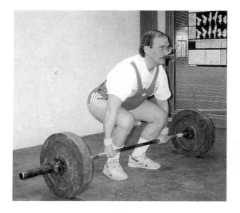

a.

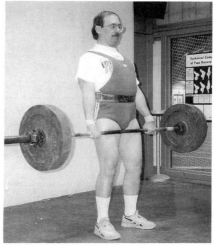

b.

FIGURE 1-5 a-b. *The dead lift.*

The Competition

The competition in both sports is conducted within certain weight, age, and gender divisions. Each of the following weight class numbers represents the upper limit for the body weight in that category. Earlier weight-lifting categories are shown in the table of 1992 world records (Table 1-1); since 1993, weightlifting body weight classes are 46, 50, 54, 59, 64, 70, 76, 83, and >83 kg for women and 54, 59, 64, 70, 76, 83, 91, 99, 108, and >108 kg for men. Power lifting body weight categories and world records are presented in Table 1-2. Competitions in both sports take place for different age groups ranging from juniors (14–21 y) to seniors (40 y and over with 5 y age categories) in both sports. Men and women now compete in both sports.

Competitive Lifts. The lifts in weightlifting and the order in which they are contested are the snatch and the clean and jerk (Figures 1-1 and 1-2).

The lifts in power lifting are contested in the following order: the squat, the bench press, and the deadlift (Figure 1-3). Weight class competitors win the competition by lifting the greatest total mass in the specified lifts using proper form as determined by meet judges. Placement in com-

TABLE 1-1. *1992 world weightlifting records (kg) for the snatch and the clean and jerk lifts. The upper limit for each body weight class is expressed in kg. The unlimited class is indicated by +.*

Class	Women, Open Group Snatch	Clean & Jerk	Class	Men, Open Group Snatch	Clean & Jerk
44	72.5	95.5	52	120.5	155.5
48	75.0	98.0	56	135.0	171.0
52	81.0	108.0	60	152.5	190.0
56	85.0	108.0	67.5	160.0	200.5
60	87.5	115.0	75	170.0	215.5
67.5	97.5	122.5	82.5	183.0	225.0
75	105.0	137.5	90	195.5	235.0
82.5	107.5	138.0	100	200.5	242.5
82.5+	113.0	143.0	110	210.0	250.5
			110+	216.0	266.0

Class	Men, Junior Open Group Snatch	Clean & Jerk	Class	Men, 40-44 Age Group Snatch	Clean & Jerk
52	118.0	155.0	52	70.0	90.0
56	132.5	170.5	56	82.5	102.5
60	148.0	188.0	60	95.5	122.5
67.5	158.5	200.0	67.5	107.5	132.5
75	170.0	211.0	75	132.5	170.0
82.5	179.0	215.0	82.5	130.0	160.5
90	183.5	225.0	90	145.0	170.5
100	200.0	240.0	100	138.0	175.0
110	205.0	250.0	110	135.0	187.5
110+	190.5	232.5	110+	152.5	180.5

Class	Men, 45-49 Age Group Snatch	Clean & Jerk	Class	Men, 50-54 Age Group Snatch	Clean & Jerk
52	65.0	87.5	52	70.0	87.5
56	85.0	105.0	56	80.0	100.0
60	90.0	110.0	60	85.0	113.0
67.5	135.0	145.0	67.5	122.5	140.0
75	130.0	160.0	75	105.0	140.0
82.5	120.0	153.0	82.5	127.5	155.0
90	130.0	167.5	90	115.0	160.0
100	140.0	162.5	100	118.0	160.5
110	135.0	175.0	110	125.0	162.5
110+	130.0	160.0	110	132.5	162.5

Class	Men, 55-59 Age Group Snatch	Clean & Jerk	Class	Men, 60-64 Age Group Snatch	Clean & Jerk
52	N.A.	N.A.	52	30.0	50.0
56	57.5	70.0	56	55.0	75.0
60	80.0	102.5	60	70.0	87.5
67.5	88.0	112.5	67.5	85.0	102.5
75	90.0	120.5	75	88.0	102.5
82.5	100.5	125.5	82.5	82.5	110.0
90	102.5	130.0	90	82.5	107.5
100	102.5	130.0	100	95.0	112.5
110	100.0	142.5	110	100.0	125.0
110+	105.0	125.0	110+	75.0	100.0

(continued)

TABLE 1-1 (Continued)

Class	Men, 65–69 Age Group Snatch	Clean & Jerk	Class	Men, 70–74 Age Group Snatch	Clean & Jerk
			52	N.A.	N.A.
			56	57.5	75.0
60	67.5	90.0	60	42.5	50.0
67.5	62.5	82.5	67.5	55.0	60.0
75	80.0	95.0	75	55.0	67.5
82.5	75.0	100.0	82.5	70.0	90.0
90	75.0	100.0	90	75.0	95.0
100	77.5	105.0	100	77.5	102.5
110	92.5	115.0	110	N.A.	N.A.
110+	72.5	95.0	110+	65.0	75.0

Class	Men, 75–79 Age Group Snatch	Clean & Jerk	Class	Men, 80–84 Age Group Snatch	Clean & Jerk
67.5	40.5	47.5	75.0	25.0	30.0
75	N.A.	N.A.	82.5	27.5	32.5
82.5	55.0	80.0			
90	N.A.	N.A.			
100	40.0	57.5			

petition is based on the lifter's "total," i.e., the sum of the best successful attempts in each of the competitive lifts. As with any sport, there are many rules regulating competition. They involve issues such as dress, supportive gear (e.g., shoes, wraps, and belts), lift technique, and competition procedures (e.g., time limits and a limit of three attempts per lift).

Development of the Sports. Olympic weightlifting and power lifting can be traced back to the "strongmen" competitions organized in the United States and Europe in the 1860s (Todd, 1978). Weightlifting is the oldest of the two strength sports, having been a part of the Olympic program for men since 1896. International weightlifting competition prior to 1972 also included a third lift, called the press (Fair, 1988). The first World Championship meet in weightlifting for women took place in 1987, and weightlifting is currently an Olympic demonstration sport for women.

While not an Olympic sport, power lifting has gained dramatically increased popularity throughout the world over the past 20 y. Power lifting is a relatively new sport, gaining Amateur Athletic Union acceptance only in the early 1960s. The first official U.S. National Power Lifting Championships for men were in 1965. Based upon memberships in national sport organizations and participation in worldwide competitions, the number of competitors in power lifting is substantially greater than in weightlifting. This popularity can be attributed to several facts: it is easier to learn the power lifting techniques, heavier weights can be lifted in compe-

TABLE 1-2. *1991 American Drug Free Powerlifting Association records (kg)*

Women's 44-kg Body Weight Class

Division	Squat	Bench Press	Deadlift
Open	130.5	77.7	145.3
Teen (14–16 y)	80.2	56.8	107.6
Teen (17–19 y)	102.7	45.1	115.9
Collegiate	130.3	55.1	130.8
Master (35–44 y)	117.7	67.6	140.3
Master (45–54 y)	122.8	72.6	145.3

Women's 47.5-kg Body Weight Class

Division	Squat	Bench Press	Deadlift
Open	137.7	77.3	149.3
Teen (14–16 y)	97.7	50.1	122.7
Teen (17–19 y)	102.6	47.5	120.3
Collegiate	118.2	52.5	132.7
Master (35–44 y)	105.2	59.1	132.7
Master (45–54 y)	132.7	77.3	149.3
Master (55–62 y)	40.0	25.0	72.6

Women's 50.5-kg Body Weight Class

Division	Squat	Bench Press	Deadlift
Open	145.5	85.1	175.4
Teen (14–16 y)	97.7	60.1	122.7
Teen (17–19 y)	120.3	72.5	142.8
Collegiate	141.3	65.1	135.3
Master (35–44 y)	132.8	75.1	152.8
Master (45–54 y)	127.8	77.7	142.8

Women's 53-kg Body Weight Class

Division	Squat	Bench Press	Deadlift
Open	160.2	87.7	166.3
Teen (14–16 y)	122.7	72.5	125.2
Teen (17–19 y)	125.2	65.1	156.8
Collegiate	142.8	72.6	156.8
Master (35–44 y)	142.7	79.5	152.8
Master (45–54 y)	113.6	56.8	147.7

Women's 55.5-kg Body Weight Class

Division	Squat	Bench Press	Deadlift
Open	162.8	90.2	170.4
Teen (14–16 y)	132.7	72.6	135.3

Women's 58.5-kg Body Weight Class

Division	Squat	Bench Press	Deadlift
Open	190.4	105.1	177.8
Teen (14–16 y)	117.7	63.6	132.8

Division	Squat	Bench Press	Deadlift
Teen (17–19 y)	147.7	88.6	165.3
Collegiate	150.3	90.2	150.0
Master (35–44 y)	142.7	77.6	150.3
Master (45–54 y)	111.4	62.6	143.2

Division	Squat	Bench Press	Deadlift
Teen (17–19 y)	162.8	87.7	160.3
Collegiate	140.2	85.1	168.9
Master (35–44 y)	167.9	82.0	160.2

Women's 63-kg Body Weight Class

Division	Squat	Bench Press	Deadlift
Open	187.8	104.5	205.3
Teen (14–16 y)	145.3	80.1	165.3
Teen (17–19 y)	165.4	87.7	175.4
Collegiate	137.8	82.7	172.9
Master (35–44 y)	170.3	102.6	182.9
Master (45–54 y)	92.7	42.6	125.3

Women's 70-kg Body Weight Class

Division	Squat	Bench Press	Deadlift
Open	200.3	110.2	228.0
Teen (14–16 y)	135.3	70.1	160.3
Teen (17–19 y)	167.9	87.6	175.4
Collegiate	137.4	75.1	168.2
Master (35–44 y)	165.3	80.1	176.1
Master (45–54 y)	75.1	35.0	85.1
Master (55–64 y)	70.1	50.1	115.2
Master (65–74 y)	70.1	40.0	107.7
Master (75–84 y)	72.6	42.5	107.7

Women's 80-kg Body Weight Class

Division	Squat	Bench Press	Deadlift
Open	210.3	110.2	213.0
Teen (14–16 y)	147.7	70.1	165.4

Women's over 80-kg Body Weight Class

Division	Squat	Bench Press	Deadlift
Open	218.0	150.0	208.0
Teen (14–16 y)	155.3	75.0	150.0

(continued)

TABLE 1-2. (Continued)

Women's 80-kg Body Weight Class

Division	Squat	Bench Press	Deadlift
Teen (17–19 y)	157.8	87.7	167.9
Collegiate	190.4	87.7	179.5
Master (35–44 y)	165.4	85.2	175.4
Master (45–54 y)	155.2	72.6	155.2
Master (55–64 y)	136.3	72.6	136.3

Women's over 80-kg Body Weight Class

Division	Squat	Bench Press	Deadlift
Teen (17–19 y)	187.9	90.9	182.8
Collegiate	182.8	75.1	192.8
Master (35–44 y)	218.0	150.0	187.9
Master (45–54 y)	154.5	70.1	163.6

Men's 52-kg Body Weight Class

Division	Squat	Bench Press	Deadlift
Open	200.0	145.9	219.0
Teen (14–16 y)	142.8	87.7	165.3
Teen (17–19 y)	177.8	115.5	170.3
Collegiate	183.0	115.9	192.8
Master (40–44 y)	159.1	88.6	181.8
Master (45–49 y)	163.8	87.7	175.4

Men's 56-kg Body Weight Class

Division	Squat	Bench Press	Deadlift
Open	245.5	145.0	248.0
Teen (14–16 y)	177.9	105.6	187.9
Teen (17–19 y)	165.3	137.7	195.0
Collegiate	187.8	127.7	207.8
Master (40–44 y)	187.9	137.8	197.9
Master (45–49 y)	156.0	82.6	177.3

Men's 60-kg Body Weight Class

Division	Squat	Bench Press	Deadlift
Open	243.0	164.8	249.5
Teen (14–16 y)	182.9	110.2	195.5
Teen (17–19 y)	202.9	130.2	230.5
Collegiate	220.5	145.2	228.0
Master (40–44 y)	197.9	120.5	187.8

Men's 67-kg Body Weight Class

Division	Squat	Bench Press	Deadlift
Open	271.6	186.4	280.6
Teen (14–16 y)	205.3	143.2	220.5
Teen (17–19 y)	232.7	147.7	243.0
Collegiate	252.6	170.3	265.5
Master (40–44 y)	233.0	167.8	250.7

Division	Squat	Bench Press	Deadlift
Master (45-49 y)	187.8	120.2	197.7
Master (50-54 y)	172.7	107.6	209.1
Master (55-59 y)	43.2	90.9	145.5
Master (60-65 y)	92.6	60.1	125.2
Master (65-69 y)	100.2	67.6	145.3

Division	Squat	Bench Press	Deadlift
Master (45-49 y)	238.0	140.2	230.5
Master (50-54 y)	230.5	135.2	215.3
Master (55-59 y)	177.8	97.6	190.3
Master (60-64 y)	155.3	122.8	205.3
Master (65-69 y)	140.2	82.6	160.3
Master (70-74 y)	77.7	70.1	125.2

Men's 75-kg Body Weight Class

Division	Squat	Bench Press	Deadlift
Open	313.9	199.9	322.2
Teen (14-16 y)	243.0	150.0	234.1
Teen (17-19 y)	257.3	185.3	262.5
Collegiate	273.0	185.3	279.8
Master (40-44 y)	252.3	197.8	281.8
Master (45-49 y)	252.8	163.5	273.1
Master (50-54 y)	225.0	145.2	253.0
Master (55-59 y)	202.8	135.2	223.0
Master (60-64 y)	197.9	122.7	240.5
Master (65-69 y)	150.2	95.1	245.5
Master (70-74 y)	127.3	38.6	220.5

Men's 82-kg Body Weight Class

Division	Squat	Bench Press	Deadlift
Open	342.8	211.8	335.7
Teen (14-16 y)	253.0	158.0	250.5
Teen (17-19 y)	279.5	182.5	303.1
Collegiate	295.5	192.8	303.1
Master (40-44 y)	295.5	183.9	296.6
Master (45-49 y)	273.0	190.4	308.0
Master (50-54 y)	236.5	160.2	259.0
Master (55-59 y)	218.2	152.3	235.5
Master (60-64 y)	172.8	138.8	215.3
Master (70-74 y)	130.2	80.1	147.7
Master (75-79 y)	110.2	47.5	107.6

(continued)

TABLE 1-2. (Continued)

Division	Men's 90-kg Body Weight Class Squat	Bench Press	Deadlift
Open	355.7	228.0	359.2
Teen (14–16 y)	234.1	155.2	250.5
Teen (17–19 y)	301.3	197.7	283.0
Collegiate	308.0	197.7	295.6
Master (40–44 y)	290.5	219.0	305.6
Master (45–49 y)	277.3	200.3	280.5
Master (50–54 y)	242.0	167.8	268.1
Master (55–59 y)	230.0	143.6	233.0
Master (60–64 y)	215.4	147.8	220.5
Master (65–69 y)	172.8	112.7	195.3
Master (70–74 y)	160.3	122.8	200.4
Master (75–79 y)	120.2	90.1	182.8

Division	Men's 100-kg Body Weight Class Squat	Bench Press	Deadlift
Open	365.7	234.1	361.1
Teen (14–16 y)	260.5	165.9	269.4
Teen (17–19 y)	300.0	185.0	306.8
Collegiate	320.6	210.4	318.1
Master (40–44 y)	324.3	233.2	320.6
Master (45–49 y)	287.3	192.9	285.0
Master (50–54 y)	285.6	180.3	303.0
Master (55–59 y)	228.0	150.3	253.0
Master (60–64 y)	215.3	122.7	220.5
Master (65–69 y)	202.9	134.1	207.9

Division	Men's 110-kg Body Weight Class Squat	Bench Press	Deadlift
Open	390.8	237.3	371.8
Teen (14–16 y)	255.5	129.5	260.5
Teen (17–19 y)	337.5	237.3	287.5

Division	Men's 125-kg Body Weight Class Squat	Bench Press	Deadlift
Open	411.8	250.9	389.1
Teen (14–16 y)	273.0	192.8	245.5
Teen (17–19 y)	325.7	228.0	278.9

Division			
Collegiate	323.0	237.3	320.5
Master (40–44 y)	348.2	227.3	338.2
Master (45–49 y)	330.7	207.9	333.2
Master (50–54 y)	283.1	182.8	273.1
Master (55–59 y)	228.0	155.2	255.5
Master (60–64 y)	197.8	122.7	233.0
Master (65–69 y)	181.8	136.4	195.5
Master (70–74 y)	160.6	135.4	139.5

Division			
Collegiate	328.2	245.5	343.2
Master (40–44 y)	390.8	250.9	318.0
Master (45–49 y)	335.7	213.6	320.7
Master (50–54 y)	278.1	187.8	270.5
Master (55–59 y)	230.5	175.1	269.1
Master (60–64 y)	181.8	190.7	181.8
Master (65–69 y)	160.3	115.2	182.9

	Men's Superheavy Class		
Division	Squat	Bench Press	Deadlift
Open	425.8	288.1	360.8
Teen (14–16 y)	343.9	203.8	301.7
Teen (17–19 y)	425.8	218.0	310.6
Collegiate	335.7	215.3	313.1
Master (40–44 y)	377.3	253.0	323.0
Master (45–49 y)	336.4	215.9	273.1
Master (50–54 y)	254.4	184.1	260.5
Master (55–59 y)	222.7	122.8	212.3

tition, and the lifts are similar to those used in typical weight training programs (Hatfield, 1981; Hatfield & McLaughlin, 1985).

The common factor in both of these sports is the extreme physiological demand for maximal force and power production from the muscles involved in each sport's competitive lifts (Garhammer, 1980; Garhammer & McLaughlin, 1980). Therefore, the primary goal for an athlete in either sport is to maximize the strength and power in the sport-specific lifts. The purpose of this chapter is to examine these two strength sports and contrast the sport demands, training programs, nutritional practices, and adaptations to training.

CHARACTERISTICS OF ELITE WEIGHTLIFTERS AND POWER LIFTERS

Not surprisingly, weightlifters and power lifters exhibit many significant similarities in anatomical and physiological characteristics. There remains great variability within certain characteristics, presumably because of differences among body weight classifications and in the caliber of the athletes that have been studied. No physiological case studies of world class weightlifters or power lifters have been reported. Thus, the upper limits of the various characteristics (e.g., muscle fiber type) for such athletes are unknown. In addition, few data are available on women weightlifters and power lifters.

Body Composition and Anthropometry

Percentage of Body Fat. The average percentage of body fat for groups of male power lifters ranges from 13 to 20% (Fahey et al., 1975; Häkkinen et al., 1984a; Kraemer et al., 1987). Male weightlifters have average body fat percentages of 8 to 12% (Fahey et al., 1975; Sprynarova & Parizkova, 1971; Stone et al., 1979; Tanner, 1964). In a study that combined the two types of lifters, the athletes had a mean of 10% body fat (Katch et al., 1980). Variation of the percent body fat within the sport appears to be related to the body mass category; the lower categories exhibit lower body fat percentages (Stone et al., 1979). This phenomenon has also been seen in wrestling and in other sports that classify competitors according to body mass (Johnson et al., 1991). Many lifters in the higher body mass categories exhibit body fat percentages similar to what might be predicted for untrained men (e.g., 16%). Empirical observations indicate that weightlifters and power lifters typically do not control their diets to modulate body fat as do body builders in preparation for competition (Newton et al., 1993). Other elite male athletes (e.g., sprinters, throwers, long distance runners, wrestlers, and gymnasts) have body compositions ranging from 3-29% fat, with the field event competitors (i.e., throwers) at the high end of the range (DeGaray et al., 1974). Athletes in other sports that also require body mass classifications (e.g., wrestlers) and/or high energy expenditures (e.g., long distance runners) exhibit lower body fat percentages (DeGaray et al., 1974).

Women power lifters across a wide variety of competitive levels average 21% body fat (Johnson et al., 1990). Skinfolds and anthropometric data indicated that women power lifters were leaner than untrained women (Bale & Williams, 1987). Stoessel et al. (1991) reported that women who were members of the 1987 Women's U.S. Weightlifting World Championship team averaged 20.4% body fat compared to 26.9% demonstrated by members of a local weightlifting club.

Body Mass, Height, and Strength. The most apparent difference between lifters and untrained individuals is muscle size. One of the perceptions in the lifting communities, especially in power lifting, has been that elite competitors have increased muscle mass to the greatest extent allowed by body height. Absolute and relative results in the snatch and the clean and jerk have been correlated to many size factors such as body height, body mass, body area, lean body mass, and body fat content (Pilis et al., 1990b). Such data have shown that no single variable appears to predominate in the explanation of strength performance. Historically, much of the research has focused upon the use of one variable—body mass—to describe strength potential. This led to the development of what has been called the "⅔ strength law," i.e., strength in weightlifting performance is proportional to body mass to the ⅔ power (Lietzke, 1956). More recently, the use of the ⅔ power function has been shown to be inaccurate in predicting strength performance in weightlifters (Croucher, 1984; Siff, 1988).

The competitive lift total relative to body mass was studied in the six best weightlifters of the various weight classes in the 1986 European Championships (Tittel & Wutscherk, 1992). The results showed that the relationship between muscular strength and body mass was best described as a non-linear function using the equation: *Total for snatch plus clean-and-jerk (kg) = 89.19 + 8.974 BM − 0.036 BM², where BM is body mass in kg* (Tittel & Wutscherk, 1992).

The contribution of body height to the weightlifting performance can be described by the equation: *Total for snatch plus clean-and-jerk (kg) = −3512 + 38.67 BH − 0.098 BH², where BH is body height in cm* (Tittel & Wutscherk, 1992).

In the multi-joint lifts used in weightlifting and power lifting, no single variable appears to completely explain strength performance. Neural factors important to the recruitment of motor units responsible for force and power production probably account for much of the non-linearity in the relationships between strength and body size (Sale, 1988).

Skeletal Muscle Fibers

Various characteristics related to muscle fiber type have been examined in male (but not female) weightlifters and power lifters. However, the muscle fiber characteristics of world and Olympic championship competitors have not been reported.

Fiber Type Percentages. The mean percentage of Type II muscle fibers in the vastus lateralis muscle sampled from either competitive male weightlifters or power lifters is 53-60% and not as high as might be expected (Häkkinen et al., 1985; 1987a; 1988b). Sample variability (10–15%) observed in the muscle fiber type percentages in lifters is similar to that in control subjects and may be due to the variation in the competitive status of the lifters examined.

The percentage of muscle fiber types in competitive lifters may not be the most representative measure of their strength capabilities. Fiber composition is not closely related to muscle strength or power production (Maughan & Nimmo, 1984; Patton et al., 1990). One might not expect a relationship between strength and the proportion of Type II muscle fibers per se because each lift is characterized by a wide range of movement velocities that require varied patterns of motor unit recruitment and therefore different magnitudes of contribution from Type I and Type II muscle fibers throughout the range of motion. Further study examining the influence of muscle fiber types and strength in competitive weightlifting and power lifting is needed. At present it is difficult to extrapolate from the results of studies using isolated joint force production and fiber types in single muscles to events occurring during integrated multi-joint force production that involve contributions from many muscles.

Cross-sectional Area of Type I and Type II Muscle Fibers. Type II muscle fibers have much larger cross-sectional areas than do Type I muscle fibers in competitive male lifters; therefore, Type II fibers predominate in the overall cross-sectional area of the intact muscle (Dudley et al., 1986; Häkkinen et al., 1985, 1987a, 1988b; Prince et al., 1976; Tesch & Karlsson, 1985; Tesch et al., 1984, 1989). For example, Tesch and Karlsson (1985) showed that the vastus lateralis of lifters contained Type II and Type I fibers with average areas of 8091 μm^2 and 5006 μm^2, respectively. In the deltoid, areas of Type II fibers (8450 μm^2) and Type I fibers (5010 μm^2) are similar to those of fibers in the vastus lateralis. The mean Type II fiber area in the vastus lateralis of power lifters was also reported to be 7900 μm^2 (Tesch et al., 1984). In competitive lifters, the high percentage (i.e., 60-90%) of the total muscle cross-sectional area comprising Type II muscle fibers helps explain how lifters, with essentially the same muscle fiber type profile as control subjects, have much greater strength.

No data are available on muscle fiber type characteristics in women lifters, but a recent study of untrained women demonstrated that the cross-sectional area significantly larger than that of the Type II musc 991). Just the opposite occurs in untrained men (T esch et al., 1984; Tesch et al., 1989). With trainin of the Type II muscle fibers in women eventually surpassed that of the Type I fibers (Staron et al., 1991). How initial muscle fiber size affects the potential for muscle size and strength increases in women requires further study.

Flexibility

Lifters display either average or above-average flexibility (Beedle et al., 1991; Leighton, 1955, 1957). The extent of the lifters' flexibility appears to be dependent on the range of movements used in the sport's training programs (Beedle et al., 1991; Chang et al., 1988). In the study by Beedle et al. (1991), who compared weightlifters, body builders, and American style football players, weightlifters had the greatest range of motion at the shoulder and elbow. It appears that flexibility can be promoted with training in the sport of weightlifting (Beedle et al., 1991; Stone & O'Bryant, 1987).

The relative importance of joint flexibility is dictated by the demands of the sport for maximal performance (Garhammer, 1982/83). Development of muscle mass for a particular competitive exercise may impair other athletic movements. In power lifters, certain movements of the arms (e.g., fully flexing the elbows of both arms and touching both forearms together) can be limited by the enlarged pectoral muscle mass needed for peak performance in the bench press. For example, Chang et al. (1988) demonstrated that power lifters had less flexibility than matched control subjects in behind-the-neck reach, shoulder flexion and extension, shoulder internal and external rotation, elbow flexion, wrist flexion, hip flexion, hip internal and external rotation, and knee flexion. On the other hand, these power lifters had greater than normal trunk flexibility as measured by the sit-and-reach test, perhaps because they train with the squat and deadlift, both of which require trunk and hamstring flexibility.

Heel contact with the floor is necessary for proper technique in the performance of the squat exercise. In many beginners, a common problem in the squat is the loss of heel contact with the floor as the lifter's thigh become parallel to the floor. In males, the primary discriminators of foot contact are torso length (33%), sit-and-reach flexibility (9.3%), femur length (8.8%), and ankle flexibility (6.9%) (A.C. Fry et al., 1988). In women, the primary discriminators of foot contact are femur length (49%) and torso length (29.8%) (A.C. Fry et al., 1991).

In certain movements, limitation of the range of motion by highly developed muscle mass may, in fact, enhance power lifting performance by reducing the distance through which the barbell must be lifted. Finally, the relative contribution of flexibility to optimal exercise technique in the competitive lifts may vary among exercises and between genders.

Muscular Strength and Power

Muscular strength and power are specific to the involved muscle groups, the type of muscle action (concentric, eccentric, and/or isometric), the velocity of the action in a dynamic test, and the joint angle in an isometric action (Knuttgen & Komi, 1992). Strength is defined as the maximal muscular force generated at a specified or predetermined velocity (Knuttgen & Kraemer, 1987). In the same manner, power assessment depends on the specific movement that is involved, and power can be defined as the product of the muscular force exerted and the distance through which the resistance is displaced, divided in turn by the duration of the movement (Knuttgen & Komi, 1992). In these sports, power can also be thought of as force times velocity. The most specific test for these athletes is their performance in the competitive lifts. Recent world weightlifting and power lifting records are shown in Tables 1-1 and 1-2, respectively.

Increases in strength are very limited in lifters who have an extensive training history. For example, following 2 y of training, only slight increases (from 272 to 280 kg) occurred in the lift total for male weightlifters who had, on average, competitive experience of 7 y (Häkkinen et al., 1988b). There was no significant group improvement in these lifters after one year of training (Häkkinen et al., 1987a).

Isometric Strength. In addition to the competitive lifts, other measures of strength and power have been reported for competitive power lifters and weightlifters. Male weightlifters with a mean body mass of 70 kg can produce over 4000 N of force (57 N·kg^{-1}) in bilateral isometric leg extension (Häkkinen et al., 1988a, 1988b); those with a mean body mass of 89 kg have produced 4539 N (51 N·kg^{-1}) in a similar test (Häkkinen et al., 1984a). A longer time is needed by power lifters than by body builders and wrestlers to reach percentages of this maximal force (53.3 vs 27.0 ms at 30%; 151.0 vs 70.5 ms at 60%; 633.3 vs 367.0 ms at 90%) or to reach certain absolute levels of force. The rates of maximal force development (26,568 N·s^{-1}) and of maximal relaxation (i.e., rate of return to resting condition) were similar to those of the other athletes (49,050 N·s^{-1}). Weightlifters have exhibited faster times than endurance athletes and controls in these types of isometric tests (Häkkinen et al., 1988b).

Differences in the force-time curves for weightlifters and power lifters may be indicative of the differences in the functional demands of the competitive lifts in the two sports. Weightlifters must generate force at a much higher velocity to produce the large power outputs required to perform the competitive lifts (Garhammer, 1993). Conversely, while force production is very high in power lifting, there is no need for high power output because the lifts allow much heavier weights to be lifted at very slow velocities of movement (Garhammer & McLaughlin, 1980). Improving the rate of force production appears to be related to the performance of ballistic muscle actions in training (Behm & Sale, 1993).

As reviewed by Maughan (1984), there is an extensive literature regarding the relationship between isolated single joint isometric strength and cross-sectional area of muscle. All of these studies have shown large individual variability but significant relationships between voluntary isometric force and cross-sectional area of muscle. Maughan (1984) has hypothesized that the reasons for the variability in this relationship include the training status of the subjects, relative proportions of different muscle fiber types, biomechanical factors, neural factors, and psychological factors.

Isokinetic Strength. Peak isokinetic torques for the flexors and extensors of the wrist and knee at 0.52 rad·s^{-1} in female power lifters (most of whom were of national caliber) were comparable to the performance of other female strength athletes when expressed relative to body mass or fat-free mass (Johnson et al., 1990). Peak torque has also been reported for male power lifters with a mean body mass of 91 kg (Sale & MacDougall, 1984). Peak torque for ankle plantar flexion was 330 Nm at 0.10 rad·s^{-1} and 165 Nm at 0.60 rad·s^{-1}; that for knee extension was 257 Nm at 0.52 rad·s^{-1} and 197 Nm at 3.14 rad·s^{-1}. Elbow extension produced 87 Nm at 0.52 rad·s^{-1} and 79 Nm at 3.14 rad·s^{-1}. When compared to 72-kg men who had no resistance training experience, the power lifters were stronger in all the tests except in plantar flexion at 0.60 rad·s^{-1}, in which both groups were similar. One might speculate that the reason for this may be that no direct training is typically performed for the plantar flexors by power lifters.

Power Production During Competitive Lifting

Olympic Weightlifting. The Olympic lifts have been extensively analyzed, and the total power output of the snatch is similar to that of the clean phase of the clean and jerk (Garhammer, 1980; 1981a; Häkkinen et al., 1984b). The power output of a lift is dependent upon the portion of the lifting movement which is analyzed. The clean portion includes the two pull phases, i.e., from the floor to the knees and from the knees until the bar reaches maximal upward velocity. The jerk portion consists of moving the bar from the finished clean position to the overhead position. As an example, a 125-kg male attempting a 260.5-kg clean and jerk lift can produce average power of 4191 W for the entire clean, including 6981 W in the second pull phase, and 4570 W during the jerk (Garhammer, 1993). Typically, the power output of the jerk is similar to that of the top pull of the snatch and of the clean (Garhammer, 1981a, 1982/83, 1985, 1991a, 1991b). In Garhammer's 1993 results, the calculation of 4570 W was relatively low for the jerk, possibly because of slower and deeper flexion of the knees used by some weightlifters in the study. The duration of the jerk in Garhammer's 1993 study was longer (320 ms) than that usually observed (180–240 ms), thus contributing to a lower power output in the jerk.

Power Lifting. A 100-kg power lifter deadlifting or squatting 375 kg would produce 1274 W or 12.7 W/kg body weight, considerably less than the power output of the clean (Garhammer, 1993). Other studies confirm this difference (Garhammer & McLaughlin, 1980). A 75-kg power lifter bench pressing 200 kg would produce 343 W or 4.6 $W \cdot kg^{-1}$. Thus, it is interesting to note that the sport called *power lifting* really does not have a high power component but rather a high force component.

Body Mass and Gender Effects on Force Production. Absolute power output tends to be greater in the heavier weight classes for male weightlifters, female weightlifters, and male power lifters (Garhammer, 1981a, 1985, 1991a, 1991b; Garhammer & McLaughlin, 1980). Women produce lower power outputs than do men relative to body mass. Women produce 21.8 $W \cdot kg^{-1}$ body weight (63% of the power for men) in the entire snatch or clean and 39.2 $W \cdot kg^{-1}$ (74% of the male value) in the jerk or the second pull during snatches and cleans.

Estimates of female power output from world record data during the three power lifts are 60 to 70% of the men's values (Garhammer, 1993). These data support previous strength comparisons of untrained men and women. For example, Laubach (1976) showed that total body strength for untrained women was 63.5% of the strength of untrained men. Upper body strength for women in various exercises ranged from 35–79% of the strength of men, and lower body strength in various exercises ranged from 57–86% of the strength of men.

Anaerobic Power and Capacity

Short-term (15–60 s) cycle ergometer tests have been used to assess the anaerobic power of lifters. Such tests are most likely inappropriate for weightlifters and power lifters because peak power outputs during lifting are produced in a fraction of a second; therefore, power estimates from tests lasting 15–60 s drastically underestimate the true power capabilities of these athletes. In a study by Häkkinen et al. (1985), power lifters produced power outputs in a 60-s test of 9.3 $W \cdot kg^{-1}$ body mass during the first 15-s interval, 7.1 $W \cdot kg^{-1}$ during the second 15-s interval, 5.1 $W \cdot kg^{-1}$ during the third 15-s interval, and 4.1 $W \cdot kg^{-1}$ during the final 15-s interval. They produced an average power of 6.4 $W \cdot kg^{-1}$ for the full 60 s and a 56% decline in power from the first to the final interval. Similarly, male weightlifters have produced power outputs of 9.2, 7.7, 5.8, and 4.5 $W \cdot kg^{-1}$ in the four intervals, respectively; average power for the 60 s was 6.8 $W \cdot kg^{-1}$ (Häkkinen et al., 1987a).

Surprisingly, these data are similar to those for non-strength trained, physically active men. In a study by Koziris & Montgomery (1992), physically active men demonstrated 10.2, 8.5, 6.0, and 5.0 $W \cdot kg^{-1}$ in the four intervals, respectively. The average power output for the 60 s was 7.4 $W \cdot kg^{-1}$ with a 51% decline from the first to the final interval. Consistent with this trend in the data for men, female power lifters (most of a national caliber) achieved a peak power output of only 486 W (7.1 $W \cdot kg^{-1}$) over 5 s and an average power of 400 W (5.8 $W \cdot kg^{-1}$) over a 30-s Wingate test (Johnson et al., 1990). Murphy et al. (1986) reported peak power values of 503 W (8.5 $W \cdot kg^{-1}$) and an average power of 334 W (5.7 $W \cdot kg^{-1}$) for 30 s in physically active but untrained women. It is unclear why power output values do not seem to be different between male and female lifters and untrained subjects. Only one study reported that male weightlifters can produce significantly higher power outputs in a short-term (15 s) cycle ergometer test when compared with untrained controls (Pilis et al., 1990a). It might be speculated that the lack of test specificity may interfere with the true expression of power output in the lifters. Alternatively, power output capabilities in these cycle ergometer tests may not be affected by the lifter's training programs.

Cardiorespiratory Function in Competitive Lifters

Aerobic Power. When tested on a cycle ergometer, male power lifters possess a relatively low aerobic power (42 $mL \cdot kg^{-1} \cdot min^{-1}$) when expressed relative to body mass (Häkkinen et al., 1984a). With similar testing, weightlifters have an aerobic power (47-50 $mL \cdot kg^{-1} \cdot min^{-1}$) that is also similar to that for untrained men (Häkkinen et al., 1987a; Lehmann & Keul, 1986). Such findings are not surprising because the aerobic requirements of both sports are minimal; oxygen consumption demands during training are less than 60% of maximal oxygen uptake (Scala et al., 1987). This lack of an aerobic stimulus from training is confirmed by data demonstrating that weightlifters and power lifters exhibit a smaller number of capillaries per muscle fiber than do non-athletes (Tesch et al., 1984).

Cardiac Dimensions. No differences were observed between lifters and non-athletic controls in the early echocardiographic studies of ventricular volume and ventricular wall thickness, whether expressed in absolute terms or relative to body surface area (Brown et al., 1983a; Longhurst et al., 1980; Menapace et al., 1982). More recent findings with sedentary controls better matched on age and body mass showed that lifters have greater left ventricular wall thickness but similar left ventricular volume (Fleck et al., 1989). Septal wall and free wall thicknesses are also greater in weightlifters than in non-athletes (Fleck, 1992). Competitive weightlifters and power lifters had normal ratios of left ventricular mass to volume, indicating that lifting had not adversely affected cardiac dimensions (Fleck, 1988; Fleck et al., 1989; Fleck, 1992). It does not appear that short-term strength training alters left ventricular cavity size (Fleck, 1988). Cross-sectional studies show that competitive lifters and highly weight-trained athletes have normal left ventricular systolic and diastolic internal dimensions and volumes, whether judged as absolute values or relative to body surface area (Fleck et al., 1989; Fleck, 1988). When cardiac dimensions are corrected for body surface area or body mass, any differences between lifters and control subjects become much less pronounced.

Acute Cardiovascular Responses to Lifting. Few data are available concerning the acute cardiovascular responses to lifting in general, and no reports have described the acute cardiovascular changes with weightlifting or power lifting competition. Heart rate and systolic and diastolic blood pressures dramatically increase with heavy resistance exercise (Fleck & Dean, 1987). During the performance of a two-legged leg press to failure at 95% of the one-repetition maximum (1 RM) in which a Valsalva maneuver was allowed, pressures of 320/250 mm Hg and a heart rate of 170 beats/min were observed (MacDougall et al., 1985). Competitive lifters typically use a Valsalva when lifting a 1 RM weight. Fleck and Dean (1987) demonstrated higher blood pressures with the use of submaximal loads (i.e., 70 and 80% of the lifters' 1 RM) performed to failure than with the 1 RM. Furthermore, trained lifters had a lower pressor response to all lifting protocols.

Large increases in intrathoracic pressures during heavy lifting decrease venous return to the heart and may subsequently decrease cardiac output. An increased intrathoracic pressure has a biphasic effect on arterial pressure, i.e., an initial dramatic rise in pressure occurs as blood in the heart and chest cavity is forced into the arterial system, and this is followed by a later fall in pressure resulting from a decreased cardiac output subsequent to a decreased venous return (Fleck, 1992). The acute development of elevated intrathoracic and intra-abdominal pressures during maximal lifting may improve strength performance by helping to stabilize the lumbar spine; these high pressures may also help to prevent back injuries.

Many competitive weightlifters rely on the development of large trunk musculature to provide external resistance rather than the use of lifting belts because the belt may interfere with lift techniques. Conversely, the majority of power lifters use weightlifting belts to help provide a barrier to push against and to provide support during the squat and deadlift exercises. The use of the weightlifting belt may augment the pressor response to weightlifting exercise, primarily through the enhancement of intrathoracic pressure during the Valsalva maneuver (Harman et al., 1988, 1989; Hunter et al., 1989).

Concentrations of Hormones in the Blood

The endocrine system can provide a physiological environment conducive to the development of muscle tissue following each heavy resistance training workout (Kraemer, 1992b). Findings that hormone responses can be differentially affected by different resistance training programs have led to the theory that certain programs may better optimize the natural anabolic environment within the body. Resting concentrations of testosterone, free testosterone, and cortisol have been used as possible markers for the anabolic/catabolic status of athletes (Busso et al., 1990). Resting concentrations of most hormones will fluctuate within a homeostatic resting range that often varies according to the training level of the athlete, the type of training being performed, and the years of training experience (Kraemer, 1992a). The involvement of a particular hormone in any physiological adaptation depends on whether or not the physiological mechanism it mediates becomes operational during the training, and the magnitude of the hormonal response is related to the intensity and the volume of exercise. The adaptations may be a function of the extent to which up- or down-regulation of the hormonal receptors in the tissue can mediate the effects of the specific hormone (Kraemer, 1992b).

Total testosterone (bound plus free) and cortisol have been used as basic measures of anabolic and catabolic status in the body, respectively (Häkkinen et al., 1987a, 1989). Resting serum total testosterone and cortisol concentrations have been examined in male weightlifters who reported no anabolic drug use. The resting concentrations of testosterone (18–30 nM) and cortisol (510–680 nM) in serum span a wide range of values over time (Häkkinen et al., 1987a, 1989). In highly trained weightlifters studied over a 2-y training period, serum total testosterone increased from 20 to 25 nmol·L^{-1}, while serum cortisol remained unchanged from an initial level of 580 nmol·L^{-1}, and the testosterone/cortisol ratio remained relatively stable (Häkkinen et al., 1988b). Sex hormone-binding globulin (SHBG) has been shown to decrease slightly from 23.0 nmol·L^{-1} to 21.2 nmol·L^{-1} over a 1-y lifting program (Häkkinen et al., 1987a). Häkkinen et al. (1988b) also showed that the total testosterone/SHBG ratio in weightlifters increased slightly from a first-year mean (4-month test intervals) of 0.96 to a second-year mean of 1.15. The testosterone/SHBG ratio was thought to provide a marker for the amount of free or *available* testosterone. The search for an effective ratio to mark the anabolic or catabolic status of the body has met with little success, perhaps because changes in circulating concentrations of two hormones cannot adequately represent the complex metabolic status of the whole body. Furthermore, the multiple roles played by most hormones make them difficult markers to interpret.

In a study indicating that the volume of training may be reflected by changes in some of the anabolic hormones, free testosterone in serum was at its lowest concentration following a high-volume phase of training (Häkkinen et al., 1989). With a reduction in the volume of training (total mass lifted) from a weekly average of 36,000 kg to 31,000 kg, increases in the concentration of serum free testosterone were observed (Häkkinen et al., 1989). Such data are consistent with the concept of periodized training, in which volume reductions are made over the course of a training cycle in an attempt to enhance the *trainability* of the athlete. In a group of weightlifters, the serum concentration of luteinizing hormone (LH) rose from 8.6 to 9.1 $U \cdot L^{-1}$, and follicle-stimulating hormone (FSH) increased from 4.2 to 5.3 $U \cdot L^{-1}$ (Häkkinen et al., 1988b). Even larger increases in FSH and LH have been reported following a 1-y lifting program (Häkkinen et al., 1987a). These increases in LH in serum are often difficult to interpret because LH concentrations are extremely pulsatile in nature and require multiple samples (e.g., every 10 min) over 2–24 h.

Some support has been provided for an association between certain endocrine variables and performance in weightlifters. Obviously, such correlational data do not prove a cause-and-effect relationship. There was a positive relationship ($r = 0.77$) between the change in the mean testosterone/cortisol ratio and the change in maximal isometric knee extensor force after 1 y of weightlifting training (Häkkinen et al., 1988b). Additionally, the mean testosterone/SHBG ratio was positively correlated ($r = 0.84$) to the change in average concentric power during the second year of training (Häkkinen et al., 1988b). This latter variable was calculated from loaded jumping performances and is presumably reflective of the overall neuromuscular ability of a weightlifter (Kauhanen et al., 1988). The change in serum testosterone/SHBG ratio has been correlated with the change in the clean and jerk lift during 2 wk ($r = 0.63$) and 4 wk ($r = 0.68$) phases of training (Häkkinen et al., 1987b). These data were used as indirect support for the concept that the minimal duration of any training element in a program (i.e., microcycles) should be between 2 and 4 wk.

There is some indication that weightlifters may have somewhat decreased levels of sympathetic activity at rest, possibly due to sympathetic stimulation during their training. Compared to untrained men, weightlifters have slightly lower plasma levels of free norepinephrine at rest (1.9 vs. 2.6 $nmol \cdot L^{-1}$) but unchanged epinephrine concentrations (0.5 $nmol \cdot L^{-1}$) (Jost et al., 1989). Values for conjugated catecholamines were also similar between weightlifters and untrained men. Jost et al. (1989) also reported that the weightlifters had lower mean platelet $alpha_2$-adrenergic receptor density (174 vs. 237 $receptors \cdot cell^{-1}$) and sensitivity (3.11 vs. 2.5 $nmol \cdot L^{-1}$) than did the untrained men, although the density and responsiveness of mononuclear leukocyte $beta_2$-adrenergic receptors were similar to those of controls (Jost et al., 1989).

It can be concluded from cross-sectional data from national caliber women weightlifters that resting levels of serum hormones (i.e., testosterone, estradiol, cortisol, and growth hormone) are not different from those of untrained women (Stoessel et al., 1991). The lack of any apparent resistance training adaptations in the resting hormonal status of women has been supported by other longitudinal resistance training studies. No significant changes have been observed in resting hormone concentrations of serum testosterone, free testosterone, cortisol, sex-hormone binding globulin, luteinizing hormone, follicle-stimulating hormone, estradiol, or progesterone (Häkkinen et al., 1990; Westerlind, et al., 1987). These studies are somewhat difficult to interpret because only single samples were obtained and because the status and the phase of menstrual cycles were not controlled. It is possible that the pulsatility of the hormones and the phase of the menstrual cycle could dramatically impact these previous findings.

Muscle Enzyme Activities

Tesch et al. (1989) have characterized the activity of several marker enzymes in the vastus lateralis for a mixed group of male power lifters and weightlifters. When compared to sedentary men, lifters on average had a lower citrate synthase activity (a marker of Krebs cycle capacity) in Type II muscle fibers and a similar activity in Type I muscle fibers. The lifters had a greater lactate dehydrogenase activity (a marker of the capacity to produce lactate from pyruvate) than did sedentary men in both Type I and Type II muscle fibers. The activity of 3-OH-acyl-CoA-dehydrogenase (a marker of lipid oxidation capacity) of lifters was similar to that of sedentary men in Type II muscle fibers but was lower in Type I muscle fibers. Myokinase activity (a marker of the capacity for ATP regeneration from ADP) in either Type I or Type II muscle fibers was similar in male lifters and sedentary men.

MECHANISMS OF STRENGTH GAINS

Exercise training protocols that increase muscular force and power capabilities rely first on altered neural activation of the involved musculature, followed later by skeletal muscle hypertrophy (Häkkinen & Komi, 1983; Moritani & de Vries, 1979; Sale, 1988). Furthermore, when hypertrophy of muscle fibers can no longer explain maximal force and power alterations in advanced stages of training, neural alterations may predominate in adaptational importance (Sale, 1988).

Many different mechanisms are available for increasing strength via the nervous system. They include increased motor unit activation, greater motor unit firing rates, increased synchrony of motor unit activation, altered activation or inhibition of antagonistic muscles, and improved movement patterns (Sale, 1988, 1992). Neural activation of skeletal muscle can be quantified by determining integrated electromyographic (IEMG) activity (Häkkinen & Komi, 1983; Sale, 1988, 1992). Increased IEMG activity is specific to the movement pattern and is associated with greater force production and increased rates of force development (Sale, 1988, 1992).

Neural adaptations can occur centrally or peripherally. Whether these changes are central and/or peripheral can be determined by comparing IEMG activity with isometric force production (i.e., the IEMG/force ratio) (Moritani & de Vries, 1979). Central and/or peripheral adaptations can also be identified by comparing forces produced by maximal voluntary and maximal electrically stimulated isometric force production (Bigland-Ritchie et al., 1978; Dudley et al., 1990).

POTENTIAL FUNCTIONAL CAUSES OF PERFORMANCE LIMITATION AND/OR IMPAIRMENT

Fatigue mechanisms in weightlifting and power lifting have yet to be fully defined. They may include both short-term neurological impairment and acute or chronic depletion of energy substrate. Overtraining or nutritional inadequacy coupled with high-intensity training sessions can lead to premature fatigue during a competition. Fatigue following the performance of a single lift does not appear to elicit any long-term deficits in performance, but inappropriate exercises, sets, and repetitions performed as a warmup prior to a competitive attempt may cause fatigue and adversely affect the attempt at a maximal lift. Typically, the preparation for a competitive attempt involves a progressive increase in the loading of multiple sets in the appropriate lift leading up to the competitive 1 RM attempt. Adequate rest (3–7 min) between maximal competitive attempts may also be important in minimizing early fatigue.

Nervous System

No direct cellular data are available regarding the resynthesis of neurotransmitters or the functional status of the neuromuscular junction after high-threshold motor unit recruitment in the competitive lifts. However, Häkkinen et al. (1988a, 1988c) have shown that the integrated electromyographic activity does decrease after a weightlifting exercise session. This suggests that repeated lifting impairs the ability to recruit high-threshold motor units and thereby limits subsequent lifting performance. An inability to recruit available motor units due to a lack of training would also contribute to performance decrements.

Muscle Phosphagens

Conceivably, an inability to sustain a sufficient rate of ATP regeneration during competition could limit performance. Significant reductions of 20 and 50%, respectively, have been observed in ATP and PCr concentrations in mixed muscle within 30 s after high-intensity, multiple-repetition resistance exercise (Tesch et al., 1986). When a brief time (e.g., 2–3 min) is allowed between lift attempts, it is likely that almost full recovery of the phosphagen pool would be accomplished prior to the next attempt. Only if heavy attempts were made inappropriately in the prep room (where competitors complete all the warm-up lifts prior to walking out on the competitive platform) would it seem reasonable to suspect that a meaningful phosphagen depletion might occur. Also, the fact that myokinase activity in Type I and Type II fibers is similar in lifters and sedentary men (Tesch, 1987) suggests that the concentration of ATP in the muscle is adequate for optimal performance and that the capacity for ATP regeneration is not challenged in these sports.

Muscle Glycogen

Tesch et al. (1986) observed a 26% decrease in glycogen in mixed muscle fibers after multiple repetitions of heavy resistance exercise. Pascoe et al. (1993), utilizing multiple sets and repetitions at 70% of the 1 RM in a single knee extension exercise to failure, also found a significant decrease in glycogen in mixed muscle fibers (-40.6 ± 2.7 mmol·kg^{-1} wet weight). Thus, decreases in muscle glycogen can occur in response to resistance exercise. The total number of repetitions performed during a meet is greater than the number of official attempts (three in each lift) made in competition. This is due to the fact that almost all lifters perform a significant number of high-intensity sets in the prep room. No data exist regarding muscle glycogen depletion in this competitive environment. Based upon the evidence from previous studies, it might be hypothesized that a significant glycogen depletion in Type II muscle fibers occurs.

Dehydration

If a competitor becomes acutely dehydrated to qualify for a lower body mass classification, it is possible that dehydration could limit performance. No data concerning this topic have been reported within the context of a weightlifting or power lifting competition. The effect of dehydration on other types of strength performance is equivocal; in some cases when wrestlers were used as subjects, there appeared to be no effects of dehydration on strength (Houston et al., 1981; Webster et al., 1990), whereas in others, strength was diminished by 10–15% at low velocities of isokinetic knee extensions (Houston et al., 1981) or by nearly 8% in isometric knee extensions (Viitasalo et al., 1987). If weight loss regimens similar to those practiced by wrestlers were used by lifters, dehydration could well be a major limiting factor. However, dehydration is not commonly practiced by lifters; when it is, the extent of dehydration is typically not as extreme as that observed in wrestlers.

BRIEF HISTORY AND CRITIQUE OF TRAINING PRACTICES

The sports of weightlifting and power lifting were both started by small, dedicated groups of lifters in the late 1800s and 1950s, respectively.

In general, training took place in local gyms and athletic clubs. The gym or club was the focal point of many lifters' social existence and leisure time. Groups of lifters would congregate, train, and exchange ideas on training. Competitions allowed lifters from many different locations to discuss their training techniques. After the competition, lifters would return to their own gyms with new ideas and workout strategies with which to experiment for the next meet. Most of these traditions and practices continue to the present.

In general, training and nutritional practices have been influenced by the habits of top lifters. A great deal of trial-and-error experimentation with different programs helps lifters find out what works best. Improved maximal strength in the competitive lifts acts as the obvious marker for the success of a program. This has led to many training fads, with many lifters adopting the techniques of the champion lifters. Communication among lifters is driven by the chase for that secret combination of factors that will make them champions. This same network of communication is also used to share experiences with performance-enhancing drugs.

Weightlifting

The fierce competition between the United States and the former Soviet Union for world influence during the Cold War greatly impacted the sport of weightlifting. In the 1950s, countries started to identify the success of their athletes with their political systems; over the years, successful training systems in weightlifting were identified by their countries of origin (e.g., "the Bulgarian system") (Garhammer & Takano, 1992). The athletic arena became a non-violent battleground between two systems of government. The United States had dominated the sport of weightlifting in the Olympics from 1948 to 1956, but in 1960, the Soviet Union won almost all of the gold medals. This started an Eastern European domination in the sport which continued through the 1992 Olympic Games. The systems of athlete development used by the Soviet and Eastern Block countries gave a new perspective on formalizing the selection and training process (Garhammer & Takano, 1992). In general, these systems formally brought together a team approach to training athletes. The team included a coach, a trainer, a physician, and appropriate scientists. Obvious rewards for success provided the motivation for winning and also for the experimental use of drugs. With the breakup of the Soviet Union and Eastern Block countries and their state-supported training systems, the potential for success in future Olympic competitions is now unclear.

The development of the training concept known as "periodization" by Matveyev (1972) represented one of the most significant advances in training program development. This training approach was based on the work of a Canadian endocrinologist, Hans Selye. Selye's studies of stress, adaptation, and death in an organism were used to construct a theoretical framework in the development of training programs used by weightlifters in the Soviet Union and Eastern Block countries. Periodization of training involves the manipulation of the intensity and the volume of the resistance exercise performed during a training cycle. Programs typically start with a phase of high-volume exercise stress at relatively low intensities and move to lower volumes of exercise using very high intensities. Periodization of resistance training is now commonly employed by lifters in most countries and has been shown to be superior to a wide variety of programs that do not provide any variation in the training stimulus (Stone et al., 1981; Stowers et al., 1983; Willoughby, 1993)

Power Lifting

Power lifting competitions continue to be dominated by North American athletes. While World Championships are conducted annually, most national sport organizations have not embraced power lifting to the same extent as they have accepted weightlifting, especially in the former Soviet and Eastern Block countries. Nevertheless, there are about 10 times as many competitors in power lifting as in weightlifting worldwide. Power lifting has flourished in North America because the lifts were identified by American-style football coaches as strength lifts, and the sport was, therefore, endorsed for use in many conditioning programs. This led to extensive participation in power lifting by athletes who had played American-style football in high school or college (Pullo, 1992).

DESCRIPTION AND CRITIQUE OF CONTEMPORARY TRAINING AND NUTRITION PRACTICES

Key Principles of Strength Training

The training programs in both weightlifting and power lifting have been based on three key principles of strength training: 1) specificity, 2) progressiveness, and 3) variety.

Specificity of Training. Movements used in training should be nearly identical to those used in competition. The two lifts used in weightlifting are biomechanically very different from those employed in power lifting (Garhammer, 1982/83; Garhammer & McLaughlin, 1980). Furthermore, the force and power characteristics of these lifts during maximal performances are also quite different (Garhammer & McLaughlin, 1980; McLaughlin et al., 1977). Very different exercises are chosen to develop strength and power in weightlifting and power lifting to satisfy the specificity principle. Training protocols emphasize the movements in the competitive lifts for each sport (Fleck & Kraemer, 1987; Stone & O'Bryant, 1987). In addition, assistance exercises are also employed to enhance the development of strength, power, and technique in the competitive lifts. The choice of the assistance exercises provides much of the variation in the exercises used in the training program. Among others, Anderson and Kearney (1982) demonstrated that the repetition maximum (RM) load (a resistance that allows only a specific number of repetitions) used in training leads to specific strength gains. Their data supported the concept of a repetition continuum for gains in strength related to the RM resistance used (i.e., lower RMs are associated with greater gain in 1 RM strength).

Progressive Overload. The concept of progressive overload was formalized in the 1940s and stressed the need for the trained musculature to be challenged with progressively greater demands that would cause physiological adaptations leading to improved strength performances (DeLorme, 1945; DeLorme & Watkins, 1948). Trainers have experimented with a host of different protocols and systems (e.g., pyramid programs, heavy sets first, multiple sets); for further reviews see Atha, 1981; Fleck & Kraemer, 1987; Kraemer et al., 1988a. Briefly, the objective of most protocols studied was to enable the athlete to lift a heavier weight each day within the context of the program for the number of repetitions prescribed. This daily progression allowed little room for variation in the loading objective for the exercise over the training period. Furthermore, most studies examined untrained college-aged subjects (typically male) during a short duration of training (4–8 weeks). Such studies, while showing that increases in strength are achieved by a variety of programs, did not give specific insights into the training programs that were considered effective for the more highly trained competitive lifters.

Variation in Training. The challenge in both weightlifting and power lifting has always been to develop a training program that allowed the lifter to peak at the time of the major competition without overtraining (Vorobyev, 1978). The principle of variation in training was established with periodization concepts from the Soviet Union and Bulgaria in the 1970s (Matveyev, 1972). This formalized a process that included different phases of training and recovery in preparing the lifter to peak for optimal performance. Variations on Matveyev's model were later developed by scientists in the United States (Stone et al., 1981; 1982).

Variation in training has been used for more than 20 y in many different ways (e.g., different lengths of loading cycles, loads used, and progressions) by power lifters and weightlifters (Hatfield, 1981; Kraemer & Baechle, 1989; Stone & O'Bryant, 1987). Just as the development and configuration of single workout protocols flourished over the 1950s, 1960s, and into the 1970s, a host of different periodization protocols for variation of the individual workouts has been developed since the middle to late 1970s. Periodized weight training has been shown to be a superior method of progression in a number of studies (Garhammer, 1979d; Stone et al., 1981, 1982; Stowers et al., 1983; Willoughby, 1993). For example, Willoughby (1993) demonstrated the superiority for maximal strength development of a periodized training program over a program based on constant resistance and sets (e.g., 3 sets of 6 RM). In this study, 92 highly trained men were randomly placed into either Group 1 (5 sets of 10 RM for 16 wk); Group 2 (6 sets of 8 RM for 16 wk); Group 3 (4 wk of 5 sets of 10 RM, 4 wk of 4 sets of 8 RM, 4 wk of 3 sets of 6 RM, and 4 wk of 3 sets of 4 RM); or Group 4 (a control group that performed no resistance exercise). No performance differences were observed among the groups before the program. After 8 wk of training, Group 3 produced significantly greater 1 RM lifts in the bench press and squat exercises than the other groups, and this advantage in performance was sustained for the remainder of the 16-wk study. Such data demonstrate that periodized training, which provides variation in resistances used, may be critical for developing maximal 1 RM lifting performance in trained subjects.

The principle of variation is based upon altering the exercises used, the intensity of the training sessions, and the volume of exercise training performed. The training program is planned before its initiation and then subtly modified if needed. The training year is broken into different training cycles (i.e., macrocycle, mesocycle, microcycle); the goals of the program are developed with specific objectives for each cycle. The macrocycle is the longest cycle (e.g., 1 y) with two or three mesocycles contained within the macrocycle. The entire program is defined by the microcycle, which typically ranges from 2–4 wk. The development of an athlete for peak performance in the Olympic Games may require the establishment of a 4-y periodized training program.

Time Course of Strength Development

When training involves heavy resistances, all muscle fibers will get larger, usually during the first 8–12 wk of training (Häkkinen et al., 1987a; Staron et al., 1991). Eventually, based upon the athlete's genetic endowment and upon the training overload, an upper limit of muscle size will be reached. This is consistent with evidence that fiber type characteristics remain remarkably stable in experienced weightlifters over training periods up to 2 y in duration (Häkkinen et al., 1987a; 1988b). Neural factors may be more important once adequate fiber size changes have been achieved (Sale, 1988). It might be hypothesized that muscle mass is more critical and neural adaptations less important in power lifting than in weightlifting because weightlifting requires the expression of force through a greater range of motion in more neurologically complicated movements.

Nutritional Practices

Consumption of large amounts of protein ($2-3 \ g \cdot kg^{-1} \cdot d^{-1}$) is common in the strength training communities (Burke et al., 1991). Chesley et al. (1992) observed that a single bout of heavy resistance exercise increased whole body protein synthesis for up to 24 h after exercise. This implies that a strength athlete may require more dietary protein than sedentary individuals. A high daily protein intake (1.6 g·kg^{-1} body mass) is more effective in retaining body protein in weightlifters than a high-carbohydrate diet, but reduced carbohydrates in the diet contribute to reduced muscular endurance (Walberg et al., 1988). Tarnopolsky et al. (1992) estimated the dietary protein requirements of strength athletes to be approximately 1.76 g·kg^{-1}·d^{-1}, compared to the currently recommended intake of protein for sedentary persons in the United States of 0.8 g·kg^{-1}·d^{-1}. Many lifters believe they need more protein in their diets than do non-lifters. However, the routine protein consumption of both athletes and non-athletes in North America is 1.5–2.5 g·kg^{-1}·d^{-1}; thus, lifters do not typically require protein supplements to meet their protein needs.

Branched chained amino acids (BCAA) have been viewed as an alternative to anabolic drugs, possibly by enhancing circulating testosterone concentrations (A.C. Fry et al., 1993). Amino acid supplementation may also influence central neurotransmitters and their regulation of circulating hormonal concentrations (Reichlin, 1992). Branched chain amino acids compete with tryptophan when crossing the blood-brain barrier. Because tryptophan is a precursor for serotonin (i.e., 5-hydroxytryptamine) in the brain and because serotonin has been linked to feelings of fatigue (Parry-Billings et al., 1990), it has been theorized that ingestion of BCAA may delay the onset of overtraining-related fatigue (Newsholme, 1990). The effectiveness of BCAA in weightlifting and/or power lifting training remains to be directly demonstrated.

Lifters using anabolic-androgenic steroids also typically ingest large quantities of protein supplements in the belief that protein supplementation is needed to support optimal muscular development with steroids (Yesalis, 1993). Such drug use has been purported to allow quicker recovery from a workout, thereby permitting the athlete to train more intensely and more often. With anabolic-androgenic steroids now illegal and banned by most sport organizing bodies in weightlifting and power lifting, athletes have started to use a variety of nutritional supplements (e.g., boron, chromium, colostrum) in the desire to find the ideal steroid replacer(s) (Burke & Read, 1988). Few scientific data are available to support the use of any of the steroid replacers. Nevertheless, trial-and-error experimentation with dietary supplements continues in the lifting communities.

Examples of Training Regimens

The following examples represent typical exercise programs and principles for weightlifting and power lifting. Such programs are based on the empirical observations of coaches and athletes who have tracked successful training programs over the years. Because there are so few scientifically based training studies using competitive lifters, anecdotal evidence from coaches and athletes provides the primary basis for training practices.

The purpose of this section is to give the reader an overview of the programs used in each sport and to highlight the different perspectives on training used in these two sports.

Weightlifting. Extensive reviews of the training protocols used by various nations have been presented by Garhammer and Takano (1992). Totten and Javorek (1988) have detailed the United States Weightlifting Federation's approach to the developmental training of weightlifters. An example of a weightlifting program is presented in Table 1-3.

Choice of Exercises. Most of the exercises used in training for Olympic lifting are related to the two competitive lifts. The major component of both lifts is the pull movement. This essentially involves pulling the weight as high as possible off the floor before the second phase of each lift. The

TABLE 1-3. *An example of a twice daily weightlifting routine*

Exercises	Sets x Repetitions at % 1 RM
Monday a.m.	
Front Squat	4 x 5 at 75%
Shoulder Shrug (snatch grip)	4 x 5 at 80%
Jerk from Rack	4 x 4 at 70%
Monday p.m.	
Power Snatch	4 x 4 at 70%
Military Press	4 x 4 at 80%
Good Morning	3 x 6 at 40% of best clean and jerk
Sit-up	3 x 30 (10 kg)
Tuesday a.m.	
Back Squat	4 x 5 at 75%
Shoulder Shrug (clean grip)	4 x 5 at 80%
Tuesday p.m.	
Power Clean	4 x 4 at 75%
Hyperextension	3 x 6 (20 kg)
Sit-up	3 x 30 (10 kg behind the neck)
Thursday a.m.	
Snatch High Pull (from floor)	5 x 4 at 85%
Pull to Knees (from floor)	4 x 4 at 85%
Snatch Pulls from Hang	4 x 4 at 75%
Thursday p.m.	
Shoulder Shrugs (snatch grip)	4 x 4 at 85%
Jerks from Rack	4 x 4 at 75%
Leg Curl	3 x 6 at 6 RM
Friday a.m.	
Clean High Pull	5 x 5 at 80%
Clean Pull to Knee (from floor)	4 x 4 at 90%
Power Clean from Hang	4 x 5 at 75%
Friday p.m.	
Back Squat	5 x 5 at 80%
Shoulder Shrug (clean grip)	4 x 4 at 85%
Leg Curl	3 x 6 at 6 RM
Sit-up	3 x 30 (10 kg behind neck)

For description of listed exercises see Stone and O'Bryant, 1987.
Note: Wednesday and Saturday are active rest days that include the performance of stretching and jumping drills. Sunday is a complete day of rest.

muscles of the thighs, hips, shoulders, and back are the major muscle groups that must be trained. In addition, each lift has a high skill component and thus requires phases within a workout that address the acquisition of lifting skills. Exercises are related to each of the competitive lifts. In addition to the complete lifts, lifts that represent portions of the total competitive lifting movements are performed. For example, hang snatches and hang cleans from the thighs, hang snatches and cleans from the knees, front squats, power snatches, and push jerks all are performed to help develop each phase of the competitive lifts. (See Stone and O'Bryant [1987] for a description of the exercises listed.)

Order of Exercises. Weightlifting workouts traditionally progress from exercises relying on large muscle groups to those primarily involving small muscle groups. However, few lifting exercises concentrate on a single isolated muscle group. Lifting exercises that are relatively complex or that require greater skill are also typically performed in the beginning of the workout to avoid the effects of fatigue on these lifts. For example, power cleans are typically performed in the beginning of a workout before front squats.

Resistance. The mass lifted is usually heavy (70–100% of 1 RM) when training is directed toward strength development in a particular lift. When exercises are considered "lead up" exercises for one of the competitive lifts, the percentage of the 1 RM is related to the competitive lift (e.g., one may use 70% of the 1 RM in the snatch for performing snatch pulls). However, when lifting technique is to be emphasized, only 40–60% of the 1 RM is used in order to limit the amount of fatigue for the movement so that multiple sets of repetitions can be performed to practice the exercise movements (Stone & O'Bryant, 1987). For beginner or novice lifters who require a greater emphasis on technique, lighter resistances (<40 % of 1 RM) may be needed. Intensity is a crucial variable in the periodization of workouts (Totten & Javorek, 1988). The loads are frequently calculated based on the lifter's best performance for the snatch and the clean and jerk. This is especially true for the primary exercises (i.e., snatch pull, clean pull, power snatch, and power clean). Load varies considerably according to training experience, individual preference, training system, and training cycle.

Number of Sets. Typically, three to six sets of each exercise are performed in a workout. The number of sets is an important determinant of the volume of exercise, and it influences both training effectiveness and the acquisition of skills. A greater number of sets allows for more practice and the acquisition of skills in each of the competitive lifts. Once the loading factor has been increased to relatively high levels (e.g., 80–85% of the 1 RM), the training stimulus of the workout can only be enhanced by increasing the volume of exercise.

Rest Periods. Because of the heavy loads and the large skill component in the lifting movements, rest periods in training for weightlifting are relatively long; this allows sufficient recovery time so that the next lift can be executed in good form. Rest periods usually range from 2–3 min between sets and between individual exercises. For lifts of 95–100% of the 1 RM, rest periods may range from 3–7 min. In an attempt to sustain high intensities, many weightlifters perform two training sessions per day (e.g., one workout in the morning and the other in the afternoon or evening with about 4–6 h between the two workouts) with little or no increase in the overall number of exercises. One might split the planned number of exercises for a particular training day into two separate workouts. This allows almost complete recovery after completion of approximately half of the day's training and enhances the intensity of the exercises performed in the second workout.

Multi-Year Planning. In weightlifting, the setting of goals begins with the planning of a 4–y training period. The major objective in training young lifters (12–16 y), should be to improve lifting technique. In more mature lifters (17–22 y), strength development is emphasized. The acquisition of skill is a crucial objective because without proper lifting techniques, loading cannot be increased, and thus training is compromised.

The Annual Plan. Within a given training year, various objectives are emphasized during particular phases or periods of training. One model of periodization is as follows:

1. Preparatory Period: This is a training phase in which the weightlifter develops general technique in the competitive lifts. This will allow the lifter to progress to the primary goal of strength improvement.
2. Contest Period: This is a phase in which the weightlifter participates in competitions. During this period, emphasis is placed on very high-intensity workouts (i.e., heavy weights and low volume of exercise) that stress technique in the competitive lifts.
3. Transition Period: This is a phase in which the weightlifter recovers after the contest period. Other modes of exercise, including basketball, volleyball, and tennis, are used to create an active rest period that does not involve weightlifting exercise.

Traditionally, the duration of these periods is highly variable and depends upon the experience of the lifter. As an example, the preparatory period for a new lifter may last as long as 8 to 10 months to allow the lifter to gain the needed motor skills to perform the lifts satisfactorily. The duration of the preparatory phase may then be slowly reduced as the lifter's performance improves. Advanced weightlifters may cycle through these different phases 2–3 times annually as competitions are available throughout the year. In the transition period, it is essential for the athlete to recover both physically and psychologically from the contest phase in order to begin the next preparatory period with enthusiasm. The transition period usually lasts 2–4 wk.

Power Lifting. Earlier publications provide further details for the many training programs used by various competitive power lifters (Hatfield, 1981; Hatfield & McLaughlin, 1985; Todd, 1978).

Choice of Exercises. In power lifting, the training emphasizes practice of the three competition lifts (core lifts). Assistance exercises are then chosen to develop the strength of these muscles that assist or stabilize prime movers for the core lifts.

Order of Exercises. The usual progression is from the larger muscle group core lifts (i.e., the competitive lifts) to the smaller muscle groups (assistance exercises). This progression helps to ensure that the practice of the competition lifts is completed before fatigue of smaller muscle groups can limit the loading of core lifts. Only empirical observations of coaches and athletes support this common practice of exercise order.

Resistance. Because the criterion of power lifting is 1 RM strength, almost all loading is heavy (i.e., 1–8 RM). Ten and 12 RM loads are used for warm-ups or when training is in a high-volume/low-intensity period. Most power lifters avoid frequent training with 1 RM loads. While the reasons for this are highly speculative and influenced by individual preferences, most lifters prefer to train with 2–6 RM and hope to see an increase in the 1 RM after a cycle of training. Since progress in the 1 RM in advanced lifters is so slow and the absolute magnitudes of increase can be very small (e.g., 1–3 kg), many athletes do not want to face such slow progress day-to-day. In training, the use of a different load for each set is popular. For example, pyramid loading involves lifting heavier and heavier resistances for each set performed (e.g., 8 RM, 6 RM, 4 RM, and 2 RM).

Number of Sets. The number of sets typically ranges from 3 to 10 for a primary exercise, followed by 3 or 4 sets of assistance exercises. Since sets determine the volume of the workout, they are used to vary the volume of exercise over a training period.

Rest Periods. In power lifting, rest periods are relatively long (e.g., 2–7 min) and are related to the intensity of the previous set of lifts; the heavier the load, the longer the rest period.

Training Styles. In addition to pyramid programming and use of multiple sets, other training styles used for power lifting commonly include the following:

1. Forced repetitions: The training partners help in the completion of the lift when failure is reached. The bench press and assistance exercises using small muscle groups are the most common exercises performed in this fashion.
2. Eccentric training: Performing only the eccentric movement with 105–110% of the 1 RM concentric load in the exercise (e.g., lower-

ing the bar down to the chest in the bench press) is commonly used when a variation in training is needed. This can cause serious delayed muscular soreness if the lifter is not familiar with this style of training.

3. Functional isometrics: This training style involves lifting a weight in an exercise until a "sticking point" occurs and the bar does not move; rather than stop, the lifter continues to exert force using an isometric muscle action. It is thought that this technique helps to eliminate sticking points within the range of motion of a competitive lift, thereby allowing the lifter to lift the mass through the full range of motion.

Periodization of Training. The periodization of training used by power lifters is very similar to that of weightlifters, i.e., the year-long program includes a preparatory period, a contest period, and a transition period. The major difference is that the amount of workout time dedicated to developing skill in the lifts is far less in training for power lifting. During the preparatory period, emphasis is not placed on technique development; therefore, the power lifter can use heavier loads earlier in the training period. Similar to the training in weightlifting, the contest period is dedicated to participation in power lifting meets, and the transition period involves lower intensity and volume to allow rest and recovery. Because the loads used in training are much heavier in power lifting, the transition period may be longer than it is for weightlifting. A typical training cycle for power lifters is shown in Table 1-4.

A sample power lifting program is shown in Table 1-5. Table 1-6 shows an 8-wk sequence of power lifting training leading up to competition.

OVERTRAINING AND IMPORTANT MEDICAL CONSIDERATIONS

There are few experimental or empirical data on overtraining that relate directly to weightlifting and even fewer to power lifting. Various investigations and reviews have used different definitions of overtrain-

TABLE 1-4. *Typical periodization training cycle for power lifting*

Microcycle Duration	Load	Frequency of Training
4 wk	10 RM	3-4 d/wk
4 wk	6 RM	4 d/wk
4 wk	3 RM	5 d/wk
4 wk	2-3 RM	6 d/wk

TABLE 1–5. *Sample power lifting program. Unless noted otherwise, all loads are expressed as a number of maximal repetitions (RM), i.e., 10 = the maximal load that can be lifted correctly ten times only (10 RM). Warm-up and stretching exercises should be performed before and after each workout.*

Monday
Bench Press: 10, 8, 6, 4, 2, 2, (a pyramid program) or periodization cycle (Table 1–4) over
        each 4-week period
Assistance Exercises
    Inclined Press: 8, 8, 8
    Press Behind the Neck: 8, 8, 8
    Triceps Extension: 8, 8, 8
    Biceps Curl: 10, 10, 10
Sit-Up (bent leg) with load: 20, 20
Crunch: 10, 10, 10
Calf Raisers: 10, 10, 10

Tuesday
Squats: 10, 8, 6, 4, 2, 2 (pyramid program) or periodization cycle (Table 1–4) over
        each 4-week period
Assistance Exercises
    Lat Pull Down: 8, 8, 8
    Seated Row: 8, 8, 8
    T-Bar Row: 8, 8, 8
    Upright Row: 10, 10, 10
    Leg Extension: 10, 10, 10
    Leg Curl: 10, 10, 10

Wednesday
Rest day, i.e., no lifting

Thursday
Bench Press (Close-Grip): 6 x 8 (easy day)
Assistance Exercises
    Inclined Bench: 8, 8, 8
    Press Behind Neck: 8, 8, 8
    Triceps Extension: 8, 8, 8
    Biceps Curl: 10, 10, 10
Sit-Ups: 20, 20, 20
Hanging Knee-Up: 10, 10, 10
Calf Raise: 10, 10, 10

Friday
Dead Lift: 10, 8, 6, 4, 2, 2 (pyramid program) or periodization cycle (Table 1–4) over each
        4-week period
Squats: 6 sets of 8 RM
Assistance Exercises
    Lat Pull Down: 8, 8, 8
    Seated Row: 8, 8, 8
    T-Bar Row: 8, 8, 8
    Leg Extension (doubles): 6, 6, 6, 6
    Leg Curl: 10, 10, 10

Saturday and Sunday
Active rest days

TABLE 1-6. Typical 8-week cycle used by powerlifters for contest preparation. Loading example: 75–80% x 5 x 8–10 = 75–80% of 1 repetition maximum (RM) x 5 sets x 8–10 repetitions per set. Assistance exercises for a competitive lift are noted by the term assistance.

Week	Monday	Tuesday	Wednesday	Thursday	Friday	Saturday
1	Bench assistance exercise 75–80% x 5 x 8–10	Squat and deadlift assistance 75–80% x 5 x 8–10	Bench assistance 75–80% x 5 x 8–10	Squat and deadlift assistance 75–80% x 5 x 8–10	Bench assistance 75–80% x 5 x 8–10	Squat and deadlift assistance 75–80% x 5 x 8–10
2	Same as week one, but cut assistance work to three sets of eight and add the competitive lifts for two sets of five at 85%–90% 1 RM.					
3	Same as week two, except drop to 2 X 8 with assistance exercises and increase to 3 x 5 x 85%–90% on the competitive lifts.					
4	Bench assistance 85% x 2 x 6–8 Bench 90–95% x 3 x 2–3	Squat and deadlift assistance 90–95% x 3 x 2–3	Bench assistance 85% x 5 x 3–5 85% x 2 x 6–8	Squat and deadlift assistance	Bench assistance 85% x 5 x 2–5 85% x 5 x 3–5	Squat and deadlift assistance 85% x 5 x 3–5
5	Same as week four. Use 3 x 3–5 for assistance work Wednesday through Saturday and add the competitive styles for 3 x 3 on Friday and Saturday.					
6	Bench competitive style 85% x 2 x 5 90% x 3 x 3	Squat and deadlift assistance to 90% x 5 x 5	Bench assistance to 90% x 5	Rest	Bench competitive style 85% x 2 x 5 95% x 3 x 3	Squat and deadlift competition style 90% x 2 x 5 95% x 3 x 3
7	Bench competitive style 90% x 2 x 5 95% x 3 x 3	Squat and deadlift competition style 90% x 2 x 5 95% x 3 x 3 98% x 2 x 2	Rest	Competitive bench same as Monday	Competitive squat and deadlift same as Tuesday	Rest
8	Bench competitive style 90% x 2 x 5 95% x 3 x 3 98% x 2 x 2	Squat and deadlift competitive style to 80% for 3 or 4 singles only	Rest	Squat, bench, and deadlift to 70% for 3 or 4 singles only	Rest	Contest: 95% x 1 98% x 1 100% x 1 each lift

ing, and this has contributed to a great deal of confusion. Overtraining is defined in this chapter as any increase in volume and/or intensity of exercise training that causes performance decrements.

A.C. Fry (1993) demonstrated that performing many 1 RM lifts during resistance training can decrease 1 RM performance. This was the first study to induce an overtraining syndrome using heavy resistance exercise. Trained subjects performed 10 maximal 1 RM machine squats each day for 2 wk. The 1 RM squat was significantly reduced in the overtrained group by 12.2 ± 3.8 kg, whereas the control group experienced no changes. Many lifters make mistakes in choosing their loads for 2–wk microcycles; the A.C. Fry study showed that such errors can cause significant performance decrements. Thus, the heavy 2–4 wk microcycles in periodized training must be carefully controlled.

A type of training excess can occur after only a few days of training; this has been termed over-reaching (Stone et al., 1991). The athlete can easily recover from over-reaching within a few days, but recovery from true overtraining may require months or even years. Over-reaching has been used as a planned phase of many training programs because it is believed to contribute to subsequent improved performances (Stone et al., 1991). This has been called a *rebound effect*. How to time an over-reaching phase in the lifter's training to produce a rebound remains a trial-and-error process because no systematic research has been published to resolve the issue. Over-reaching may actually be an early stage of overtraining. This means that lifters must be very careful when experimenting with over-reaching in their training programs.

Overtraining may involve alterations in a number of physiological systems (Brown et al., 1983b; Stone et al., 1991). Two distinct types of overtraining syndromes have been proposed: a sympathetic (i.e., Basedowian) syndrome and a parasympathetic (i.e., Addisonoid) syndrome (R.W. Fry et al., 1991; Stone et al., 1991). The sympathetic syndrome includes increased sympathetic activity at rest, whereas the parasympathetic syndrome includes decreased sympathetic activity with enhanced parasympathetic tone at rest and during exercise. Parasympathetic overtraining is uniquely characterized by low resting heart rates, rapid heart rate recovery after exercise, hypoglycemia during exercise, decreased maximal plasma lactate during exercise, and decreased serum catecholamine concentrations at rest and during exercise (Kuipers & Keizer, 1988). It is believed that the sympathetic syndrome develops before the parasympathetic syndrome and is predominant in younger subjects who train for speed and/or power (R.W. Fry et al., 1991; Stone et al., 1991). All overtraining may eventually result in the parasympathetic syndrome. Changes in autonomic nervous system function could account for numerous physiological responses to an overtraining stress.

INJURIES AND ANABOLIC DRUG USE

Injuries from competitive lifting are relatively rare when proper exercise techniques are used in the exercises. It has been estimated that the forces acting on the lumbar spine are 30 to 40 times the normal compression created by body mass alone (Granhed et al., 1987). This force exceeds the predicted fracture threshold of vertebral bone. The spinal column and the knee joints are the most susceptible to injury during competitive training. Almost all weightlifters complain of pains in the lumbar region during competition (Kotani, 1971). Spondylolysis rates of 18–30% have been reported in weightlifters and power lifters (Kulund, 1978; Goertzen et al., 1989). In contrast to these findings, Krahl (1975) found that degenerative disc lesions, spondylolyses, and osteochondroses rarely occur in world class lifters.

To withstand great forces, the lumbar spine must virtually act as a solid block of bone, and this is reflected in an elevated bone mineral content in lifters (Conroy et al., 1992). Despite such great forces acting on the back, intervertebral disc prolapses are rare in lifters (Jaros & Chech, 1965). Problems with discs may be more problematic for older athletes (i.e., > 50 y). Granhed and Morelli (1988) observed less space between the vertebrae in more than 50% of former lifters.

Male lifters have greater knee stability than control subjects as measured by joint tightness (Chandler et al., 1989). Power lifters were tighter than the controls on the anterior drawer test, which evaluates the stability of the anterior cruciate ligament, whereas both power lifters and weightlifters were tighter on the quadriceps active drawer test, which evaluates the anterior or posterior laxity of the knee joint. Overuse problems in the knee joint are common and thought to be due to a high volume of loading stress (Chandler et al., 1989). The complaints are related to the femoropatellar joint, e.g., patellar chondromalacia and patellar tracking problems, and are often traced to improper squatting technique. Overuse and acute trauma injuries in the shoulder and elbow joints are also seen in competitive lifting. These are due to heavy loading in training and competition as well as accidental mistakes in lifting techniques. In rare cases, muscle tears or ruptures can occur.

Anabolic Drug Use

A detailed discussion of anabolic drugs is beyond the scope of this chapter. Nevertheless, anabolic drug use to enhance muscle size and strength has been a part of both weightlifting and power lifting for almost 40 y. U.S. weightlifters were introduced to the idea that anabolic drugs might improve strength performance in 1954 at the world weightlifting championships, when the U.S. team physician was reportedly told by his

Soviet counterpart that the Soviets were taking testosterone (Yesalis, 1993).

In 1958, Ciba Pharmaceutical Company released Dianabol (methandrostenolone), and experimentation with this drug began soon thereafter. Through word of mouth, the reputation of the drug for enhancing muscle mass and strength was spread. By the 1964 Olympics, anabolic-androgenic steroids were being used by almost all Olympic athletes in the strength sports (Yesalis, 1993). It has been estimated that over 88% of elite power lifters use anabolic steroids (Yesalis, 1993). The potential health hazards of such drug use were not dramatic enough to discourage proliferation. New federal laws make it illegal to possess or distribute anabolic steroids for non-medical use. Sports governing bodies discourage anabolic drug use with comprehensive drug testing programs, especially for Olympic-related competitions, that include penalties of exclusion from future competitions for positive test results.

Drug testing became a routine part of Olympic sports in the 1980s. The international governing body in power lifting could not finance a drug testing program comparable to that for the Olympics. This resulted in a split in the power lifting governance structure to include drug-free power lifting associations (e.g., American Drug Free Power Lifting Association). While new drug-free power lifting associations supported the idea of clean competitions, no funding was available for extensive drug testing to verify the drug-free status of the competitors.

Another anabolic agent that has gained great popularity in recent years is a substance called Clenbuterol, which is a beta$_2$ agonist (essentially an antihistamine). It is classified as both a stimulant and an anabolic agent and is banned by the International Olympic Committee. Its use is thought to promote an increase in muscle mass, but no controlled human studies have confirmed this hypothesis. Clenbuterol reduces body fat, but changes in lean tissue mass remain controversial. Side effects, including headaches, restlessness, insomnia, and tremor are observed in roughly 15% of the subjects who use Clenbuterol. With the increased availability of growth hormone and other growth-promoting drugs, concerns persist that anabolic drug use in weightlifting and power lifting may expand even further.

SUGGESTED DIRECTIONS FOR FUTURE RESEARCH

The following are some of the general questions on weightlifting and power lifting that should be investigated:

- What physiological mechanisms influence physical and psychological recovery from weightlifting and power lifting training sessions?
- What are effective restoration methods (e.g., whirlpool baths,

massage, hot or cold packs, etc.) that might enhance recovery between training sessions?
- What improvements can be made in the current training practices related to the periodization of training?
- What are the neural, muscle fiber, and endocrine adaptations that occur with training for weightlifting and power lifting?
- What are the causes and markers of overtraining in power lifting and weightlifting?
- What is the role of neural inhibition in limiting maximal lifting performance?
- What are the physiological characteristics of elite world champion and Olympic level competitors in weightlifting and power lifting?
- What is the duration of time needed to observe a performance rebound after a period of over-reaching during a training cycle?
- What are the effects of dehydration on the performance of competitive lifts?
- How can various nutritional strategies be used to optimize training and competitive lifting performance?
- What factors contribute to injury in weightlifting and power lifting?
- What are the relationships of anthropometric variables to lifting performances?

SUMMARY

Weightlifting and power lifting require unique strength and power capabilities for elite performance. Few data on physiological profiles are available from world champion competitors. A combination of factors appears to be important for an optimal biological predisposition for championship performance. These factors include a large cross-sectional area of fast twitch fibers in the muscles involved, body and limb lengths optimal for lifting mechanics in the competitive lifts, the genetic predisposition to avoid injuries consequent to the high-intensity training, and a psychological disposition to tolerate the rigors of training. Inadequate energy stores in the muscle and excessive motor demands might limit performance in competition. Training techniques have evolved less as a result of controlled scientific investigations and more by emulating the methods of the top lifters or national coaches. Although there is scientific support for the idea that the athletes need greater protein intake than that recommended for sedentary persons, weightlifters, power lifters, and even most untrained individuals usually consume more than enough protein in their normal diets; protein supplements are probably unnecessary. Other nutritional strategies (e.g., high carbohydrate intake) for improving lifting performance remain relatively poorly studied. Anabolic drug use is rampant in these sports, and steps to respond to this problem have been taken; their effectiveness remains to be determined. Overtraining can become a serious problem in strength training. The major injuries in these sports appear to be related mostly to technical mistakes made in training.

ACKNOWLEDGMENTS

The preparation of this chapter was supported in part by a grant from the Robert F. and Sandra M. Leitzinger Research Fund in Sports Medicine for the Center for Sports Medicine at the Pennsylvania State University.

BIBLIOGRAPHY

Anderson, T., and J.T. Kearney (1982). Effects of three resistance training programs on muscular strength and absolute and relative endurance. *Res. Quart. Exerc. Sport*, 53:1–7.

Atha, J. (1981). Strengthening muscle. In: D.I. Miller (ed.) *Exercise and Sport Science Reviews, Vol. 9*. Philadelphia: Franklin Institute, pp. 1–73.

Bale, P., and H. Williams (1987). An anthropometric prototype of female power lifters. *J. Sports Med.* 27:191–196.

Beedle, B., C. Jessee, and M.H. Stone (1991). Flexibility characteristics among athletes who weight train. *J. Appl. Sport Sci. Res.* 5:150–154.

Behm, D.G., and D.G. Sale (1993). Intended rather than actual movement velocity determines velocity-specific training response. *J. Appl. Physiol.* 74:359–368.

Bigland-Ritchie, B., D.A. Jones, G.P. Hosking, and R.H.T. Edwards (1978). Central and peripheral fatigue in sustained maximum voluntary contractions of human quadriceps muscle. *Clin. Sci. Mol. Med.* 54:609–614.

Blomstrand, E., P. Hassmén, B. Ekblom, and E.A. Newsholme (1991). Administration of branched-chain amino acids during sustained exercise—effects on performance and on plasma concentration of some amino acids. *Eur. J .Appl. Physiol.* 63:83–88.

Brown, R.L., E.C. Frederick, H.L. Falsetti, E.R. Burke, and A.J. Ryan (1983b). Overtraining of athletes—a round table. *Phys. Sportsmed.* 11:93–110.

Brown, S., R. Byrd, M.O. Jayasinghe, and D. Jones (1983a). Echocardiographic characteristics of competitive and recreational weight lifters. *J. Cardiovasc. Ultrasonograph.* 2:163–165.

Burke, L.M., R.A. Gollan, and R.S.D. Read (1991). Dietary intakes and food use of groups of elite Australian male athletes. *Int. J. Sport Nutr.* 1:378–394.

Burke, L.M., and R.S.D. Read (1988). Food use and nutritional practices of elite Olympic weightlifters. In: S. Trunswell and M.L. Wahlqvist (eds.) *Food habits in Australia*. Melbourne: Rene Gordon, pp. 112–121.

Busso, T., K. Häkkinen, A. Parkarinen, C. Carasso, J.R. Lacour, P.V. Komi, and H. Kauhanen (1990). A systems model of training responses and its relationship to hormonal responses in elite weightlifters. *Eur. J Appl. Physiol.* 61:48–54.

Chandler, T.J., G.D. Wilson, and M.H. Stone (1989). The effect of the squat exercise on knee stability. *Med. Sci. Sports Exerc.* 21:299–303.

Chang, D.E., L.P. Buschbacher, and R.R. Edlich (1988). Limited joint mobility in power lifters. *Amer. J. Sports Med.* 16:280–284.

Chesley, A., J.D. MacDougall, M.A. Tarnopolsky, S.A. Atkinson, and K. Smith (1992). Changes in human muscle protein synthesis after resistance exercise. *J. Appl. Physiol.* 73:1383–1388.

Conroy, B.P., W.J. Kraemer, C.M. Maresh, and G.P. Dalsky (1992). Adaptive responses of bone to physical activity. *Med. Exerc. Nutr. Health* 1:64–74.

Croucher, J.S. (1984). An analysis of world weightlifting records. *Res. Quart. Exerc. Sport* 55:285–288.

DeGaray, A.L., L. Levine, and J.E.L. Carter (1974). *Genetic and anthropological studies of Olympic athletes*. London: Academic Press.

DeLorme, T.L. (1945). Restoration of muscle power by heavy-resistance exercises. *J. Bone Joint Surg.* 27:645–667.

DeLorme, T.L., and A.L. Watkins (1948). Techniques of progressive resistance exercise. *Arch. Phys. Med. Rehab.* 29:263–273.

Dudley, G.A., R.T. Harris, M.C. Duvoisin, B.M. Hather, and P. Buchanan (1990). Effect of voluntary vs. artificial activation on the relationship of muscle torque to speed. *J. Appl. Physiol.* 69:2215–2221.

Dudley, G.A., P.A. Tesch, S.J. Fleck, W.J. Kraemer, and T.R. Baechle (1986). Plasticity of human muscle with resistance training (abstract). *Anat. Rec.* 214:4.

Fahey, T.D., L. Akka, and R. Rolph (1975). Body composition and VO₂max of exceptional weight trained athletes. *J. Appl. Physiol.* 39:559–561.

Fair, J.D. (1988). Olympic weightlifting and the introduction of steroids: A statistical analysis of world championship results, 1948–1972. *Intl. J. Hist. Sport* 5:96–114.

Fleck, S.J. (1988). Cardiovascular adaptations to resistance training. *Med. Sci. Sports Exerc.* 20:S146–S151.

Fleck, S.J. (1992). Cardiovascular response to strength training. In: P.V. Komi (ed.) *Strength and Power in Sports*, Oxford: Blackwell Scientific Publications, pp. 305–315.

Fleck, S.J., J.B. Bennett III, W.J. Kraemer, and T.R. Baechle (1989). Left ventricular hypertrophy in highly strength trained males. In: T. Lubich, A. Venerando, and P. Zeppilli (eds.) *Proceedings of the 2nd International Conference on Sports Cardiology, Vol. 2*. Bologna: Aulo Gaggi Pub., pp. 302–311.

Fleck, S.J., and L.S. Dean (1987). Resistance-training experience and the pressor response during resistance exercise. *J. Appl. Physiol.* 63:116–120.

Fleck, S.J., and W.J. Kraemer (1987). *Designing Resistance Training Programs*. Champaign, IL: Human Kinetics Publishers.

Fry, A.C. (1993). Physiological responses to short-term high-intensity resistance exercise overtraining. (Unpublished Ph.D. dissertation). University Park, PA: The Pennsylvania State University.

Fry, A.C., T.J. Housh, R.A. Hughes, and T. Eyford (1988). Stature and flexibility variables as discriminators of foot contact during the squat exercise. *J. Appl. Sport Sci. Res.* 2:24–26.

Fry, A.C., W.J. Kraemer, K.W. Bibi, and T. Eyford (1991). Stature variables as discriminators of foot contact during the squat exercise in untrained females. *J. Appl. Sport Sci. Res.* 5:77–81.

Fry, A.C., W.J. Kraemer, M.H. Stone, B.J. Warren, J.T. Kearney, C.M. Maresh, C.A.Weseman, and S.J. Fleck (1993). Endocrine and performance responses to high volume training and amino acid supplementation in elite junior weightlifters. *Int. J. Sport Nutr.* 3:306–322.

Fry, R.W., A.R. Morton, and D. Keast (1991). Overtraining in athletes, an update. *Sports Med.* 12:32–65.

Garhammer, J. (1979a). Biomechanical comparison of the U.S. Team with divisional winners at the 1978 World Weightlifting Championships. (Unpublished report to the U.S. National Weightlifting Committee).

Garhammer, J. (1979b). Longitudinal analysis of highly skilled Olympic weightlifters. In: J. Terauds (ed.) *Science in Weightlifting*. Del Mar, CA: Academic Publ., pp. 79–88.

Garhammer, J. (1979c). Performance evaluation of Olympic weightlifters. *Med. Sci. Sports* 11:284–287.

Garhammer, J. (1979d). Periodization of strength training for athletes. *Track Tech.* 74:2398–2399.

Garhammer, J. (1980). Power production by Olympic weightlifters. *Med. Sci. Sports Exerc.* 12:54–60.

Garhammer, J. (1981a). Biomechanical characteristics of the 1978 world weightlifting champions. In: A. Morecki, K. Fedelus, K. Kedzior, and A. Wit (eds.) *Biomechanics VII-B*. Baltimore: University Park Press, pp. 300–304.

Garhammer, J. (1981b). Force-velocity constraints and elastic energy utilization during multi-segment lifting/jumping activities (abstract). *Med. Sci. Sports Exerc.* 13:96.

Garhammer, J. (1982) and (1983). Unpublished Elite Weightlifting Project Biomechanics Reports. (Submitted to the Sports Medicine Div., U.S. Olympic Committee, and the U.S. Weightlifting Federation, One Olympic Plaza, Colorado Springs, CO 80909-5764).

Garhammer, J. (1985). Biomechanical profiles of Olympic weightlifters. *Int. J. Sport Biomech.* 1:122–130.

Garhammer, J. (1991a). A comparison of maximal power outputs between elite male and female weightlifters in competition. *Int. J. Sport Biomech.* 7:3–11.

Garhammer, J. (1991b). Maximal human power output capacity and its determination for male and female athletes (abstract). In: *Book of Abstracts*. Proceedings of the XIII International Congress on Biomechanics, University of Western Australia, Perth. pp. 67–68.

Garhammer, J. (1993). A review of power output studies of Olympic and powerlifting: Methodology, performance prediction, and evaluation tests. *J. Strength Cond. Res.* 7:76–89.

Garhammer, J., and T. McLaughlin (1980). Power output as a function of load variation in Olympic and power lifting (abstract). *J. Biomech.* 3:198.

Garhammer, J., and B. Takano (1992). Training for weightlifting. *Strength Power Sports* 5:357–381.

Goertzen, M., K. Schöppe, G. Lange, and K.P. Schulitz (1989). Verletzungen und uberlastungsschäden bei bodybuildern and powerlifters. *Sportverl. Sportschad.* 3:32–36.

Granhed, H., R. Jonson, and T. Hansson (1987). The loads on the lumbar spine during extreme weight lifting. *Spine* 12:146–149.

Granhed, H., and B. Morelli (1988). Low back pain among retired wrestlers and heavy weight lifters. *Am. J. Sports Med.* 16:530–533.

Häkkinen, K, M. Alen, and P.V. Komi (1984a). Neuromuscular, anaerobic, and aerobic performance characteristics of elite power athletes. *Eur. J. Appl. Physiol.* 53:97–105.

Häkkinen, K., H. Kauhanen, and P.V. Komi (1984b). Biomechanical changes in the Olympic weightlifting technique of the snatch and clean and jerk from submaximal to maximal loads. *Scand. J. Sports Sci.* 6:57–66.

Häkkinen, K., K.L. Keskinen, M. Alen, P.V. Komi, and H. Kauhanen (1989). Serum hormone concentrations during prolonged training in elite endurance-trained and strength-trained athletes. *Eur. J. Appl. Physiol.* 59:233–238.

Häkkinen, K., and P.V. Komi (1983). Electromyographic changes during strength training and detraining. *Med. Sci. Sports Exerc.* 15:455–460.

Häkkinen, K., P.V. Komi, M. Alen, and H. Kauhanen (1987a). EMG, muscle fiber and force production characteristics during a 1 year training period in elite weight-lifters. *Eur. J. Appl. Physiol.* 56:419–427.

Häkkinen, K., A. Pakarinen, M. Alen, H. Kauhanen, and P.V. Komi (1987b). Relationships between training volume, physical performance capacity, and serum hormone concentrations during prolonged training in elite weightlifters. *Int. J. Sports Med.* 8:61–65.

Häkkinen, K., A. Pakarinen, M. Alen, H. Kauhanen, and P.V. Komi (1988a). Daily hormonal and neuromuscular responses to intensive strength training in 1 week. *Int. J. Sports Med.* 9:422–408.

Häkkinen, K., A. Pakarinen, M. Alen, H. Kauhanen, and P.V. Komi (1988b). Neuromuscular and hormonal adaptations in athletes to strength training in two years. *J. Appl. Physiol.* 65:2406–2412.

Häkkinen, K., A. Pakarinen, M. Alen, H. Kauhanen, and P.V. Komi (1988c). Neuromuscular and hormonal responses in elite athletes to two successive strength training sessions in one day. *Eur. J. Appl. Physiol.* 57:133–139.

Häkkinen, K., A. Pakarinen, H. Kyrolainen, S. Cheng, D.H. Kim, and P.V. Komi (1990). Neuromuscular adaptations and serum hormones in females during prolonged power training. *Int. J. Sports Med.* 11:91–98.

Häkkinen, K, P. Rahkila, and M. Alen (1985). Anaerobic power during the course of one-minute strenuous muscular performance. *J. Hum. Studies* 11:237–250.

Harman, E.A., P.M. Frykman, E.R. Clagett, and W.J. Kraemer (1988). Intra-abdominal and intra-thoracic pressure during lifting and jumping. *Med. Sci. Sports Exerc.*, 20:195–201.

Harman, E.A., R.M. Rosenstein, P.N. Frykman, and G. Nigro (1989). Effects of a belt on intra-abdominal pressure during weightlifting. *Med. Sci. Sports Exerc.*, 21:186–190.

Hatfield, F.C. (1981). *Powerlifting: A scientific approach.* Chicago: Contemporary Books.

Hatfield, F.C., and T.M. McLaughlin (1985). Powerlifting. In: T.K. Cureton (ed.) *Encyclopedia of Physical Education, Fitness, and Sports, Vol. 4.* Reston, VA: American Association for Health, Physical Education, Recreation and Dance, pp. 587–593.

Houston, M.E., D.A. Marrin, H.J. Green, and J.A. Thomson (1981). The effect of rapid weight loss on physiological functions in wrestlers. *Physician Sportsmed.* 9:73–78.

Hunter, G.R., J. McGuirk, N. Mitrano, P. Pearman, B. Thomas, and R. Arrington (1989). The effects of a weight training belt on blood pressure during exercise. *J. Appl. Sport Sci. Res.* 3:13–18.

Jaros, A., and J. Chech (1965). Die wirbeläule bei gewichtebern. *Beitr. Orthop.* 12:653–660.

Johnson, G.O., T.J. Housh, D.R. Powell, and C.J. Ansorge (1990). A physiological comparison of female body builders and power lifters. *J. Sports Med. Phys. Fit.* 30:361–364.

Johnson, G.O., T.J. Housh, W.G. Thorland, C.J. Cisar, R.A. Hughes, and J.M. Schilke (1991). Preseason body composition of high school wrestlers according to age and body weight. *J. Appl. Sport Sci. Res.* 5:11–15.

Jost, J., M. Weiß, and H. Weicker (1989). Comparison of sympatho-adrenergic regulation at rest and of the adrenoceptor system in swimmers, long-distance runners, weight lifters, wrestlers and untrained men. *Eur. J. Appl. Physiol.* 58:596–604.

Kamen, G., P. Taylor, and P.J. Beehler (1984). Ulnar and posterior tibial nerve conduction velocity in athletes. *Int. J. Sports Med.* 5:26–30.

Katch, V.L., F.I. Katch, R. Moffatt, and M. Gittleson (1980). Muscular development and lean body weight in body builders and weight lifters. *Med. Sci. Sports Exerc.* 12:340–344.

Kauhanen, H., K. Häkkinen, and P.V. Komi (1988). Changes in biomechanics of weightlifting and neuromuscular performance during one year training of elite weightlifters. In: D.A. Winter, R.W. Norman, R.P. Wells, K.C. Hayes, and A.E. Patla (eds.) *Biomechanics IX*, Champaign, IL: Human Kinetics Publishers.

Knuttgen, H.G., and P.V. Komi (1992). Basic definitions for exercise. In: P.V. Komi (ed.) *Strength and Power in Sports.* Oxford: Blackwell Scientific Publications, pp. 3–6.

Knuttgen, H.G., and W.J. Kraemer (1987). Terminology and measurement in exercise performance. *J. Appl. Sport. Sci. Res.* 1:1–10.

Kotani, P.T. (1971). Studies of spondylolysis found among weight lifters. *Br. J. Sports Med.* 6:4–10.

Koziris, L.P., and D.L. Montgomery (1992). Power output and peak blood lactate concentration following intermittent and continuous cycling tests of anaerobic capacity. *Sport Med. Train. Rehab.* 3:289–296.

Kraemer, W.J. (1990). Physiological and cellular effects of exercise training In: W.B. Leadbetter, J.A. Buckwalter, and S.L. Gordon (eds.) *Sports–induced Inflammation.* Park Ridge, IL: American Academy of Orthopaedic Surgeons, pp. 659–676.

Kraemer, W.J. (1992a). Endocrine responses and adaptations to strength training. In: P.V. Komi (ed.) *Strength and Power in Sports.* Oxford: Blackwell Scientific Publications, pp. 291–304.

Kraemer, W.J. (1992b). Hormonal mechanisms related to the expression of muscular strength and power. In: P.V. Komi (ed.) *Strength and Power in Sports.* Oxford: Blackwell Scientific Publications, pp. 64–76.

Kraemer, W.J., and T.R. Baechle (1989). Development of a strength training program. In: F.L. Allman and A.J. Ryan (eds.) *Sports Medicine*, 2nd Ed. Orlando, FL: Academic Press, pp. 113–127.

Kraemer, W.J., M.R. Deschenses, and S.J. Fleck (1988a). Physiological adaptations to resistance exercise: implications for athletic conditioning. *Sports Med.* 6:246–256.

Kraemer, W.J., S.J. Fleck, and M. Deschenes (1988b). A review: factors in exercise prescription of resistance training. *National Strength Cond. Assoc. J.* 10:36–41.

Kraemer, W.J., B.J. Noble, M.J. Clark, and B.W. Culver (1987). Physiologic responses to heavy-resistance exercise with very short rest periods. *Int. J. Sports Med.* 8:247–252.

Krahl, H. (1975). Aspekte der tauglichkeisbeurteilung im leistungssport. *Orthop.Praxis* 11:56–61.

Kuipers, H., and H.A. Keizer (1988). Overtraining in elite athletes, review and directions for the future. *Sports Med.* 6:79–92.

Kulund, D.M. (1978). Olympic weight-lifting injuries. *Phys. Sportsmed.* 6:111–118.

Laubach, L.L. (1976). Comparative muscular strength of men and women: A review of the literature. *Aviat. Space Environ. Med.* 47:534–542.

Lawrence, J.H., and C.J. DeLuca (1983). Myoelectric signal versus force relationship in different human muscles. *J. Appl. Physiol.* 54:1653–1659.

Lehmann, M., and J. Keul (1986). Free plasma catecholamines, heart rates, lactate levels, and oxygen uptake in competition weight lifters, cyclists, and untrained control subjects. *Int. J. Sports Med.* 7:18–21.

Leighton, J. (1955). Instrument and technique for measurement of range of joint motion. *Arch. Phys. Mental Rehab.* 36:571–578.

Leighton, J. (1957). Flexibility characteristics of three specialized skill groups of champion athletes. *Arch. Phys. Mental Rehab.* 38:580–583.

Lietzke, M.H. (1956). Relation between weightlifting totals and body weight. *Sci. Amer.* 124:486–487.

Longhurst, J.C., A.R. Kelly, W.J. Gonyea, and J.H. Mitchell (1980). Echocardiographic left ventricular masses in distance runners and weight lifters. *J. Appl. Physiol.* 48:154–162.

MacDougall, J.D., D. Tuxen, D.G. Sale, J. R. Moroz, and J. R. Sutton (1985). Arterial blood pressure response to heavy resistance exercise. *J. Appl. Physiol.* 58:785–790.

Matveyev, L.P. (1972). *Periodisienang das Sportlichen Training* (translated into German by P. Tschiene with a chapter by A. Kruger). Berlin: Beles and Wernitz.

Maughan, R.J. (1984). Relationship between muscle strength and muscle cross-sectional area: Implications for training. *Sports Med.* 1:263–269.

Maughan, R.J., and M.A. Nimmo (1984). The influence of variations in muscle fiber composition on muscle strength and cross-sectional area in untrained males. *J. Physiol.* 351:299–311.

McLaughlin, T.M., C.J. Dillman, and T.J. Lardner (1977). A kinematic model of performance in the parallel squat by champion powerlifters. *Med. Sci. Sports* 9:128–133.

McLaughlin, T.M., T.J. Lardner, and C.J. Dillman (1978). Kinetics of the parallel squat. *Res. Q.* 49:175–189.

McLaughlin, T.M., and N. Madsen (1984). Bench press techniques of elite heavyweight powerlifters. *National Strength Cond. Assoc. J.* 6:44, 62–65.

Menapace, F.J., W.J. Hammer, T.F. Ritzer, K.M. Kessler, H.F. Warner, J.F. Spann, and A.A. Bove (1982). Left ventricular size in competitive weight lifters: An echocardiographic study. *Med. Sci. Sports Exerc.* 14:72–75.

Moritani, T., and H.A. de Vries (1979). Neural factors versus hypertrophy in the time course of muscle strength gain. *Am. J. Phys. Med.* 58:115–130.

Murphy, M.M., J.F. Patton, and F.A. Frederick (1986). Comparative anaerobic power of men and women. *Aviat. Space Environ. Med.* 57:636–641.

Newsholme, E.A. (1990). Effects of exercise on aspects of carbohydrate, fat, and amino acid metabolism. In: C. Bouchard, R.J. Shephard, T. Stephens, J.R. Sutton, and B.D. McPherson (eds.) *Exercise, Fitness, and Health*, Champaign, IL: Human Kinetics Publishers, pp. 293–308.

Newsholme, E.A., I.N. Acworth, and E. Blomstrand (1975). Amino acids, brain neurotransmitters and a functional link between muscle and brain that is important in sustained exercise. *Adv. Myochem.* 1:127–133.

Newton, L.E., G. Hunter, M. Bammon, and R. Roney (1993). Changes in psychological state and self-reported diet during various phases of training in competitive bodybuilders. *J. Strength Cond. Res.* 7:153–158.

Parry-Billings, M., E. Blomstrand, N. McAndrew, et al. (1990). A communicational link between skeletal muscle, brain, and cells of the immune system. *Int. J. Sports Med.* 11(Suppl. 2):S122–S128.

Pascoe, D.D., D.L. Costill, W. J. Fink, R.A. Robergs, and J.J. Zachwieja (1993). Glycogen resynthesis in skeletal muscle following resistive exercise. *Med. Sci. Sports Exerc.* 25:349–354.

Patton, J.F., W.J. Kraemer, H.G. Knuttgen, and E.A. Harman (1990). Factors in maximal power production and in exercise endurance relative to maximal power. *Europ. J. Appl. Physiol.* 60:222–227.

Pilis, W., J. Langfort, A. Zajac, and J. Wojtyna (1990a). Changes of anaerobic power after propranolol administration in weight-lifters and non-trained students. *Biol. Sport* 7:287–296.

Pilis, W., J. Langfort, R. Zarzeczny, A. Zajac, and J. Wojtyna (1990b). Morphological and physiological characteristics of top weight lifters. *Biol. Sport* 7:113–128.

Prince, F.P., R.S. Hikida, and F.C. Hagerman (1976). Human muscle fiber types in power lifters, distance runners and untrained subjects. *Pflugers Arch.* 371:161–165.

OLYMPIC WEIGHTLIFTING AND POWER LIFTING   **49**

Pullo, F.M. (1992). A profile of NCAA division I strength and conditioning coaches. *J. Appl. Sport Sci. Res.* 6:55–62.

Reichlin, S. (1992). Neuroendocrinology. In: J.D. Wilson and D.W. Foster (eds.) *William's Textbook of Endocrinology*, Philadelphia: W.B. Saunders, pp. 135–219.

Sale, D.G. (1988). Neural adaptation to resistance training. *Med. Sci. Sports Exerc.* 20 (suppl.):S135–S145.

Sale, D.G. (1992). Neural Adaptation to strength training. In: P.V. Komi (ed.) *Strength and Power in Sports.* Oxford: Blackwell Scientific Publications, pp. 249–265.

Sale, D.G., and J.D. MacDougall (1984). Isokinetic strength in weight-trainers. *Eur. J. Appl. Physiol.* 53:128–132.

Scala D., J. McMillan, D. Blessing, R. Rozenek, M. Stone (1987). Metabolic cost of a preparatory phase of training in weight lifting: a practical observation. *J. Appl. Sport Sci. Res.* 1:48–52.

Siff, M.C. (1988). Biomathematical relationship between strength and body mass. *J. Res. Sport Phys. Educ. Rec.* 11:81–92.

Sprynarova, S., and J. Parizkova (1971). Functional capacity and body composition in top weight-lifters, swimmers, runners, and skiers. *Int. Z. Angew. Physiol.* 29:184–194.

Staron, R.S., M.J. Leonardi, D.L. Karapondo, E.S. Malicky, J.E. Falkel, F.C. Hagerman, and R.S. Hikida (1991). Strength and skeletal muscle adaptations in heavy-resistance-trained women after detraining and retraining. *J. Appl. Physiol.* 70:631–640.

Stoessel, L., M.H. Stone, R. Keith, D. Marple, and R. Johnson (1991). Selected physiological, psychological and performance characteristics of national-caliber U.S. Women weightlifters. *J. Appl. Sport Sci. Res.* 5:87–95.

Stone, M.H., D. Carter, D.P. Smith, and T. Ward (1979). Olympic weightlifting: physiological characteristics. In: J. Terauds (ed.) *Science in Weightlifting.* Del Mar, CA: Academic Publ., pp. 45–54.

Stone, M.H., R.E. Keith, J.T. Kearney, S.J. Fleck, G.D. Wilson, and N.T. Triplett (1991). Overtraining: A review of the signs, symptoms and possible causes. *J. Appl. Sports Sci. Res.* 5:35–50.

Stone, M.H., and H.S. O'Bryant (1987). *Weight Training: A Scientific Approach.* Minneapolis: Burgess.

Stone, M.H., H.S. O'Bryant, and J. Garhammer (1981). A hypothetical model for strength training. *J. Sports Med. Phys. Fit.* 21:342–351.

Stone, M.H., H.S. O'Bryant, J. Garhammer, J. McMillan, and R. Rozenek (1982). A theoretical model of strength training. *National Strength Cond. Assoc. J.* 4:36–39.

Stowers, T.J., D. McMillan, D. Scala, V. Davis, D. Wilson, and M. Stone (1983). The short-term effects of three different strength-power training methods. *National Strength Cond. Assoc. J.* 5:24–27.

Tanner, J.M. (1964). *The Physique of the Olympic Athlete.* London: Allen and Unwin.

Tarnopolsky, M.A., S.A. Atkinson, J.D. MacDougall, A. Chesley, S. Phillips, and H.P. Schwarcz (1992). Evaluation of protein requirements for trained strength athletes. *J. Appl. Physiol.* 73:1986–1995.

Tesch, P.A. (1987). Acute and long-term metabolic changes consequent to heavy resistance exercise. *Med. Sci. Sports Exerc.* 26:67–89.

Tesch, P.A., E.B. Colliander, and P. Kaiser (1986). Muscle metabolism during intense heavy resistance exercise. *Eur. J. Appl. Physiol.* 55:362–366.

Tesch, P.A., and J. Karlsson (1985). Muscle fiber types and size in trained and untrained muscles of elite athletes. *J. Appl. Physiol.* 59:1716–1720.

Tesch, P.A., A. Thorsson, and B. Essen-Gustavsson (1989). Enzyme activities of FT and ST muscle fibers in heavy-resistance trained athletes. *J. Appl. Physiol.* 67:83–87.

Tesch, A., A. Thorsson, and P. Kraiser (1984). Muscle capillary supply and fiber type characteristics in weight and power lifters. *J. Appl. Physiol.* 56:35–38.

Tittel, K., and H. Wutscherk (1992). Anthropometric factors. In: P.V. Komi (ed.) *Strength and Power in Sports.* Oxford: Blackwell Scientific Publications, pp. 180–196.

Todd, T. (1978). *Inside Powerlifting.* Chicago: Contemporary Books.

Totten, L., and I. Javorek (1988). General physical training for the weightlifter. *US Weight Lifting Federation Coaching Manual*, Vol. 2. (U.S. Weightlifting Federation, One Olympic Plaza, Colorado Springs, CO 80909-5764).

Tüsch, C., and S.P. Ulrich (1974). Wirbelsäule und Hochleistungssport. *Sportarzt. Sportmed.* 9:206–208.

Viitasalo, J.T., H. Kyrolainen, C. Bosco, and M. Alen (1987). Effects of rapid weight reduction on force production and vertical jumping height. *Int. J. Sports Med.* 8:281–285.

Vorobyev, A.N. (1978). *A Textbook on Weightlifting* (translated by J. Brice). Budapest: International Weightlifting Federation.

Walberg, J.L., M.K. Leidy, D.J. Sturgill, D.E. Hinkle, S.J. Ritchey, and D.R. Sebolt (1988). Macronutrient content of a hypoenergy diet affects nitrogen retention and muscle function in weight lifters. *Int. J. Sports Med.* 9:261–266.

Webster, S., R. Rutt, and A. Weltman (1990). Physiological effects of a weight loss regimen practiced by college wrestlers. *Med. Sci. Sports Exerc.* 22:229–234.

Westerlind, K.C., W.C. Byrnes, P.S. Freedson, and F.I. Katch (1987). Exercise and serum androgens in women. *Phys. Sportsmed.* 15:87–94.

Willoughby, D.S. (1993). The effects of mesocycle-length weight training programs involving periodization and partially equated volumes on upper and lower body strength. *J. Strength Cond. Res.* 7:2–8.

Yesalis, C.E. (1993). *Anabolic Steroids in Sport and Exercise.* Champaign, IL: Human Kinetics Publishers.

DISCUSSION

KNUTTGEN: You have suggested that when performing the three Olympic lifts repetitively during a conditioning workout, the lifts should not be carried out to failure. Is part of your concern related to the athlete being exposed to injury from the falling weight?

KRAEMER: Injury prevention is certainly a concern, but the ability to maintain appropriate technique is also important. Several groups of muscles are used in each of these lifts; if one group becomes fatigued early, the lifting technique will be adversely affected so that loads for subsequent lifts will be less than optimal for training adaptations.

KNUTTGEN: There are many published studies pertaining to the strength training of what we might call the average person or average athlete in a variety of sports. What is the relevance of these studies done with volunteers to the elite weightlifter and power lifter?

KRAEMER: We can gain some information from the average athlete or untrained individual, but extrapolating principles learned from studying such persons to elite athletes is probably unjustified. For example, it is not clear how much we can learn about weight training for an elite athlete who trains with 350 kg in the squat by studying someone who trains with 100 kg. To understand the physiology of competitive lifters, we need to examine them directly.

CLARKSON: Will you please expand on your discussion of how neural inhibition may be involved in limiting lifting performance?

KRAEMER: Central and peripheral neural mechanisms can inhibit the activation of motor units and thereby limit the maximal recruitment of all the available fibers for a particular movement. Psychological factors are probably often involved such inhibitory mechanisms during competition; this is sometimes called "bombing" by the lifters if they fail to complete all three attempts at a lift they have previously accomplished in training and end up with a zero score in the competition. Such inhibition may involve excessive levels of catecholamines generated by the stress of competition, but the exact mechanism is unclear.

CLARKSON: With regard to health issues in lifters, are there any data showing negative effects of anabolic steroids on the cardiovascular systems of lifters? Are there long-term cardiovascular consequences of maintaining such a large muscle mass when the lifters' athletic careers are completed?

KRAEMER: Some case studies suggest that anabolic steroids may have detrimental effects on cardiac structure and function. Position stands published by the National Strength and Conditioning Association and the American College of Sports Medicine describe the potential adverse side effects associated with chronic use of steroids, including the negative effects on blood lipid profiles. Nevertheless, many of these effects appear to be reversible, and the health implications of chronic anabolic steroid cycling remain unknown. Still, heart, liver, kidney, and connective tissue are all negatively affected.

We know very little about detraining in those with large muscle masses. A particularly important issue is how well an athlete who has been routinely consuming 10,000 kcal daily for years can cut back to 2,000–3,000 kcal daily.

LAMB: Why don't lifters get down to 5 or 6% body fat by dietary restriction to qualify for the lowest possible body weight classification?

KRAEMER: I don't know, but it may be related to the fact that lifters typically perceive themselves to be weak if they don't consume lots of food energy. This may be a purely psychological issue.

HORSWILL: Isn't there a point in the unlimited weight class for weightlifters at which additional body fat is beneficial from a mechanical point of view?

KRAEMER: Large amounts of abdominal body fat, typical of many famous super heavyweight weightlifters in the 1960s and 1970s, was found to interfere with optimal technique in pulling the weight up from the floor. Heavyweight lifters in the 1980s and 1990s have found that by increasing the muscle mass, especially in the back and trunk musculature, they could bring the bar closer to the body and create more lifting power. This approach may not be effective in power lifting because of the different biomechanical properties of power lifting.

HORSWILL: Are there differences in the regional fat of elite and non-elite lifters? Is it possible that elite lifters have more upper body fat, which may reflect androgen differences in the two groups?

KRAEMER: That is possible, but as far as I know, there are no data to suggest such a thing.

GISOLFI: Could you clarify the role of dehydration to make lower weight classes in these athletes?

KRAEMER: Lifters typically do not lose more than about 2% of their body weights by acute dehydration to make a lower body weight class. The common belief is that a greater extent of dehydration will be detrimental to performance.

EKBLOM: What is the role of the trunk musculature in minimizing injury to the spine when these athletes lift up to 500 kg?

KRAEMER: Trunk musculature is very important for both injury prevention and lifting performance. Increased abdominal strength allows for greater pressures to be developed in the vertical lifts and thereby helps to stabilize the spine. The improved stabilization associated with greater intra-abdominal and intrathoracic pressures improve the performance of the lifts as well. In a similar fashion, lifting belts provide an artificial barrier to push against during the lift, thereby enhancing performance. The current trend is for increased training emphasis on the trunk musculature.

KANTER: It has been said that lifters' hearts in some respects may resemble those of people in long-standing hypertension. Are there any studies that justify this assertion? Also, there are suggestions of a decreased capillary-to-fiber ratio in the hearts of lifters. Should this concern us? Finally, are there any longevity studies on power lifters?

KRAEMER: Although a few reports have characterized the weightlifter's heart as having some commonalities with the hypertensive heart, this characterization doesn't hold up if comparisons are made with the appropriate controls matched for age and body weight. There is no systematic evidence of a pathologic effect of chronic heavy resistance training.

As cardiac muscle fibers enlarge, there will be a decrease in the volume densities of capillaries and mitochondria simply because of the increased size of the muscle fibers without a corresponding proliferation of capillaries and mitochondria. However, despite mitochondrial and capillary dilutions, there is no evidence that hypertrophied skeletal or cardiac muscle leads to a reduced $\dot{V}O_2$max or to any long-term health risk.

I know of no reports of longevity in lifters. I think the greatest concern would be for the super heavyweights, who carry a tremendous amount of total body weight and consume an enormous amount of energy on a daily basis.

BAR-OR: Duncan MacDougall observed extremely high arterial blood pressures, e.g, up to 350 mm Hg, in those doing heavy weightlifting. Should this be of concern? Also, are there any known effects of chronic weightlifting on arterial pressure at rest?

KRAEMER: Anecdotally, I have never seen anybody faint while lifting under competitive conditions; also, I have not seen any research demonstrating such a phenomenon in controlled circumstances. It seems to me these high pressures demonstrate the plasticity of a cardiovascular system able to tolerate such pressures. No data have demonstrated negative changes in resting blood pressures as a result of resistance training.

EICHNER: There is an article on weightlifters' blackout a couple of decades ago in *Lancet*. Also, Paul Thompson and colleagues in the past year in *Med. Sci. Sports Exerc.* reported that resting blood pressure was slightly higher in anabolic steroid-using body builders than in normals.

BAR-OR: Would you allow an adolescent known to have hypertension to participate in power lifting or weightlifting?

KRAEMER: I would rely on a physician's clinical judgement.

HAGERMAN: Middle distance runners can have very high blood pressures during training and competition, too. I suppose in runners the pressure is mostly a function of greater preload and cardiac output as opposed to greater afterload in lifters.

EICHNER: The difference in runners is that in contrast to lifters, the diastolic pressure doesn't go up; there wouldn't be nearly the theoretical risk for "blow out" in runners.

KRAEMER: It is possible that some of the blackout symptoms are related not so much to blood pressure, but rather to severe systemic stress associated with blood lactates of 21 mM or more. Another consideration is whether or not the lifters experiencing blackouts were anabolic steroid users; the steroids may have caused the problems. In one study, Fleck and Dean showed that maximal lifts do not elevate blood pressure as much as sets performed to failure with 70–80% of the one repetition maximum.

COYLE: It's often assumed that Type II fibers are superior for weight-lifting. But as you've mentioned, that hasn't been well studied; the few biopsy data that are available show quite a large range in fiber types among lifters. For example, Costill in the 1970s found that Mac Wilkins, a world-class shot putter and Olympic champion in the discus in 1976, had 67% Type I fibers in his gastrocnemius muscle. In power lifting, where the contractions are very slow, there is no reason to think that fast twitch fibers would be superior to slow twitch fibers; these two fiber types are equal in their isometric tension-generating ability. What is known about the time-to-peak tension during those very powerful moves in the second pull phase? Are these times out of the velocity ranges and time-to-peak tension ranges of slow twitch fibers?

KRAEMER: Performance in the discus is primarily a function of the ability to generate rotational torque; the movement technique and limb lengths may be more important to performance than fiber type profile. The multi-joint lifts require complex motor recruitment patterns. It may be that high-threshold, fast twitch motor units are important only at certain limited ranges of motion within a competitive lift. I don't know of any data from competitive lifters that describe the time-to-peak tension involved in these lifts. This type of work certainly needs to be done.

2

Physiology and Nutrition for Sprinting

Clyde Williams, Ph.D.

George Gandy, M.Sc.

INTRODUCTION

Sprinting is the simplest of all sporting contests. It is an event that in its elemental form needs nothing more than starting and finishing lines. The prize goes to the athlete who crosses the finishing line first. Sprinting holds such a central place in sport that it is not surprising that the earliest records of the ancient Olympic Games give prominence to an outstanding sprinter. Coreobus won the sprint event in the ancient Olympics of 776 BC. The sprinters ran the length of the stadium, called a stade, which was about 192 m. There were two other races in the ancient Olympic Games, the *diaulos*, which was two lengths of the stadium (384 m), and a longer race over about 24 stades (4615 m) (Durant, 1961).

Of course, even if the length of the stadium was not exactly the same in each of the city states of ancient Greece, this was of little concern because the prize went to the fastest runner. In this one respect the modern Olympic Games shares the same principle with the games of Greek antiquity. It is the fastest athlete on the day who wins the prize and not necessarily the athlete who sets a new world record during periods between the Games. This is one reason why the Olympic gold medal holds such an unique place in the minds of spectators and athletes alike. World records punctuate the progress of the event, but it is for a gold medal that sprinters earn lasting recognition as well as their places in the record books (Table 2-1).

Records are a relatively new phenomenon. They emerged when accurate and reliable forms of timekeeping became available. Electronic timing was introduced in 1968 and has since become the standard method of timekeeping in all major sprint championships. A claim for a new world record is scrutinized rigorously, and competitors are aware that they should ensure that the competition and conditions are acceptable to the International Amateur Athletics Federation (IAAF) before attempting to set a new record. The IAAF not only establishes a strict set of conditions for timing an event but also considers the nature of the track before recognizing new records. The current world records for the sprint are shown in Table 2-2.

In contrast to the encyclopedic quantity of the literature on endurance running, the literature on sprinting is relatively small. Even so, most of the available information on sprinting tends to focus on 100-m running, with a considerable emphasis on the biomechanics of this event. There is, unfortunately, even less published information on 200-m and 400-m racing. Nevertheless, the aim of this chapter is to provide the

TABLE 2-1. *World record breakers for the 100-m sprint*

Name	Time (s)	Year
Ben Johnson	9.79 °°	1988
Carl Lewis	9.86	1991*
Leroy Burrell	9.90	1991*
Calvin Smith	9.93	1983*
Jim Hines	9.95	1968
Armin Hary	10.0	1960
Willie Williams	10.1	1956
Jesse Owens	10.2	1936

(* Records set at non-Olympic events; °° Record disallowed)

TABLE 2-2. *Current world sprint records*

Distance	Men			Women	
	Time (s)	Sprinter		Time (s)	Sprinter
100-m	9.86	C. Lewis		10.49	F. Griffith-Joiner
200-m	19.72	P. Mennea		21.34	F. Griffith-Joiner
400-m	43.26	H. Reynolds		47.6	M. Koch

reader with an overview of the essential physiological features of sprinting and, where possible, provide information on the contribution that nutrition does and may make to this event. Under the heading of Sprint Training we have provided some historical reflections, from a coach's perspective, of the development of sprint training, along with an overview of current approaches to sprint training.

CHARACTERISTICS OF ELITE SPRINTERS

Body Composition

Sprinters are heavier and more muscular than other track athletes. Elite male sprinters have heights ranging from 1.57 m to 1.90 m and body weights which range from 63.4 kg to 90.0 kg (Koshla, 1978). Female sprinters are generally shorter and lighter than male sprinters. They range in height from 1.57 m to 1.78 m and fall in the weight range of 51.0 kg to 71.0 kg (Koshla & McBroome, 1984). Height or, more importantly, leg length has an obvious influence on stride length of sprinters. During a 100-m race, elite sprinters, both men and women, take between 44 and 53 strides to cover the distance (Moravec et al., 1988). This amounts to stride rates of about 4.23 to 5.05 m/s. For example, in the 1987 World Athletics Championships in Rome the eight men in the 100-m final averaged 45.7 strides to complete the race at a stride frequency of 4.6 strides/s (Moravec et al., 1988). The average values for stride rates and stride lengths for the

TABLE 2-3. *Mean stride rate, stride length, and reaction times for the four fastest sprinters in the 100-m final at the 1991 World Athletics Championships in Tokyo (Ae et al., 1992)*

Variable	Carl Lewis	Leroy Burrell	Dennis Mitchell	Linford Christie
Stride rate (strides/s)	4.51	4.40	4.70	4.55
± SD	0.30	0.33	0.21	0.32
Stride length (m)	2.37	2.41	2.25	2.33
± SD	0.41	0.38	0.38	0.38
Reaction times (ms)	140	120	90	126

four fastest sprinters in the 100-m final in 1991 Tokyo World Athletics Championship are shown in Table 2-3.

As might be expected, tall sprinters have longer stride lengths and slower stride rates than shorter sprinters, who have smaller stride lengths but faster stride rates. However, it is interesting to note that women sprinters of the same height, leg length, and stride length as male sprinters record times for the 100-m that are about 1 second slower than the performances of men. This difference is attributed to the slightly slower stride frequency of the female sprinters (Hoffman, 1972).

Muscle Fiber Composition

The early biopsy studies on elite athletes showed that sprinters tend to have larger proportions of the fast-contracting, fast-fatiguing fibers (Type IIb) than the slow-contracting, slow-fatiguing fibers (Type I) (Gollnick et al., 1972). The ratio of fast to slow muscle fibers is also greater for sprinters than it is the general population of men and women of similar ages (Costill et al., 1976). In this respect sprinters share similar fiber characteristics with other power athletes (Thorstensson et al., 1977; Gregor et al., 1981; Staron et al., 1984; Tesch & Karlsson, 1985). Although the skeletal muscles of other elite power athletes and sprinters share the same characteristically high proportion of fast twitch fibers it is unlikely that this fiber composition is a result of strength training per se. However, strength training in preparation for sprinting may cause a shift in fiber composition from Type II b to Type IIa fibers (Tesch, 1992) but not from slow to fast twitch (Type I to Type II). Of course, it is not only the fiber composition that influences sprinting speed but also the number of fibers and their recruitment during exercise. Esbjornsson and colleagues (1993) examined the relationships between muscle fiber composition and anaerobic power output during cycle ergometer exercise. They concluded that the anaerobic power output was directly related to the percentage of Type II fibers in the vastus lateralis muscles and to the potential for anaerobic metabolism (as reflected by the activity of the enzymes lactate dehydrogenase and phosphofructokinase), "with no sex differences in this relationship."

Muscular Strength

The large muscle mass that is characteristic of elite sprinters contributes to their running success because it allows them to generate great forces quickly. The generation of high forces is essential during the start of a race, and it is particularly important during the section of the race when sprinters reach their maximum speeds and have only the briefest contact with the track. The leg strength of sprinters is greater than that of distance runners (Maughan et al., 1983; Hakkinen & Keskinen, 1989) and of the general population (Barnes, 1981). Compared to strength-trained athletes, who record higher absolute forces during isometric strength tests, sprinters have faster times for any given absolute isometric load, which may reflect the nature of their muscle fiber composition and their innervation rates (Hakkinen & Keskinen, 1989). However, many of the strength-testing methods are, unfortunately, non-specific for athletes in general and sprinters in particular. Therefore, it is not surprising that strong correlations are not always reported between various measures of strength and sprinting performance (Farrar & Thorland, 1987).

One of the recent exceptions is a study of the isokinetic leg strengths of a group of sprinters. An isotonic profile was developed for each runner by recording his or her responses to a progressive isotonic load using a Lido dynamometer. Each runner performed a series of leg extensions against progressively higher loads. Peak power was calculated along with average peak velocity for quadriceps and hamstring muscles (Mahler et al., 1992). The isotonic peak power output thresholds for these muscles were derived from plotting peak power output against workload over a range of loads. The strongest correlation was between 100-m performance times and the isotonic peak power output threshold ($r = 0.957$) for the hamstrings. Mahler and colleagues (1992) concluded that this result is consistent with the fact that the hamstrings are the limiting muscle group during sprinting (Mahler et al., 1992). Ideally, strength measurements on sprinters should be made while these athletes are performing movements that are part of the running action; this has not yet been accomplished. Of course, another view is that while a certain level of strength is essential for successful sprinting, it is not a determinant of sprinting success (Farrar & Thorland, 1987).

Flexibility

Flexibility exercises are just as important in training programs for modern sprinters as they are in training programs for gymnasts. the reasonable assumption made by coaches is that flexibility training will help sprinters improve stride lengths and generate maximal power during brief contact between the driving leg and the ground. However, this view is based on perceived wisdom rather than on the results of well-controlled trials. Therefore, it is difficult to be prescriptive about the amount of flexibility training that should be undertaken. It is also a common belief that good flexibility, over a wide range of movements, will also provide some protection against injury during training and competition, but again there is no body of literature to either support or deny this view. Part of the explanation for the lack of reliable research on this topic is the difficulty in measuring flexibility in a reliable and accurate way. It is an even more complex problem to assess the influence of flexibility training on running. These are problems clearly in need of research.

Movement Speed

Sprinters, by definition, move quickly. The world's elite male sprinters achieve maximal running velocities of at least 11.0 m/s, and the females achieve maximal velocities of 10.0 m/s or better. It would be reasonable to assume that elite sprinters have nerve conduction velocities that are faster than non-sprinters. Casabona et al. (1990) used surface electrodes and electrical stimulation to assess neural conduction velocities in sprinters; they provided evidence that these athletes have faster conduction velocities than do strength-trained athletes. There also appears to be a good correlation between neural conduction velocity and the relative area of Type II muscle fibers, i.e., the greater the relative Type II fiber area, the greater the conduction velocity (Sadoyama et al., 1988).

A comparison of the patellar tendon reflex characteristics of endurance-trained and sprint-trained athletes showed that the sprinters exhibited greater peak force, faster time to peak force, and faster reflex latency following stimulation than did the endurance athletes (Koceja & Kamen, 1988). These differences may reflect differences in muscle-tendon stiffness, but they may also reflect differences in neural organization. However, Radford and Upton (1976) concluded that sprinters were not distinguished by differences in neural organization. Nevertheless, they did show that sprinters were better than non-sprinters at coordinating arms and legs rapidly while running on the spot and that the sprinters were faster at tapping tasks. Therefore, the circumstantial evidence suggests that the functional organization of the neuromuscular system in sprinters may be different from that of endurance athletes and sedentary people.

Being able to run fast is only a precondition for successful sprinting; it is not the determinant of success during competition among athletes of similar abilities. The 100-m sprint is made up of several sections, and is not, as the casual observer might conclude, a simple race between gun and tape (Table 2-4) (Radford, 1990). Sprinters have different strengths; some may be slow starters but have the ability to sustain their maximal speeds to the finish line, whereas others may be fast starters and fade toward the end. Nevertheless, the elite sprinter must be able to achieve maximal effi-

TABLE 2-4. *Approximate times for sections of a 100-m sprint (Radford, 1990)*

Stage	Men (10.0 s)	Women (11.0 s)
Reaction to gun	0.1-0.3	0.1-0.3
Drive off blocks	0.3-0.4	0.3-0.4
Acceleration	5.5-7.0	5.0-6.0
Maximum speed	1.5-3.0	1.5-2.5
Deceleration	1.0-1.5	1.5-2.5

ciency over each section of the race if he or she seeks to cross the finishing line ahead of the competition.

In the 100-m sprint, reaction time would appear to be important because it is essential that runners respond rapidly to the starter's pistol. Nevertheless, athletes will often record different reaction times, even in the same competition, depending upon whether they are running in heats or in finals. The reaction times become slower as the distances are extended from 100 m to 400 m. However, the overall performances of sprinters are hardly affected by slight changes in their speeds of reaction to the starter's signal (Atwater, 1982; Moravec et al., 1988). This may not be the case, however, for the world's elite sprinters.

Knowing the fastest reaction times of world class sprinters allows manufacturers of electronic timing systems to electronically program the starting blocks to the starter's gun so a false start will register if a runner moves before 0.1 s has elapsed. But this value is an arbitrary one, and the final decision about a false start rests with the official starter.

Sprinters must be able to generate large forces rapidly against their starting blocks to accelerate effectively. This requires considerable strength, flexibility, and coordination. Acceleration is the longest stage of the 100-m sprint; thereafter, the sprinter tries to maintain maximum speed for as long as possible. The traditional view of the kinetics of sprinting over 100 m is that maximum speed is normally achieved about 40 m into the race. For most sprinters, the challenge is then to maintain their speeds for the remainder of the 100-m race.

In the 1987 World Athletic Championships in Rome the finalists in the men's 100-m sprint reached their maximum speeds at distances of between 50 m and 60 m, and they were able to maintain those speeds for the remainder of the race. In the women's 100-m final, the sprinters achieved their maximum velocities at about the same distances as the men but appeared unable to sustain their running speeds for the rest of the race. An analysis of the performances of the two fastest men in the race, namely Johnson (9.83 s) and Lewis (9.93 s), shows that Johnson had a faster average stride rate while Lewis had a longer average stride length (Moravec et al., 1988). It seems that Johnson won the race in the first 20 m when his contact time with the ground and his flight phase were less than those of

Lewis, because after 20 m these factors were the same for both athletes, as were their average running velocities (Moravec et al., 1988).

In contrast, the peak velocities of the four fastest men in the 100-m final of the 1991 Tokyo World Athletic Championships were achieved between 70 and 80 m into the race, which is unique in top class sprinting (Table 2-5). They also appeared to be able to increase their running speeds over the last 10 m of the race. Elite sprinters are able not only to achieve high running velocities, but also to maintain those velocities throughout the race.

Anaerobic Power and Capacity

Sprinting involves a maximal rate of energy expenditure that must be matched by a rapid rate of energy resynthesis. The terms *anaerobic power* and *anaerobic capacity* are commonly used to describe exercise performances of maximal intensity and brief duration that, of necessity, rely mainly on anaerobic biochemical events to generate energy rapidly. The external work achieved by an athlete during maximal exercise on a cycle ergometer or treadmill is often used as a way of describing anaerobic power (Bouchard et al., 1982).

In biochemical terms, anaerobic power describes the rate of ATP resynthesis by a series of non-oxidative reactions in skeletal muscles. The two principal anaerobic sources for ATP resynthesis are (1) phosphocreatine (PCr) and (2) non-oxidative degradation of glycogen to lactate (anaerobic glycogenolysis). In theory, the maximal anaerobic capacity can be calculated from the size of the PCr and glycogen stores in active muscles. In practice, however, not all the available PCr and glycogen can be used to replace ATP. Nevertheless, biopsy samples of the quadriceps muscles before and after brief high-intensity exercise provide data for the calculation

TABLE 2–5. *Speeds over 10-m sections of the 100-m final for the four fastest sprinters in the 100-m final at the 1991 World Athletics Championships in Tokyo (Ae et al., 1992)*

| Distance | Speed (m/s) | | | |
	Carl Lewis	Leroy Burrell	Dennis Mitchell	Linford Christie
10 m	5.31	5.46	5.56	5.41
20 m	9.26	9.43	9.35	9.43
30 m	10.87	10.99	10.75	10.87
40 m	11.24	11.36	11.36	11.24
50 m	11.90	11.49	11.49	11.76
60 m	11.76	11.63	11.49	11.63
70 m	11.90	11.49	11.63	11.63
80 m	12.05	11.90	11.63	11.76
90 m	11.49	11.24	11.36	11.11
100 m	11.63	11.49	11.24	11.36
Finishing times (s)	9.86	9.88	9.91	9.92

of the rate of ATP resynthesis, i.e., anaerobic power, from an analyses of the changes in PCr and glycolytic metabolites (Sahlin & Henriksson, 1984). For example, when a 6-s maximal sprint was performed on a mechanically braked cycle ergometer, the rate of ATP resynthesis was calculated to be between 10.4 and 13.4 mmol·kg^{-1} dry material (dm)·s^{-1} (Boobis et al., 1987; Gaitanos et al., 1993). These values are close to the predicted maximal value of 17 mmol·kg^{-1} dm·s^{-1} for ATP resynthesis in human skeletal muscle (McGilvery, 1975).

Phosphocreatine and anaerobic glycogenolysis contribute almost equally to energy production during 6 s of sprint cycling. Although muscle has sufficient glycogen to contribute to energy production, it is the loss of PCr that causes a fall in power output (Boobis et al., 1987; Gaitanos et al., 1993).

Estimates of anaerobic capacity can also be made from an analysis of the PCr and glycogen stores before and after maximal exercise. Values ranging from 258 to 387 mmol ATP/kg dm (60–90 mmol ATP/kg wet weight [ww]) in muscle have been reported in studies that have used electrical stimulation of skeletal muscle (Spriet et al., 1987), single leg exercise (Bangsbo et al., 1993), or two leg cycling (Medbø & Tabata, 1993). In sprints up to 200 m, anaerobic power is more critical than anaerobic capacity because in short sprints the rate of ATP production is all-important; in a 400-m sprint, the capacity for ATP production also becomes important.

Non-invasive methods of assessing anaerobic power and capacity are, for obvious reasons, more attractive than those that rely on the muscle biopsy procedure. One non-invasive method currently receiving considerable attention is based on the oxygen deficit concept (Hermansen, 1969; Medbø et al., 1988; Saltin, 1990). Oxygen deficit describes the difference between the oxygen cost of exercise and the actual oxygen utilized in performing that activity. The most familiar illustration of oxygen deficit is the mismatch at the beginning of submaximal exercise between the observed rate of oxygen uptake and the calculated oxygen cost of the activity. The deficit in aerobic energy provision is covered by the non-oxidative resynthesis of ATP from PCr and anaerobic glycogenolysis.

Using the oxygen deficit concept, the anaerobic contribution to energy production can be estimated by determining the actual amount of oxygen consumed by the athlete during maximal exercise and then subtracting this value from the calculated oxygen cost of the exercise. The oxygen cost of maximal exercise can be estimated by assuming that the linear relationship between oxygen uptake and a wide range of submaximal exercise intensities holds true during exercise beyond those intensities that elicit maximal oxygen uptake (Medbø et al., 1988). Having calculated the oxygen cost of the exercise from this linear relationship, the total cost of the period of maximal activity is the product of this value and exercise time. Not everyone agrees that this assumption about the linearity of the oxygen cost of exercise can be made with confidence (Olesen, 1992; Saltin, 1990). Nevertheless, Medbø et al. (1988) determined values for maximal accumulated oxygen deficit during exercise intensities that caused fatigue in 0.5–3.0 min. The results suggest that maximal accumulated oxygen deficit is achieved during 2–3 min of maximal exercise and ranges from 50–90 mL O_2/kg body weight. The maximum rate of anaerobic energy production i.e., anaerobic power, can be obtained by dividing the maximal accumulated oxygen deficit by the exercise duration. Values for maximal accumulated oxygen deficit and, therefore, maximal anaerobic power may also be expressed in biochemical terms by assuming that 1 mmol of oxygen is equivalent to 6.5 mmol of ATP (Medbø et al., 1988).

The determination of maximal accumulated oxygen deficit is reproducible, and there are strong correlations between values for sprinters and their performance times during races over 100 m ($r = -0.88$; $P < 0.01$) and 400 m ($r = -0.82$; $P < 0.01$) (Ramsbottom et al., unpublished observations). Similar results have been reported by Scott and colleagues (1991), but they found only a weak correlation between maximal accumulated oxygen deficit and 400-m times for their 12 subjects ($r = -0.57$).

The maximal accumulated oxygen deficit for sprinters is about 30% higher than the values for endurance trained runners, but there appears to be no difference in the values between endurance runners and untrained people (Medbø & Burgers, 1990) or among a wide range of other elite athletes (Bangsbo et al., 1993). Therefore, there is a prima facie case to accept maximal oxygen deficit as a reproducible physiological characteristic of an individual and as a measure of the maximal rate of anaerobic energy production.

Sprinting is a physical expression of anaerobic energy production. In mechanics, power is the instantaneous product of force and velocity, but in athletic terms power may be viewed as the product of strength and speed. Sports scientists have considered several methods for measuring maximal power output in athletes (Bar-Or, 1987; Bouchard et al., 1982; Lakomy, 1986, 1987; Vandewalle et al., 1987). The most frequently used method involves cycling at maximal speed against a predetermined external resistive load for 30–40 s. This test of maximal power output is generally referred to as the Wingate Anaerobic Test (WAnT) (Bar-Or, 1987). Values for peak power, mean power, and end power output can be determined during maximal exercise when a mechanically braked cycle ergometer is coupled to a microcomputer (Lakomy, 1986). A fatigue index can also be calculated from the differences between peak and end power outputs (Figure 2-1).

There are clear differences between the power outputs of sprinters and endurance runners when they complete the WAnT procedure (Figure 2-2; Bogdanis personal communication). Sprinters and power athletes generate greater peak power, but they also have a more marked onset of

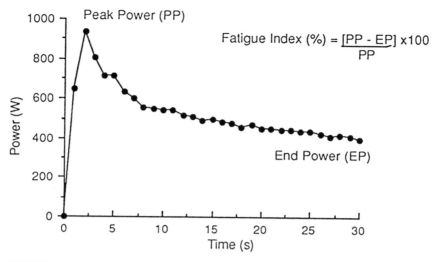

FIGURE 2-1. *Power output during a 30-s Wingate Anaerobic Test (WAnT) on a cycle ergometer*

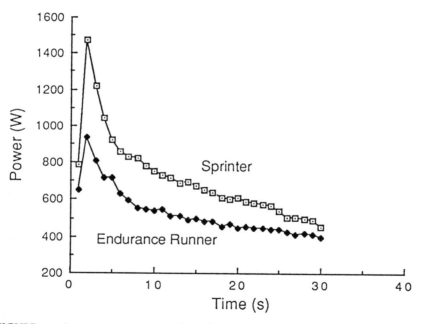

FIGURE 2-2. *Power outputs of a sprinter and an endurance athlete during a 30-s Wingate Anaerobic Test on a cycle ergometer*

fatigue than do endurance athletes. Thus, this test provides scientists with the opportunity to study the power outputs of different populations of athletes in an attempt to describe more precisely the physiological characteristics of elite athletes and those aspiring to join their ranks. For example, Denis and colleagues (1992) compared the peak power outputs of 100-m sprinters and 800-m runners using the WAnT procedure during cycling. Twelve runners cycled for 45 s (rather than the usual 30 s), and the peak power outputs of the sprinters and middle-distance runners were 1006 W (14.8 ±1.4 W/kg) and 796 W (11.9 ±1.6 W/kg), respectively. The average peak power output of the sprinters was, as might be expected, higher (P<0.01) than the value for the middle-distance runners. However, there was no difference between the total work done by the two groups of runners. The mean peak power output of 1.06 kW achieved by the sprinters was clearly greater than that achieved by the middle-distance runners. These values, however, were probably even higher than those reported (Denis et al., 1992) because the calculation of the peak power outputs did not take into consideration the work done to accelerate the flywheel of the cycle ergometer (Lakomy, 1986). Nevertheless, the WAnT procedure used to compare groups in this way clearly demonstrated differences in the peak power output of sprinters. Furthermore, the study also identified differences in the metabolic responses. It is only when the results are used to make comparisons with those obtained in other studies that the work done during acceleration of the ergometer flywheel must be included in the calculations of power output (Lakomy, 1986).

Another approach to studying the anaerobic power output of sprinters is based on the use of a non-motorized treadmill. When a non-motorized treadmill is interfaced with a microcomputer, the running speed and horizontal component of force (and hence power output) can be assessed (Figure 2-3) (Lakomy, 1987). Figure 2-4 shows the changes in power output during a 30-s sprint on an instrumented non-motorized treadmill (Lakomy, 1987). Peak, mean, and end power outputs, as well as a fatigue index, can be calculated for runners during this sprint version of the WAnT procedure.

Using this system, the power outputs of sprinters and sprint-trained sportsmen and sportswomen have been determined. The power output values obtained for trained athletes during sprint running for 30 s are about 150–200 W lower than those obtained during sprint cycling, using the same WAnT procedure (Cheetham et al., 1987). The reason for this difference is that during sprint running only the horizontal component of force is used to calculate power output values. Furthermore, peak and mean speeds achieved on the sprint treadmill are approximately 80% and 75%, respectively, of those achieved during 30 s of free running on a track (Lakomy, 1987). Nevertheless, the method provides the opportunity to

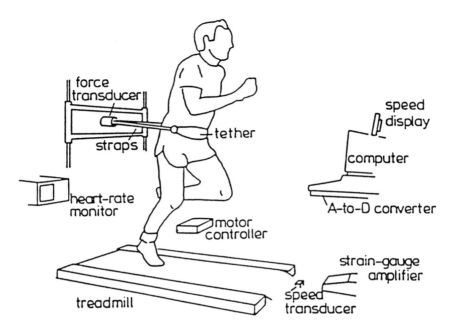

FIGURE 2-3. *Schematic diagram of a non-motorized treadmill adapted to measure the power outputs of sprinters (Lakomy, 1987)*

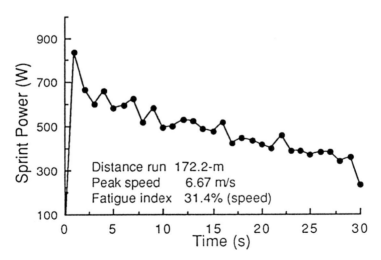

Distance run   172.2-m
Peak speed   6.67 m/s
Fatigue index   31.4% (speed)

FIGURE 2-4. *Power output of an athlete during a 30-s maximal sprint on a non-motorized treadmill (Lakomy, 1987)*

study the physiological responses to sprinting, even if the absolute speeds are lower than those achieved during free sprinting (Cheetham et al., 1986; Nevill et al., 1989). Furthermore, this method measures one of the essential products of strength training, namely, functional power output during sprinting. Therefore, it has the potential to complement the more traditional methods of assessing the strength of sprinters.

Aerobic Power

The maximal oxygen uptakes ($\dot{V}O_2$max) of sprinters and strength athletes are often not different from those of sedentary people (Neuman, 1988). In some cases, however, the values for sprinters are higher than those of the normal population but less than those of endurance athletes (Barnes, 1981). Values for sprinters range from about 48–55 mL·kg^{-1}·min^{-1} for men and 43–50 mL·kg^{-1}·min^{-1} for women, though in absolute terms (L/min), $\dot{V}O_2$max may be larger for sprinters, who tend to have greater muscle mass and body weight, than for sedentary people. The nature of sprint training is such that it does not promote as large an increase in $\dot{V}O_2$max as does endurance training. Furthermore, the genetic influences that give elite sprinters a high proportion of fast twitch fibers reduce their potential to develop an exceptionally large capacity for oxygen transport.

POTENTIAL LIMITATIONS TO PERFORMANCE

Metabolic Events During Sprinting

There are, unfortunately, only a few studies on the metabolic responses to sprinting. In one such study on 100-m racing, Hirvonen et al. (1987) illustrated the importance of PCr. They obtained muscle samples, using the percutaneous muscle biopsy procedure, from a group of seven sprinters before and after they completed several sections of a 100-m race. Each sprinter ran 100 m as fast as possible and also completed runs of 40 m, 60 m, and 80 m, before and after which muscle biopsies were obtained. Half of the resting PCr concentration (21.7 mmol/kg ww or 45.2 mmol/kg dm) was used up during the vigorous warm-up before each race over the intermediate distances. Nevertheless, taken as a whole, the PCr values show that most of this substrate was used during the first 5–6 s of the race (Figure 2-5). These authors concluded from the constant rate of lactate accumulation that the contribution of glycogenolysis was constant throughout the sprint and that the fall in PCr concentrations was the reason the sprinters were unable to maintain their maximal running speeds for the latter part of the race (Hirvonen et al., 1987).

Blood lactate concentrations have been determined for 400-m sprinters taking part in international level competitions. Mean post-exercise blood lactate concentrations of 20.1 mmol/L were generated during several 400-m races by four national level sprinters. There was a strong cor-

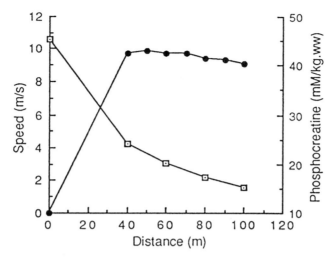

FIGURE 2-5. *Speed (closed circles) and muscle phosphocreatine (PCr) concentrations (squares) during a simulated 100-m track race (Hirvonen et al., 1987)*

relation (r = 0.85; P<0.05) between post-race blood lactate concentrations of the male sprinters and their performance times for the 400-m races (Lacour et al., 1990). Based upon post-race blood lactate concentrations and several assumptions about muscle metabolism, the authors calculated the energy cost of the 400-m race to be approximately 110 mL O_2/kg (0.274 mL·kg^{-1}·m^{-1}).

In another study on 400-m sprinting, some of the changes in substrate metabolism in the skeletal muscles were reported (Hirvonen et al., 1992). Split times were recorded for each 100-m of a 400-m race on an indoor 200-m track. The sprinters were subsequently required to run the intermediate distances in the same times as they had recorded during their 400-m time trials. The time for the 400-m was 51.9 ± 0.7 s (mean ± SE), whereas individual times for these six sprinters during the competitive season ranged from 47.5 to 50.5 s. Muscle biopsies were obtained from the vastus laterali muscles before and after each sprint and analyzed for PCr and muscle lactate concentrations.

The PCr concentrations during the 400-m time trials are shown in Figure 2-6, along with the speeds for each 100 m. As can be seen, the most rapid fall in PCr values occurred during the first 100 m of the 400-m time trial. The largest decrease in running speed, however, occurred from 200 m onward, but this was accompanied by only a modest further decrease in PCr concentrations.

The accumulation of muscle lactate after 200 m was double the value recorded after the first 100 m (Figure 2-7) and reflects a significant in-

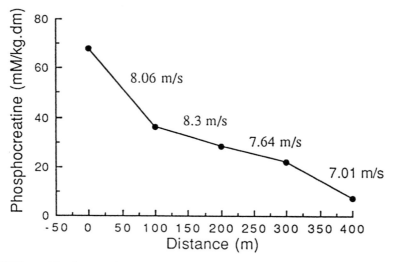

FIGURE 2-6. *Phosphocreatine (PCr) concentrations in muscle at various running speeds during a simulated 400-m track race (Hirvonen et al., 1992)*

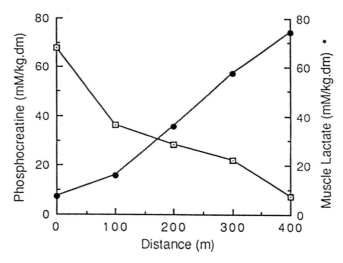

FIGURE 2-7. *Phosphocreatine (closed circles) and lactate concentrations (squares) in muscle during a simulated 400-m track race (Hirvonen et al., 1992)*

crease in the contribution of anaerobic glycogenolysis to energy production. Changes in muscle lactate concentration between 200 and 300 m were similar to those that occurred over the previous 100 m. The rate of accumulation of muscle lactate over the last 100 m was, however, somewhat lower than that during the previous 200 m. Blood lactate concentrations increased in parallel, but at lower values, with the changes in muscle lactate concentrations. Lactate accumulation in muscle achieved its maximal value after 35 s of sprinting, whereas the equivalent value for blood lactate accumulation was achieved after about 27 s of sprinting (Hirvonen et al., 1992).

Studies using a non-motorized treadmill simulate track running performances in the controlled environment of a laboratory, but this procedure does not exactly reproduce sprint performance on a track. Nevertheless, even though the performances during sprint running in the laboratory are less than those achieved on a track, the metabolic responses to sprinting in both situations appear to be similar. For example, when seven national level sprinters (10.6–11.0 s for 100 m, 21–22 s for 200 m, and 48–50 s for 400 m) completed 30 s of maximal sprinting on a non-motorized treadmill and on an all-weather track, the distances covered on the treadmill and the track were 186.7 ± 4.41 m and 248.0 ± 13.1 m (mean $\pm$ SD), respectively (P<0.01) (Lakomy, 1987). Blood lactate concentration at the end of the treadmill and track runs were 16.8 and 15.2 mmol/L and were not significantly different. There was also no difference between the blood glucose concentrations at the end of the 30 s of treadmill and track sprinting (6.4 ± 1.1 mmol/L and 6.2 ± 1.0 mmol/L, respectively) nor in heart rates of approximately 198 beats/min (Lakomy, Okilo, and Williams, unpublished observations).

Therefore, as a first approximation, a 30-s sprint on a non-motorized treadmill is equivalent to a 200-m race on a track (Lakomy, 1987). This laboratory approach to the study of sprinting allows us to gain some insight into the metabolic responses to running at maximal speeds. For example, when a 30-s maximal sprint was performed by eight active, but non-sprint-trained people, the peak blood lactate concentration (5 min post-sprint) was 14.5 mmol/L (Nevill et al., 1989). The intense metabolic challenge of sprinting in this experiment was also reflected by the fall in venous blood pH from 7.38 to 7.15 and in muscle pH from 7.02 to 6.82. Muscle lactate concentration increased from 3.9 to 82 mmol/kg dm. The PCr concentrations decreased from 79.0 to 25.1 mmol/kg dm, which represents a decrease of 68% (Nevill et al., 1989). Costill and colleagues (1983) recorded even lower values (6.63 ± 0.27; mean $\pm$ SEM) for muscle pH in four runners at the end of a 400-m sprint. Post-exercise blood pH and blood lactate concentrations were, nevertheless, similar for sprint treadmill running in the experiment by Nevill et al. (1989) and for the 400-m track time trial reported by Costill's group (1983).

The physiological demands of the 30-s maximal sprint were such that the oxygen uptake was 15.4 mL/kg, which was equivalent to 27% of the runners' $\dot{V}O_2$max values (Nevill et al., 1989). Heart rates approached 175 beats/min but did not reach maximum values (192 beats/min) during the sprint. The 30 s of treadmill sprinting also produced large endocrine responses. Plasma adrenaline concentrations increased 600%, from 0.2 to 1.4 nmol/L, and plasma noradrenaline increased by 509%, from 2.2 to 13.4 nmol/L. In addition, the sprint stimulated a large increase in the concentration of the opioid, beta-endorphin, from less than 0.5 to 10.2 pmol/L (Brooks et al., 1988).

The contribution of anaerobic glycogenolysis to energy production during the 30-s sprint was calculated from an analysis of the changes in muscle glycogen, lactate, pyruvate, and PCr concentrations (Nevill et al., 1989). Anaerobic glycolysis contributed 52.3% to ATP resynthesis, whereas the degradation of PCr and the muscle's limited ATP store contributed half this amount, i.e., 26.2%. The aerobic contribution to energy production during the 30-s sprint, calculated from the oxygen uptake values during the sprint, was 21.5%. The 200-m track performance time for these subjects was 29.34 s (Nevill et al., 1989). Therefore, these responses to treadmill running may be regarded as similar to what might be expected in response to a 200-m track race.

Analyses of the changes in glycogen, ATP, and PCr in single muscle fibers after a similar 30-s treadmill sprint confirmed the importance of PCr in energy production during maximal exercise. For example, muscle biopsy samples obtained from the vastus laterali of six active young men before and after a 30-s treadmill sprint showed that the Type II fibers had higher PCr and glycogen concentrations before exercise than the Type I fibers (Figures 2-8, 2-9). But after the sprint, the PCr values were lower in the Type II fibers than in the Type I fibers. Phosphocreatine and glycogen concentrations decreased by 94% and 27%, respectively, whereas the

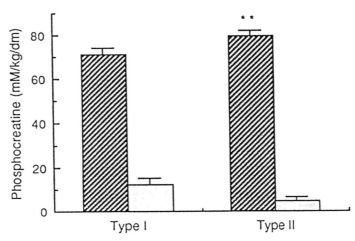

FIGURE 2-8. *Phosphocreatine concentrations in Type I and in Type II muscle fibers before (dark bars) and after (light bars) a 30-s sprint on a non-motorized treadmill (Greenhaff et al., 1992)*

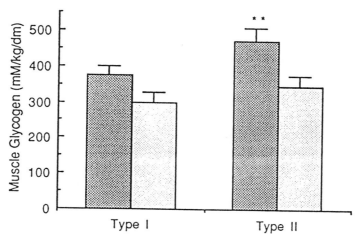

FIGURE 2-9. *Muscle glycogen concentrations in Type I and in Type II muscle fibers before (dark bars) and after (light bars) a 30-s sprint on a non-motorized treadmill (Greenhaff et al., 1992)*

ATP concentration declined by only 21% (Figure 2-10). Peak power output was 885 W, and by the end of the sprint, power output had declined by 65% (Greenhaff et al., 1992). The subjects with the highest pre-exercise PCr concentrations in Type II fibers had the smallest decrease in power output during the 30 s sprint (r = 0.93; P<0.01) (Greenhaff et al., 1992).

Influence of Sprint Training on Energy Production

In order to understand the reasons for training-induced improvements in sprint performance, sports scientists have focused on possible limitations in energy supply to working muscles. In one of the few studies of sprint training effects on muscle metabolism and performance, Nevill and colleagues (1989) reported an improvement in 50-m and 200-m track times of eight subjects (four men and four women) after 8 wk of training. Training involved two 30-s treadmill sprints twice weekly and one session weekly of 10 x 6-s sprints with recovery intervals of 54 s between sprints. Once a week the training group also completed 2–5 runs on a motorized treadmill, each run lasting 2 min, at speeds equivalent to 110% of each runner's V̇O₂max.

Training improved the average 50-m track times of the training group from 7.72 s to 7.55 s, and their 200-m times decreased from a pre-training value of 31.11 s to 29.65 s. These changes represented improvements of 2% and 4.7% for the 50-m and 200-m races, respectively, whereas there were no improvements in the performance times of the control group of runners. Performances of the training group on the sprint treadmill also improved after training. Their peak power output increased from 606 W to 681 W, an improvement of 12% (P<0.05), whereas there was no signif-

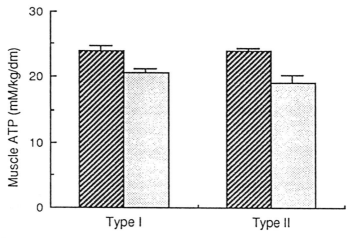

FIGURE 2-10. *ATP concentrations in Type I and in Type II muscle fibers before (dark bars) and after (light bars) a 30-s sprint on a non-motorized treadmill (Greenhaff et al., 1992)*

icant change in their mean power output (378 W before and 399 W after training).

Analyses of pre- and post-training biopsy samples from the quadriceps of the subjects before and after a 30-s treadmill sprint provided a good description of the metabolic changes accompanying the improvements in sprint treadmill and track performances (Nevill et al., 1989). The training-induced 12% increase in peak power output was accompanied by a 20% increase in muscle lactate concentration and an equivalent increase in the rate of ATP resynthesis from anaerobic glycogenolysis. However, the post-sprint decrease in muscle pH was not affected by training. This suggests that training increased the buffering capacity of muscle, but this hypothesis was not confirmed by biochemical analysis of muscle buffering capacity (Nevill et al., 1989). Still, an increase in buffering capacity of muscle has been reported as one of the products of high-intensity training (Sharp et al., 1986).

Even though peak power output increased as a consequence of sprint training, there was no increase in the concentration of PCr in resting muscle (Nevill et al., 1989). This study showed that muscle metabolism adapted to the sprint training by increasing energy production from anaerobic glycolysis to support an increased peak power output. This may have been the consequence of a training-induced increase in the activity of phosphofructokinase (PFK) or even an increase in the proportion of Type IIa fibers (Jacobs et al., 1987).

The main focus of metabolic research on sprinting has been on changes in energy production as a consequence of sprint training. However, changes in other biochemical/physiological systems also contribute to improvements in performance. For example, sprint training increases skeletal muscle Na^+-K^+ ATPase concentrations and improves K^+ regulation during exercise (McKenna et al., 1993). The central role of K^+ in physiological regulation is such that alterations in its responses to exercise will have widespread influences, not the least of which are effects on the processes involved in excitation-contraction coupling in skeletal muscles.

Metabolic Limitations

Fatigue during sprinting is associated with a reduction in PCr stores in skeletal muscle to critically low values. Hirvonen and colleagues (1992) reported PCr concentrations of 1.7 mmol/kg ww of muscle (7.3 mmol/kg dm) at the end of a 400-m race. Similarly, at the end of a 30-s treadmill sprint, the PCr concentrations in Type I and Type II fibers were 12.2 and 5.0 mmol/kg dm, respectively. Muscle glycogen concentration decreased by 27% in the Type II fibers and by only 20% in Type I fibers (Greenhaff et al., 1992). These results are similar to those obtained by histochemical analyses of glycogen depletion in different muscle fiber populations during 30 s of maximal cycling exercise (Vøllestad et al., 1992). Therefore, even at fatigue there was sufficient glycogen in both populations of fibers to support energy production. Furthermore, the ATP content of muscle fibers decreased by only 20% after the 30-s treadmill sprint (Figure 2-10) (Greenhaff et al., 1992).

The explanation for why muscle is unable to exploit the available substrate for energy production has yet to be established. However, Hultman et al. (1987) suggested that when the PCr stores are exhausted, muscle is prevented from generating force by the increasing amounts of H^+, P_i, and even free Mg^{2+} ions—all products of the highly stimulated metabolism in the working muscles. They suggest that the accumulation of these products inhibits cross-bridge recycling between actin and myosin filaments in muscle and hence suppresses activation of the contractile system. Therefore, once the PCr stores are insufficient for rapid resynthesis of ATP, the continuing high rate of anaerobic glycogenolysis generates by-products that not only inhibit glycolysis, but, more importantly, prevent the use of the available ATP by impairing the excitation-contraction process (Hultman et al., 1987). Regardless of the precise mechanism, it seems clear that when there is a marked reduction in intramuscular PCr stores, even though glycogen is readily available, the glycogen cannot be used quickly enough to sustain the high rates of ATP utilization required for maximal exercise.

Low concentrations of PCr and ATP may also induce an increased activity of the purine cycle, leading to a further decrease in the available pool of adenine nucleotides and an increase in ammonia concentrations, first in muscle and later in plasma (Tullson & Terjung, 1990). Thus, plasma ammonia concentrations increase during sprinting (Schlicht et al., 1990). It has been postulated that high concentrations of ammonia in plasma may contribute to the onset of fatigue by adversely affecting the central nervous system (Banister & Cameron, 1990). This may be the case during 400-m running and during repeated shorter sprints during training, but it is probably not a factor during a 100-m race.

Mechanical Limitations

An increase in running speed is achieved by an increase in stride length and in stride frequency. The ability to increase stride length is progressively limited as runners approach maximal speeds; eventually, an increase in speed can only be achieved by increasing stride frequency (Hay, 1985). At maximal speeds the contact time with the track is reduced; thus, the opportunity to develop greater driving force to improve or maintain forward velocity diminishes. These mechanical factors may contribute as much to limiting sprinting speed as the biochemical events leading to ATP resynthesis in the muscles.

Air resistance also contributes to the sprinter's inability to sustain maximal velocity throughout a race. Therefore, sprinting on tracks located at high altitude give the athlete a significant advantage (Davies, 1980).

The nature of the running track also influences sprinting speed. Comparisons of contemporary sprint times with those established in earlier periods must take into account that some records were set on cinder tracks. Not only did the quality of such tracks change with weather conditions, but the number of races that preceded a given sprint also influenced the times achieved during the competition. For example, the sprint relays are traditionally held at the end of the track races; thus, in the days before synthetic tracks, the relay team frequently had to contend with a running surface that was rutted and slippery. It is remarkable that in the final of the 4 x 100-m relay race in the 1964 Tokyo Olympics, Bob Hayes recorded a world best time of 8.86 s for the last 100 m on a cinder track.

There appear to be fast tracks around the world on which sprinters frequently record their best times. Tracks must be suitable for several types of races; very hard tracks favor the sprinters but are disadvantageous to the 10,000-m runners because of their potential to cause injury. The International Amateur Athletics Federation (IAAF) has laid down clear guidelines for track surfaces, and only approved tracks are normally considered as venues for international and world championship races. The fast times achieved in the 1991 World Athletics Championship in Tokyo have been attributed to the fast track in the Japanese National Stadium. Six men ran the 100-m in less than 10 s, and two sprinters beat the former world record of 9.90 s. Carl Lewis and Leroy Burrell ran the 100-m in 9.86 and 9.88 s, respectively; the previous record was 9.9 s. It has been reported that the Tokyo track did not conform with the specifications laid down by the IAAF, so the performances of these sprinters both in the 100-m and in the long jump may be partly explained by the hard track on which they were achieved. The difference in track surfaces is offered as one explanation for the differences in sprint performances of the same six runners when they competed in the 1992 Olympics in Barcelona (Table 2-6). This observation, if it does nothing else, serves to highlight the multiplicity of factors that can influence the outcome of races in which the competitors are closely matched. This is especially true when the races are between the world's elite sprinters. In some of these elite races, the differences in finishing times are so close that they are unmeasurable, even with the best technology.

NUTRITIONAL INFLUENCES ON SPRINTING

Dietary Aspects and Food Intake

Unlike distance runners, the dietary habits of sprinters have not attracted wide attention from nutritional scientists. This may reflect sprinters' attitudes about the links between nutrition and performance. For example, before competition, Linford Christie, who won the Olympic gold medal in Barcelona for the 100-m and won the same race at the 1993 World Athletics Championships in Stuttgart, eats whatever he is given (Forbes, 1993). His interest in food is hedonistic; he does not consider it an integral part of his training program. However, his habitual diet is West Indian and is thus high in fruit and other carbohydrate-containing foods.

There is a long-held belief among sprinters and other power athletes that improvements in strength can be enhanced by consuming a diet high in meat. But the available evidence suggests that the protein requirements of sprinters and strength athletes can be met by a daily intake of 1.2–1.7 g of protein per kg of body weight (bw) (Lemon & Proctor, 1991). Even endurance runners, who are not normally concerned about their protein consumption, achieve daily protein intakes of about 1.5–1.6 g/kg bw (Williams, 1993). Still, the message athletes often receive is that they

TABLE 2-6. *Performance times of sprinters who competed in the 100-m finals at both the 1991 World Athletics Championships in Tokyo and the 1992 Barcelona Olympics (Temple, 1993)*

Sprinter	Times (s)	
	Tokyo, 1991	Barcelona, 1992
L. Burrell (USA)	9.88	10.10
D. Mitchell (USA)	9.91	10.04
L. Christie (UK)	9.92	9.96
F. Fredericks (Nam)	9.95	10.02
R. Stewart (Jam)	9.96	10.22
B. Surin (Can)	10.14	10.09

should eat more than the recommended amounts of protein "just in case" (Hatfield, 1987).

Nutrition scientists recommend diets made up of a wide variety of foods to ensure that all needs for energy, vitamins, and minerals are satisfied. Carbohydrates should contribute at least 50% of daily energy intake, whereas less than 35% should be obtained from fat, and the remainder should be provided by protein.

Athletes are advised to obtain 60–70% of their daily energy intake from carbohydrate and about 12% from protein (Devlin & Williams, 1991), but only endurance athletes come close to achieving these recommendations (Williams, 1993). This is not surprising, because training for endurance events requires high daily energy expenditures. Therefore, the carbohydrate stores of the endurance athlete must be adequate to meet the demands of daily long-distance training runs. Unfortunately, the food intake of sprinters is not well documented; what information is available is often included under the heading of "track athletes." Short and Short (1983) reported that the track athletes had a daily energy intake of approximately 4,000 kcal, which was similar to that of the body builders in their study of university sportsmen and women.

Carbohydrate Loading and Sprinting

Carbohydrate loading is a nutritional strategy used by endurance athletes in preparation for competition. It is not a practice to be recommended for sprinters because muscle glycogen stores are not limiting for sprints, even during races over 400 m (Hirvonen et al., 1992). Circumstantial evidence from laboratory studies on maximal exercise of brief duration supports this conclusion. For example, Wootton and Williams (1984) showed that carbohydrate loading did not improve peak or mean power outputs of athletes during 30 s of maximal cycle ergometer exercise using the WAnT procedure or during a second 30-s maximal test performed 15 min later.

A study of single muscle fibers obtained from human biopsies before and after a 30-s sprint on a non-motorized treadmill provides some explanations for the failure of carbohydrate loading to influence performance (Greenhaff et al., 1992). In this investigation, the small (20% and 27%) reductions in glycogen concentrations in Type I and Type II muscle fibers, respectively, showed that the maximal sprinting exercise made relatively modest demands on glycogen stores (Greenhaff et al., 1992). In terms of substrate availability, the decrease in running speed was more closely linked to the 83% and 94% declines in PCr concentration in Type I and Type II fibers, respectively, than to the decrease in glycogen stores (Greenhaff et al., 1992).

In recent research studies, some attempt has been made to be prescriptive about the amount of carbohydrate that should be eaten to replenish muscle glycogen stores. For example, a diet containing about 8 to 10 g of carbohydrate per kilogram of body weight is sufficient to replace muscle glycogen stores after daily 1 h training sessions (Pascoe et al., 1990; Sherman & Wimer, 1991).

On the other hand, Sherman et al. (1993) reported that a daily carbohydrate intake of only 5 g/kg bw was as effective in replacing muscle glycogen during a week of training as was a carbohydrate intake of 10 g/kg bw (Sherman et al., 1993). Runners completed 1 h of treadmill running at 75% $\dot{V}O_2$max each day followed by 5 x 60-s sprints at speeds corresponding to each person's $\dot{V}O_2$max. At the end of the week of training, the group on the high-carbohydrate diet (10 g/kg bw) and the group on the moderate carbohydrate diet (5 g/kg bw) performed two performance tests 5 min after the last training run. The performance tests required the subjects to run to exhaustion twice at speeds corresponding to 80% $\dot{V}O_2$max, with a 5-min recovery between runs. Even though the muscle glycogen concentrations of the runners on the moderate carbohydrate diet were 30–36% lower than those on the high-carbohydrate diet at the end of the week of training, their performance times were not different. Therefore, the glycogen stores of the runner on the moderate carbohydrate diet were adequate to cover the energy demands of the prescribed training and the performance tests. These results could be used to argue that, although glycogen stores will be enhanced, performance may not always be improved by chronically consuming a diet that is high in carbohydrate.

When athletes must exercise to exhaustion on a daily basis, rather than complete a fixed amount of activity, they may require a high, rather than a moderate, carbohydrate intake. Fallowfield and Williams (1993) reported that athletes could reproduce a 90-min treadmill run only when carbohydrate intake during the previous 22.5-h recovery period was increased from 6 to 9 g/kg bw. Without the additional carbohydrate intake, the runners in this study ran about 15 min less than during the previous day's training session. However, it is worth noting that the training session involved constant pace running, whereas sprint training involves repeated brief periods of high-speed running.

Currently, there is little information on the glycogen demands of repeated bouts of high-intensity exercise. In one study, Gaitanos et al. (1993) had subjects perform 10 x 6-s maximal sprints on a cycle ergometer; the sprints were loaded according to the WAnT procedure and were separated by 30-s recovery intervals. Only about half the muscle glycogen used during the first sprint was used during the tenth sprint. Accordingly, there appeared to be a trend towards a reduced use of glycogen as the exercise session continued. The authors concluded that there was an increased contribution to energy production from aerobic metabolism as exercise time increased (Gaitanos et al., 1993). Nevertheless, these results do not deny the need for sprinters in training to consume adequate amounts of carbohydrates in their daily diets, especially because a high-carbohydrate diet is recommended for everyone as a means of reducing the risk of early coronary artery disease.

In a recent study, sprinters simulated a training session for 90 min, including a mixture of sprints with long and short recovery periods (during which they jogged or walked) (Nicholas and Williams, unpublished observations). Only the sprinters who increased carbohydrate intake to 10 g/kg during a 24 h recovery period were able to reproduce their training performances on the following day. Therefore, even though there is no reason to recommend carbohydrate loading per se for sprinters preparing for competition, they should not neglect the carbohydrate content of their diets, and they should consume at least the amounts recommended by health professionals.

Dietary Supplements and Sprinting

Protein and Amino Acids. The dietary supplements that appear to be most popular among sprinters are protein powders and amino acids, usually used to enhance diets that are already high in meat and meat products. Sprinters and strength athletes who take amino acid supplementation usually do so in an attempt to stimulate an increased release of human growth hormone. Arginine and ornithine are particularly popular amino acids because they are believed to have anabolic effects through their ability to stimulate a biologically significant increase in the plasma concentration of human growth hormone (Hatfield, 1987; Williams, 1989). However, recent research studies have failed to substantiate the view that amino acid supplementation enhances performance or increases the serum concentrations of human growth hormone. In 11 competitive weight lifters, Fogelholm et al. (1993) examined the effects of 4 d of dietary supplementation with a combination of L-arginine, L-ornithine, and L-lysine (2 g/d divided into two daily doses) on 24 h serum concentrations of growth hormone. They found no effect of the supplement on the three daily peaks in serum growth hormone concentrations nor on the serum insulin concentrations.

Lambert et al. (1993) also studied the influences of amino acid supplementation on the serum growth hormone concentrations of seven male body builders. The amino acid supplementation consisted of 2.4 g of arginine/lysine mixture and 1.85 g of ornithine/tyrosine mixture. These commercially available supplements were given in doses recommended by the manufacturers. The results of this study showed that these low-dose supplements had no detectable influence on the serum growth hormone concentrations of the body builders.

In another study, which examined the possible influences of amino acid supplementation on strength performance after 7 d of heavy resistance training, Fry et al. (1993) enlisted the help of 28 male participants at a junior age group U.S. national weightlifting training camp. The weight-lifters were assigned to a protein group or a placebo group after having been matched according to body weights and lifting ability. A double-blind procedure was adopted in assigning a commercially available amino acid supplement to one group and lactose capsules to the placebo group. The amino acid supplement (2.4 g), which contained a mixture of all 20 amino acids, and the placebo were taken by the two groups before their three daily meals for 7 d. In addition, the weightlifters also took 2.1 g of branched-chain amino acids (L-leucine, L-isoleucine, and L-valine), L-glut-amine, and L-carnitine before each training session, whereas the placebo group took additional lactose capsules. Serum growth hormone, testoste-rone, and cortisol concentrations were measured at 7 a.m. and imme-diately before an exercise testing session, 5 min after the testing session, and again 10 min later. There were no differences between the two groups in their hormonal responses to the exercise tests. The authors concluded that 7 d of amino acid supplementation did not alter resting or exercise-induced changes in serum growth hormone, testosterone, or cortisol con-centrations, and there were no measurable improvements in performance. An unexpected finding in this study was that the week of heavy training produced hormonal and performance decrements suggesting that the weightlifters were showing early signs of the overtraining syndrome.

What is usually overlooked by strength athletes and sprinters is that even brief periods of high-intensity exercise will produce significant in-creases in the concentration of circulating growth hormone. For example, a 30 s-maximal sprint on a non-motorized treadmill produced a 14-fold increase in plasma growth hormone in sprint-trained athletes and a 6-fold increase in endurance-trained athletes. The growth hormone concentra-tions of the sprinters were still about 11 times higher (44.9 ± 27.0 mU/L) than pre-exercise values (4.0 ± 2.0 mU/L) after an hour of recovery (Ne-vill et al., 1993). Therefore, training per se is probably more effective than amino acid supplements as a stimulus for releasing growth hormones.

Unfortunately, dietary supplementation is not limited to protein and amino acids. There is an extensive variety of commercially available sup-plements, many of which are too bizarre for serious consideration (Hat-field, 1987; Williams, 1989). There is little evidence to support nutritional supplementation of a diet that contains a wide range of foods that are of sufficient quantity to cover the energy needs of athletes in training (Clarkson, 1990; Van Der Beek, 1990).

Bicarbonate Loading. A significant reduction in muscle pH will dis-rupt intracellular function. Therefore, it is not surprising that an increase in muscle lactate and the accompanying increase in hydrogen ions and de-crease in pH have long been regarded as principal contributors to the onset of fatigue. Removal of hydrogen ions from muscle as quickly as pos-sible is a logical strategy to delay the onset of fatigue. Animal studies have demonstrated that perfusing contracting skeletal muscle with alkalotic blood (pH ~ 7.5) increases the rate of lactate release from muscle and perfusing with acidotic blood (pH ~ 7.1) decreases it (Heigenhauser & Jones, 1991). Extending the concept to humans performing prolonged heavy exercise in the laboratory has provided, on balance, equally positive results (Heigenhauser & Jones, 1991).

Applying this principle to track racing, Kindermann et al. (1977) increased the blood buffering capacity of 10 young men before they ran a 400-m time trial. They received a bicarbonate infusion about 2 h before the race, and blood pH increased to 7.5. There was no improvement in the performance times for the 400-m (control: 62.4 ± 4.1 s vs bicarbonate: 62.6 ± 4.9 s) as a result of elevating the pre-race buffering capacity of this group of subjects. The authors concluded that a reduction in pH may not be such a central influence on the fatigue process as previously believed (Kindermann et al., 1977).

In contrast, Goldfinch and colleagues (1988) reported a 1.52-s improvement in 400-m performance time for a group of six runners who ingested a bicarbonate solution an hour before the race. Their subjects ran the 400-m on three occasions, including a control trial without any treatment (58.46 ± 2.49 s). After the bicarbonate treatment (400 mg/kg bw), the 400-m time was 56.94 ± 2.25 s, whereas after the placebo treatment (calcium carbonate), it was 58.63 ± 2.25 s. A similar performance benefit has also been shown for 800-m running by Wilkes et al. (1983), who reported a 2.9-s improvement in performance (control: 2:05.8 ± 0:02.2 vs alkalosis: 2:02.9 ± 0:01.9 min:sec) when runners drank a bicarbonate solution (300 mg/kg bw) before the race. In both studies, the subjects were experienced but not elite runners; it would be interesting to know whether or not similar improvements in performance times could be achieved by elite sprinters.

The improvements in running performance over 400 m and 800 m were attributed to the increased blood buffering capacity as a consequence of ingesting a bicarbonate solution before these races. The same performance benefits appear to be achievable in laboratory studies of high-intensity, short duration exercise (Matson & Tran, 1993). However, there are no definitive studies on the influences of bicarbonate loading on sprinting performance over 100 to 200 m. Furthermore, inducing alkalosis before races does not appear to be a widespread practice among sprinters. One of the reasons may be that elite sprinters have tried it, found it to be ineffective, and have conveyed their results to others by word of mouth. Another important consideration is that drinking a concentrated bicarbonate solution an hour or two before competition may cause gastrointestinal discomfort; vomiting is not an uncommon response to this treatment.

Creatine Supplementation. The central role of PCr in the rapid resynthesis of ATP in skeletal muscle during maximal exercise of short duration is now widely acknowledged, if not fully understood. Sprinting draws upon the PCr stores in skeletal muscle; as PCr is depleted, running speed decreases (Hirvonen et al., 1992). Therefore, it is not surprising that ways of enhancing pre-exercise PCr concentrations have been sought. Creatine is found mainly in skeletal muscles; dietary intake is obtained from meat and fish products. Supplementation of the diet with 20–30 g of creatine monohydrate daily for 5 d increases the total creatine content and the PCr concentrations in human quadriceps muscle (Harris et al., 1992). Daily exercise during the period of supplementation enhances the uptake of creatine into skeletal muscles. Thus, the PCr concentration in skeletal muscle that had been exercised during 4 d of creatine supplementation increased from 81.9 ± 5.6 to 103.1 ± 6.2 mmol/kg dm. The largest increases in PCr were recorded in a vegetarian subject and in those who had low PCr values before supplementation (Harris et al., 1992).

A daily creatine supplementation of 20–30 g for 5 d delays the onset of fatigue during intense intermittent exercise with short recovery periods (Balsom et al., 1993; Greenhaff et al., 1993). Creatine supplementation also improves interval track running performance, as reported by Harris et al. (1993); they studied university middle-distance athletes who consumed either a placebo or 30 g/d of creatine for 6 d. Time trials on the track before and after the 6-d diet manipulation required the athletes to complete four 300-m runs at speeds corresponding to 90–95% of their best performances; each run was followed by a recovery period of 4 min. These runners also had to complete four 1000-m runs under the same conditions but with 3-min recovery intervals between runs. The reduction in the final 300-m run time after the 6-d supplementation period was greater for the creatine group (−0.7 ± 0.3 s) than for the placebo group (−0.3 ± 1.5 s). The best 1000-m time was also significantly faster for the creatine supplementation group (−5.5 ± 1.55 s) than for the placebo group (−1.6 ± 0.67 s) (Harris et al., 1993). The authors did not report changes in PCr concentrations as a result of the creatine supplementation.

In light of the improvements in performance following creatine supplementation, it is surprising that sprint training does not seem to increase PCr concentrations in human muscle (Nevill et al., 1989). Furthermore, as of this writing there are no reports of performance benefits of creatine supplementation for 100-m or 200-m sprinters. However, there is no shortage of anecdotal evidence about the contribution of creatine supplementation to gold medal performances in the Barcelona Olympic Games.

In summary, although it has not yet been proven, creatine is the dietary supplement that appears to have the greatest potential to enhance sprint performance. The available evidence suggests that creatine is effective in enhancing performance during repeated periods of high-intensity exercise when there are only short recovery periods between bouts of exercise. Thus, creatine supplementation may be most valuable in supporting sprint training rather than as a pre-competition ergogenic aid.

SPRINT TRAINING

Historical Aspects of Sprint Training

The contention that "sprinters are born, not made" was undoubtedly consistent with sprint training methods throughout the first half of this century and beyond. In fact, for many years, engaging in any serious training was often frowned upon, and the association of Harold Abrahams with a professional coach, Sam Mussabini, in preparation for competition for the 1924 Olympic 100-m gold medal, was itself very much against the tide of contemporary opinion.

Loader (1960), a sprinting product of the first half of the century, exemplified the opinion of the time in asserting that "Running is not an affair of applied mechanics or economic necessity, but an expression by the human body of rhythm and grace and strength," and "About other branches of athletics I would not be so dogmatic, but about sprinting I would say that you are either a sprinter, or you aren't." The fundamental attributes of top sprinting ability undoubtedly have a substantial basis in genetics, and therein lies an implicit and continuing challenge to coaching. Henry Carr, the 1960 Olympic 200-m champion, modestly suggested that "a little natural ability" with "desire" were the main requirements for success (Aitken, 1992). Although effective training, up to a point, surely existed, and some sprinters did undoubtedly work hard at it, coaches formerly lacked the insights and sophistication of methods available today. In the past, out-of-season activity (for as long as eight months) consisted of mainly non-specific, only moderately demanding exercise, often including involvement in another sport. Beginning in early season, sprint running and starting practice was usually regarded as sufficient training for ensuing competitions.

Weight training and body conditioning exercises (calisthenics) were used by some, but with only a crude understanding of their specific application to sprinting. For example, Carr avoided using weights out of concern that he might become "bigger and more bulky" and develop shorter muscles (Aitken, 1992). The rare sprinter keen enough to train seriously in the winter, and able to keep pace, would often be goaded into joining the distance running fraternity to "get in the miles." Too much of this type of training could lead to the transformation of potentially good sprinters into mediocre cross-country runners. Other sprinters with potential often found they preferred their off-season sports and gave up track running completely.

The success of the Soviet Union and other Eastern Bloc nations in the 1952 Olympic Games sparked greater worldwide interest in the potential for national investment in developing training theory and creating more systematic, structured approaches to training. A highly publicized focus on Eastern Bloc training achievements involved the build-up to Valery Borzov's double victory at the Munich Olympics in 1972 (Kozlova, 1972), but by far the greatest returns for the Eastern Bloc countries were from their women athletes, especially those of the former German Democratic Republic. During this era, the United States coaching establishment certainly had opinions on training, but they thrived by using more short-term arrangements, including the recruitment of promising secondary school sprinters onto university teams and the exploitation of their talents in a hotbed of student competition. As a result, the U.S. continued to dominate the world scene in men's sprinting—almost exclusively with black athletes—from the 1960s forward.

The acceptance of the notion that sprinters should train systematically and specifically, in and out of season, grew in the 1950s and 1960s, but at different rates in different countries. In Britain, weight training, circuit training and hill sprints were increasingly used for general pre-season conditioning, giving way to the practice of starting techniques and actual sprints on the track as the competitive season approached. There was some awareness of a need to train for strength, stamina, suppleness, skill, and speed, but there was as yet no greatly sophisticated insight into the interrelationships among these factors, or into their specific influences on performance. There was also tacit agreement that psychological factors could be important, but there was little attempt outside individual initiative to capitalize on implicit possibilities for manipulating psychological variables (Brightwell & Packer, 1965).

By the 1960s and 1970s newer insights were emerging, mainly from the Eastern Bloc countries, with active and passive stretching routines the rule rather than the exception for sprinters, alongside the associated evolution of plyometric exercises and drills. For example, the successful Polish sprinter Irena Szevinska was noted for her commitment to impressive bounding routines. Pietro Mennea, the Olympic 200-m champion in 1980 and still the world record holder at 200 m, was another who invested heavily in plyometric conditioning. Meanwhile, 100-m winner Allan Wells employed twice-daily, out-of-season strength training along with speedball work, as the sprinting world became increasingly aware of the potential gains to be made from supplementary conditioning programs. Specificity became a much-preached gospel in the 1960s, but the detailed physiology and mechanics of sprinting were insufficiently understood to ensure the precise and appropriate implementation of the specificity principle. Nevertheless, progress was made toward applying the specificity principle and refining old and new training methods.

When Matveyev presented his findings on "Peaking and Periodization" in 1965, he was really describing what top athletes were already doing (Dick, 1991). Indeed Abrahams, from as early as 1924, was said with retrospective wisdom to be "a good example of a runner who timed his condition perfectly for the big occasion" (Quercetani, 1965). But by labeling and identifying component parts of the overall training cycle, Matveyev also provided the basis for more systematic planning for training and competition with better evaluative possibilities. His work has been as influential as that of Harre (1982), who defined more precisely the components of fitness and pointed the way for development of special event skills from a base of more general fitness qualities.

Current Training Methods for Sprinters

Current training methods are more comprehensive and systematic than older ones, although few of the newer methods could be termed revolutionary. Serious sprinters typically train almost year-round for about 2 h/d. For the most successful, the sport has become the equivalent of full-time employment. There is a wealth of advice from sport scientists clarifying the role of the central nervous system in motor unit recruitment, the elastic responses of muscle tissue, the optimal utilization of energy sources, the relaxation of antagonist muscles, the psychological influences such as willpower and concentration, the rapidity of cue selection (Kraaijenhof, 1990), and the interrelationships of all of these factors with training and performance. This undoubtedly has had a considerable effect. However, the extent to which current training methods can be scientifically substantiated is still incomplete. There remains a critical need for scientifically derived data to be communicated to coaches in relatively simple and practical terms.

The International Athletic Foundation's scientific program has provided quickly available and easily interpreted biomechanical information on sprint events at recent World Championships and Olympic Games. Such data have included reaction times, acceleration characteristics indicated by time over the first 30 m, maximum velocity achieved over successive 10-m segments, and "speed endurance," derived from times for sections in the final stage of each race (Table 2-5). With such information, model performance profiles may be constructed as targets for individual athletes.

Tellez and Doolittle (1984), long involved in the training of Carl Lewis, found that reaction time contributes only 1% to 100-m performance; time to clear the starting blocks, 5%; acceleration, 64%; maintenance of maximal velocity, 12%; and reduction of deceleration, 12%. These figures, in conjunction with individual profiles derived as described above, can clearly indicate which particular aspects of sprinting ability are in need of emphasis. Table 2-7 illustrates how they can also point to the employment of the training forms likely to be specifically effective. These training forms themselves represent a mixture of empiricism (weight training, circuit training, running workouts, etc.) as well as a growing scientific understanding of processes and effects.

One aspect of sprinting and related training activity that has been a focus of continuing attention is the starting position and initial response to the firing of the pistol. Many leading British sprinters employ a method closely akin to the *medium* start commended by somewhat rudimentary research that emerged in the 1950s. This method is characterized by 30-40 cm separation of the feet (side view) and 90 and 120 degree angles of front and rear knees, respectively, in the *set* position. Others, including leading Americans, have preferred to have the feet separated by only 10-20 cm (*bunch* start) and to have the feet withdrawn further behind the start line (*rocket* start) with a view to achieving a greater horizontal force component in the initial drive. Raising the hips to high levels and/or lowering the shoulders (by bending the elbows slightly or by increasing the distance between the hands) seems likely to encourage a greater contribution from the hip extensors (gluteals) in the starting action. The importance of both the knee and hip extensor muscles in all aspects of sprinting cannot be overstated, and strengthening these muscles as well as practicing variations in starting technique are central to all training programs. *Roll-over* starts from a supine position are often practiced in order to develop reactive ability and to encourage athletes to stay low in the early strides, although the need for the latter was perhaps called into question by the supreme effectiveness of Ben Johnson's starting method, which was characterized by an explosive drive into an early upright position.

The particular features of a training program indicative of a successful modern approach are as follows: 1) a very substantial investment in aerobic development during the first three months of the program, primarily by using repetition sessions on a grass surface covering about 5000 m in total distance; 2) great attention to the details of running technique from the initiation of the program; 3) extensive use of plyometric sprinting drills; 4) the employment of water power workouts to provide variety and to protect the body from impact stresses; and 5) a blending of and careful progression in the type of workouts used throughout the year.

Training Programs for Sprinters

Thorough planning is a prerequisite for a successful program of sprint training. Such planning must take into account medium (whole season), long-term (perhaps up to 4 y), and short-term (7–14 d) objectives, and accommodate the age, gender, previous experience, and circumstances of the individual athlete. Obviously, the longer-term aspects of planning will be expressed in more general terms, but great detail in shorter-term scheduling is highly desirable. Training is typically organized in weekly, biweekly, or monthly cycles, each of which will include a blend and balance of work units or sessions, ensuring carefully graduated progression and maintenance of qualities (e.g, strength, flexibility) already developed, while seeking enhancement of other qualities (e.g., speed, endurance) and providing sufficient, but not excessive, time for recovery and regeneration (Fry et al., 1992a). This approach not only attempts to produce the maximum adaptations to training but also attempts to avoid overtraining (Fry et al., 1992b).

Training cycles and units will fit in rationally as functional components of either a single-periodized year (6–7 months of general/specific preparation, 4–5 months of competition, and one month of transition/recuperation) or a double periodized year which consists of two single periods having phases half as long as that described for the single periodized year. With indoor competition now readily available in winter, a double-periodized year is much the more popular with most sprinters because they have two competitive seasons each year. The broad framework on which a program for a 100/200-m sprinter might be based and organized in a double-periodized year is shown below.

Phase 1: General Preparation 1 (10–12 weeks)
1. Ease gradually into full training routine.
2. All-round body conditioning using weights, circuit training, and stretching routines.
3. Work on technical aspects of sprinting at 70–80% maximum effort.
4. Aerobic work, including 3.2–5 km runs 2–3 times per week and/or Fartlek and/or track work, e.g., 1) 6 x 200 m (200 m jog recovery) or 2) up to 4 km of repeated sets of 100 m jog, 100 m relaxed striding, 100 m walk, and 100 m fast striding.
5. Regular inclusion of alternative training methods, such as running in water, ergometer cycling, aerobics, or yoga.

Phase 2: Competition Preparation 1 (4 weeks)
1. Maintenance of full training routine.
2. More specific conditioning work using weights and stage training with emphasis on leg power and resilience, and continuing daily mobility program.
3. Development of technique using drills and starting practice (5–8 repetitions up to 40 m with 3–5 min recovery intervals).
4. Continuation of some aerobic training, but giving way to speed/speed-endurance work, e.g., 3 sets of 3 x 90 m building up speed and/or clock sessions of 60, 90, 120, 150, 120, 90, and 60 m (walk back) and/or time trials at 60, 150, and 250 m.
5. Associated Performance Tests (see under Evaluation below).
6. Less regular use of alternative training.

Phase 3: Indoor Competitions (4–8 weeks)
1. Reduction in training routine to promote adequate recovery and sharpness for explosive efforts.

2. Use of lighter weights and faster movements during resistance training, mini-circuits, and full mobility routines with the aim of maintaining qualities already achieved.
3. Continuation of technical work but specifically geared to competitions.
4. Acceleration and maximum speed sessions (facilities and weather permitting), as indicated in Table 2-7.
5. Use of massage and whirlpool if available.

Phase 4: General Preparation 2 (6–8 weeks)

As for previous general conditioning phase but without need to ease into full routine; less emphasis on aerobic aspects and more on increasing strength-endurance via heavier loadings and more specific muscle group targeting in weight training and stage training; introduction of more demanding hill repetitions (12–25 s duration); increase of track session volumes, e.g., 6 x 300 m (500 jog) and/or sets of 4 x 30, 4 x 40, 4 x 50, 4 x 60, 4 x 50, 4 x 40, and 4 x 30 m (1–1.5 min recovery intervals); and inclusion of harness work or tire towing.

Phase 5: Competition Preparation 2 (4–5 weeks)

1. Speed-endurance sessions on track, e.g., 2–4 sets of 3–4 repetitions at 90–150 m (1–1.5 min between runs and 5–10 min between sets), and/or clock sessions (50–150 m) on grass or road inclines.
2. Great emphasis on gradual increase of speed via types of work specified in Table 2-7 (special preparation training).
3. Strength-endurance maintenance via less frequent, lighter, faster,

---

TABLE 2-7. *Specific training drills for 100-m sprinters*

Starting Action: Practice squats, leg presses, reaction exercises, individual starts from blocks with pistol signal, and starts in competition with teammates.

Acceleration: Practice power cleans; bounding routines for up to 5 strides; repeated uphill accelerations, harness work, and tire towing over distances of 30–40 m; measure distance covered in 10 strides to improve technique; and time 10-m sections of 40-m sprints.

Pick-up (knee lift phase): Practice keeping knees high while sprinting from 3 x 60 m to 6 x 100 m; practice long bounding strides, e.g., from 3 x 40 m to 6 x 60 m; practice rebound strides over hurdles; and practice depth jumps.

Maximum Velocity: Practice increasing speed gradually (wind-up) or in stages (build-up) at distances up to 80 m; practice movement frequency routines from 2–10 s; spring 4–6 x 20–40 m with flying starts; practice towed running, downslope sprinting, and wind-assisted sprinting; and practice timing of 10-m sections of the final 40–80 m of 100-m sprints.

Holding Form for Final 20 m: Sprint, float, and sprint over continuous 30-m sections or for 2–3 sets of 3–4 repetitions of 60 m, 30 m, and 60 m; perform circuit and stage training; perform weight training with sets of 10–20 repetitions; and practice fast endurance runs of 4 x 120 m, with 8–10 min recovery intervals.

and more specific weight training exercises and/or mini-circuits tailored to individual needs and other training demands.
4. Practice on starting techniques and considerable emphasis on speed drills.
5. Daily mobility routine maintained.
6. Associated performance tests (see below under Evaluation).
7. High-quality work on sprint-specific weight training exercises such as power cleans and snatches.
8. Occasional use of alternative training methods.

Phase 6: Outdoor Competitions 1 (4 weeks)
1. Similar to Phase 3 but retaining speed-endurance work from Phase 4 and including an enhanced speed component (possible use of downhill, towed, or wind-assisted sprinting and transition drills).
2. Work on particular aspects of sprinting needing attention, e.g., acceleration, holding form, etc..
3. Conduct 3-5 competitions used as an extension of training and as a form guide rather than as an end in themselves.

Phase 7: Outdoor Competitions 2 (8–12 weeks)
1. Participate in 10–15 races planned with the aim of producing personal best performances in selected important competitions.
2. Training to be scheduled around races; primary emphasis on ensuring speed and sharpness. Sample training session for men: 5 x 30 m plus 6 x 60 m, with senior men's target times (see Table 2-7) for 30 m and progressing from 7.20 s to 6.40 s for 60 m. Recovery intervals must be adequate to ensure high technical quality. Training sessions for women would use similar distances and repeats, but times would be adjusted appropriately. This work should be supported by continuance of mobility work and less frequent sessions of maintenance weight training or (as used by Linford Christie) mini-circuits to assist retention of strength and strength-endurance.
3. The best training at this time is competitive sprint racing along with adequate recovery, including massage and frequent rest days, plus a minimum of training aimed at maintaining previously developed fitness qualities.

Phase 8: Transition Period (4–6 weeks)
1. Rest and recovery from the season.
2. Evaluation of training over the previous year.
3. Establish future plans.

Evaluation of Training Efficacy

Kraaijenhof (1990) proposed scientific monitoring of training through muscle biopsies, blood and/or urine analyses, measurement of neurotransmitters (noradrenaline and dopamine), and testing for vitamin and/or mineral deficiencies, food allergies, and metabolic functioning. However, this level of sophisticated evaluation is not yet widely available. Fortunately, the experienced coach is well able to derive much invaluable feedback concerning an athlete's form and well-being from observation of competitive performances and achievement in certain standard training sessions.

Performance tests are often incorporated into training programs to indicate training status and degree of progress towards perceived targets. For instance, by 1968 Valery Borzov (Borzov, 1984) had achieved 3.7 s for 30 m from a crouch start, 2.7 s for 30 m with a flying start, and 6.6 s for 60 m from a crouch start and was seeking a 0.1 s improvement in each of these events, which, according to his advisors, was necessary to achieve a time of 10.0 s and the 1972 Olympic title at 100 m. Other measurements, together with the performance levels thereby inferred, have been proposed by Tabatschnik (1983) and are presented in Table 2-8.

Whatever the methods employed, evaluation should be an ongoing process that incorporates regular revisions of plans within cycles, and even at times within single training sessions. Effective training requires that the coach and athlete be able to adjust quickly on the basis of experience. It may frequently be preferable for coaches to use results from familiar, simple, rapid, and readily understandable tests than to await more complex data dependent on the sophisticated analyses of external experts.

In the final analysis, the best performance results may well emerge, as they apparently did in the case of Borzov, out of a blending of empirical knowledge and contemporary scientific methods. The success of training along these lines rests on two basic assumptions: 1) that scientific methods remain within the limits set by the rules of the sport's governing bodies, rather than being intended to outwit them, and 2) that, giving due regard

TABLE 2-8. *Approximate standards for performance of ancillary skills for sprinters aiming to achieve various 100-m times*

Ancillary Skill	Goal for 100 m			
	10.70 s	10.50 s	10.20 s	10.00 s
Sprint 30 m (crouch start) (s)	4.1-4.2	4.0-4.1	3.8-3.9	3.7-3.8
Sprint 30 m (flying start) (s)	2.90-3.00	2.80-2.90	2.75-2.80	2.70
Max. sprint velocity (m/s)	10.86	11.11	11.62	11.90
Sprint 150 m (s)	15.7	15.2	14.8	14.7
Sprint 300 m (s)	35.2-36.2	34.0-35.0	32.4-33.2	32.0-32.4
Standing long jump (m)	2.85-2.90	2.90-3.00	3.00-3.10	3.00-3.10
Standing triple jump (m)	8.60-8.80	8.90-9.20	9.30-10.00	9.30-10.00
10 hops (standing start) (m)	33-34	34-35	35-36	35-36

to the importance of genetic endowment, athletes of appropriate potential are initially selected or fortuitously become involved in the training process. Otherwise, even the most enlightened and persistent training endeavors may fail.

MEDICAL CONSIDERATIONS

Overtraining

One of the threats to the performances of sprinters is overtraining. Unlike distance runners who train almost entirely by running, sprinters undertake a variety of different types of training. Strength training, for instance, is a central element in a sprinter's training program. Inherent in any strength training program is the risk of serious injury during heavy weight training. This risk increases when athletes are tired, often as a consequence of training too frequently. The heavy dynamic exercises performed by sprinters in training may also lead to disruption of the structural organization of those skeletal muscle fibers carrying the greatest burden during training. Friden and colleagues (1988) reported that the fine structure of muscle samples obtained from the vastus lateralis muscles of strength-trained sprinters had a significantly greater degree of disruption than samples from a group of sprinters who had not undertaken similar heavy training for the study. Interestingly, the sprinters who acted as control subjects also had a certain amount of fine structure disruption, which was probably the consequence of their long-term sprint training. Sprint training often involves a large component of eccentric exercise (e.g., plyometric exercises or drills) that has been shown to cause muscle soreness, fiber damage, and delayed glycogen repletion (Costill et al., 1990). Even when carbohydrate intake is increased after eccentric exercise training, glycogen repletion is slower during the days that follow than it is when the mode of exercise is mainly concentric (Doyle et al., 1993). Therefore, the type of exercises during the early phase of training should be chosen carefully, and the principle of progression should be implemented so that recovery between training sessions is not delayed (Fry et al., 1992a).

Overtraining is another risk facing an athlete who is committed to a very demanding and time-consuming training program. This condition is manifest as a lack of enthusiasm for training and excessive tiredness, often accompanied by a decrease in food intake and an inability to sleep soundly. Endurance athletes are susceptible to the so-called overtraining syndrome, whereas sprinters appear to be less so. Nevertheless, there is an increasing body of evidence to suggest that overtraining may also lead to a reduction in the efficacy of the athlete's immune system (immunosuppression) (Sharp, 1993; Tvede et al., 1993).

Anabolic Steroids

In the search for greater strength gains from training, some sprinters attempt to increase their muscle bulk by taking anabolic steroids. This practice is banned by the International Olympic Committee (IOC), not simply on the grounds that it may give an athlete an unfair advantage in competition, but more importantly because of the health risks associated with drug abuse of this kind. The most publicized steroid case in sport was that of Ben Johnson, who won the Olympic gold medal and the world record for the 100-m sprint at the 1988 Olympic Games in Seoul. He was found to have traces of the anabolic steroid stanozolol in his urine during the postrace examination of competitors. His record of 9.79 s for the 100-m was declared null and void, he was disqualified from the race, and the gold medal was recalled. Four years later in Barcelona another sprinter, Jason Livingston, was disqualified because traces of the same anabolic steroid were found in his urine during the pregames examination of Olympic competitors.

Controversy raged in Barcelona about Clenbuterol. Sprint and power athletes around the world claimed it was used simply as a medication for asthma, whereas the IOC Medical Commission ruled that it has anabolic effects. The direct and circumstantial evidence clearly indicate that drug taking, to a greater or lesser extent, is part of the preparation for competition of some athletes. Most of the drug use is based at best on perceived wisdom (Philips, 1991) and at worse on ignorance. There are no reports of scientific experiments on the effects of anabolic steroid use on sprinting performance, and space does not allow a comprehensive review of the effects of steroid use on strength and lean body mass, and the potential adverse side effects. The reader is directed to earlier reviews on these subjects by Lombardo et al. (1991) and Stone (1993).

DIRECTIONS FOR FUTURE RESEARCH ON SPRINTING

Most sprint training methods are based on empirical knowledge of the coaching fraternity. Therefore, there is a need for well-controlled training studies on sprinting. For example, the types of studies undertaken by Hirvonen and colleagues (1987, 1992), in which they measured changes in energy substrates before and after sprint races, need to be extended to include measurements before and after training. Although considerable information can be obtained about sprinting from laboratory studies using cycle ergometers, more specific forms of exercise must be developed if we are intent on completely understanding the metabolic demands of sprinting. One of the questions that requires a clear answer is whether or not sprint training increases the buffering capacity of skeletal muscles and, if it does, is this related to a training-induced ability to maintain maximum speed for as long as possible in the 100-m sprint? It is also unknown if the rate of ATP production and/or the rate of ATP utilization limits the maintenance of maximal speed during sprinting. This question leads naturally to studies on ways of enhancing the concentration of PCr in muscle, including the use of creatine supplementation as an ergogenic aid for sprinters.

Strength is an essential element is sprinting, but there is need to define the contribution of an increase in strength to improved sprinting speed. Part of the reason for this gap in knowledge is that the methods of measuring strength are dictated by the design of commercially available equipment, none of which is well-suited to measuring sprint-specific strength. Such equipment should be developed.

Flexibility is a contributory component to sprinting success, but reliable and reproducible methods of measuring dynamic flexibility have yet to be developed. It is only when well-accepted methods of measuring sprint-specific flexibility become available that answers to the question about the contribution of improved flexibility to improved sprint performance will emerge.

Although there have been excellent descriptive studies of the biomechanics of sprinting, there is a lack of prescriptive studies in which analyses are translated into performance changes.

Nutritional principles must be translated into nutritional strategies using foods that are palatable and commonly available so that no obstacles are placed in the way of these athletes during their pursuit of good and effective nutritional practices. In this way the nutritional myths that surround strength and sprint training will be laid to rest. Well-controlled studies are required to provide clear evidence of the success that is achievable from the combination of a quality training program supported by good nutritional practices.

SUMMARY

Sprint running appears to involve only minimal skill, but it is actually a complex activity that involves a host of finely tuned biochemical, neurological, mechanical, and psychological events. Sprinting challenges energy metabolism to replenish ATP in working muscle at the fastest possible rates. Limitations to this process are manifest as a reduction in running speed towards the end of the race. The weight of available evidence suggests that when skeletal muscle PCr concentrations are reduced during sprinting, then speed also begins to decline because glycogenolysis cannot generate ATP fast enough to cover the energy needs of working muscles. At the elite level, the ability to run at high speeds is an obvious precondition for successful sprinting, but it is not necessarily a determinant of a winning performance. Starting technique and the ability to control form, acceleration, and speed in discrete portions of the race are all important considerations to winning races.

Training methods for improving sprinting performance have benefitted to a certain extent in recent years from scientific studies of sprint performance. In particular, the use of periodized training schedules, plyometric exercises, and improved starting techniques can be traced to scientific analysis. Nevertheless, most of the current training techniques of elite sprinters are based on anecdotes about how the current champions are training and on empirical evidence collected over the years by individual coaches and sprint athletes. More research is required to establish a firmer base for sprint training.

BIBLIOGRAPHY

Ae, M., A. Ito, and M. Suzuki (1992). The men's 100 metres. *New Studies Athletics* 7:47–52.

Aitken, A. (1992). *More Than Winning*. Lewes, England: Temple House Books.

Atwater, A.E. (1982). Kinematic analyses of sprinting. *Track Field Quart. Rev.* 82:12–16.

Balsom, P.D., B. Ekblom, K. Soderlund, B. Sjodin, and E. Hultman (1993). Creatine supplementation and dynamic high-intensity intermittent exercise. *Scand. J. Med. Sci. Sports* 3:143–149.

Bangsbo, J., L. Michalsik, and A. Petersen (1993). Accumulated O_2 deficit during intense exercise and muscle characteristics of elite athletes. *Int. J. Sports Med.* 14:207–213.

Banister, E.W., and B.J.C. Cameron (1990). Exercise-induced hyperammonemia: peripheral and central effects. *Int. J. Sports Med.* 11(suppl. 2):S129–S142.

Bar-Or, O. (1987). The Wingate Anaerobic Test. An update on methodology, reliability and validity. *Sports Med.* 4:381–394.

Barnes, W.S. (1981). Selected physiological characteristics of elite male sprint athletes. *J. Sports Med. Phys. Fit.* 21:49–54.

Boobis, L.H., S. Brooks, M.E. Cheetham, and C. Williams (1987). Effect of sprint training on muscle metabolism during high-intensity treadmill running in man (abstract). *Proc. Phys. Soc.* 390:1.

Borzov, V. (1984). Training procedures in sprinting. *Mod. Ath. Coach* 22:15–17.

Bouchard, C., A.W. Taylor, and S. Dulac (1982). Testing maximal anaerobic power and capacity. In: J.D. MacDougal, H.A. Wenger, and J.H. Green (eds.) *Physiological Testing of the Elite Athlete*. Ottawa: Mutual Press, Ltd., pp. 61–74.

Brightwell, R., and A. Packer (1965). *Sprints, Middle-Distance and Relay Running*. London: Nicholas Kaye.

Brooks, S., J. Burrin, M.E. Cheetham, G.M., Hall, T. Yeo, and C. Williams (1988). The responses of the catecholamines and B-endorphin to brief maximal exercise in man. *Eur. J. Appl. Physiol.* 57:230–234.

Casabona, A., M.C. Polizzi, and V. Perciavalle (1990). Differences in H-reflex between athletes trained for explosive contractions and non-trained subjects. *Eur. J. Appl. Physiol.* 61:26–32.

Cheetham, M., L.H. Boobis, S. Brooks, and C. Williams (1986). Human muscle metabolism during sprint running. *J. Appl. Physiol.* 61:54–60.

Cheetham, M.E., R.J. Hazeldine, A. Robinson, and C. Williams (1987). Power output of rugby forwards during maximal treadmill sprinting. In: T. Reilly, A. Lees, K. Davids, and W.J. Murphy (eds.) *Science and Football, Vol. 1.* Liverpool, England: E. & F.N Spon, pp. 206–210.

Clarkson, P.M. (1990). Minerals: exercise performance and supplementation in athletes. *J.Sports Sci.* 9:S91–116.

Costill, D.L., A. Barnett, R. Sharp, R.J. Fink, and A. Katz (1983). Leg muscle pH following sprint running. *Med. Sci. Sports Exerc.* 15:325–329.

Costill, D.L., J. Daniels, W. Evans, W. Fink, G. Krahenbuhl, and B. Saltin (1976). Skeletal muscle enzymes and fiber composition in male and female track athletes. *J. Appl. Physiol.* 40:149–154.

Costill, D.L., D.D. Pascoe, W.J. Fink, R.A. Roberts, S.I. Barr, and D. Pearson (1990). Impaired muscle glycogen resynthesis after eccentric exercise. *J. Appl. Physiol.* 69:46–50.

Davies, C.T.M. (1980). The effects of wind assistance and resistance on the forward motion of a runner. *J. Appl. Physiol.* 48:702–709.

Denis, C., M. Linossier, D. Dormis, S. Padilla, A. Geysant, J. Lacour, and O. Inbar (1992). Power and metabolic responses during supramaximal exercise in 100-m and 800-m runners. *Scand. J. Med. Sci. Sports* 2:62–69.

Devlin, J.T., and C. Williams (1991). Foods, nutrition and sports performance; a final consensus statement. *J. Sports Sci.* 9(Suppl):iii.

Dick, F.W. (1991). *Training Theory* (3rd ed.). London: British Amateur Athletics Board.

Doyle, A.J., W.M. Sherman, and R.L. Strauss (1993). Effect of eccentric and concentric exercise on muscle glycogen replenishment. *J. Appl. Physiol.* 74:1848-1855.

Durant, J. (1961). *Highlights of the Olympics: From Ancient Times to the Present.* London: Arco Publications.

Esbjornsson, M., C. Sylven, I. Holm, and E. Jansson (1993). Fast twitch fibres may predict anaerobic performance in both females and males. *Int. J. Sports Med.* 14:257-263.

Fallowfield, J.L., and C. Williams (1993). Carbohydrate intake and recovery from prolonged exercise. *Int. J. Sport Nutr.* 3:150-164.

Farrar, M., and W. Thorland (1987). Relationship between isokinetic strength and sprint times in college age men. *J. Sports Med. Phys. Fit.* 27:368-372.

Fogelholm, G.M., H.K. Naveri, K.T.K. Kiilavuori, and M.H.A. Harkonen (1993). Low dose amino acid supplementation: no effect on serum growth hormone and insulin in male weightlifters. *Int. J. Sports Nutr.* 3:290-297.

Forbes, L. (1993). Linford Christie. *Observer Magazine,* March 7, p. 53.

Friden, J., J. Seger, and B. Ekblom (1988). Sublethal muscle fibre injuries after high tension anaerobic exercise. *Eur. J. Appl. Physiol.* 57:360-368.

Fry, A.C., W.J. Kraemer, M.H. Stone, B.J. Warren, J.T. Kearney, C.M. Maresh, C.A. Weseman, and S.J. Fleck (1993). Endocrine and performance responses to high volume training and amino acid supplementation in elite junior weightlifters. *Int. J. Sports Nutr.* 3:306-322.

Fry, R.W., A.R. Morton, and D. Keast (1992a). Periodisation of training stress—a review. *Can. J. Sports Sci.* 17:234-240.

Fry, R.W., A.R. Morton, and D. Keast (1992b). Periodisation and the prevention of overtraining. *Can. J. Sports Sci.* 17:241-248.

Gaitanos, G.C., C. Williams, L.H. Boobis, and S. Brooks (1993). Human muscle metabolism during intermittent maximal exercise. *J.Appl. Physiol.* 75:712-719.

Goldfinch, J., L. McNaughton, and P. Davies (1988). Induced metabolic alkalosis and its effects of 400-m racing time. *Eur. J. Appl. Physiol.* 57:45-48.

Gollnick, P.D., R.B. Armstrong, C.W. Saubert, K. Piehl, and B. Saltin (1972). Enzyme activity and fiber composition in skeletal muscle of untrained and trained men. *J. Appl. Physiol.* 33:312-319.

Greenhaff, P.L., A. Casey, A.H. Short, R. Harris, K. Soderlund, and E. Hultman (1993). The influence of oral creatine supplementation on muscle torque during repeated bouts of maximal voluntary exercise in man. *Clin. Sci.* 84:565-571.

Greenhaff, P.L., M.E. Nevill, K. Soderlund, L. Boobis, C. Williams, and E. Hultman (1992). Energy metabolism in single muscle fibres during maximal sprint exercise in man (abstract). *J. Physiol.* 446:528P.

Gregor, R.J., V.R. Edgerton, R. Rozenek, and K.R. Castleman (1981). Skeletal muscle properties and performance in elite track athletes. *Eur. J. Appl. Physiol.* 47:355-364.

Häkkinen, K., and K.L. Keskinen (1989). Muscle cross-sectional area and voluntary force production characteristics in elite strength and endurance trained athletes and sprinters. *Eur. J. Appl. Physiol.* 59:215-220.

Harre, D. (1982). *Principles of Sport Training: Introduction to the Theory and Methods of Training.* Berlin: Sportverlag.

Harris, R.C., K. Soderlund, and E. Hultman (1992). Elevation of creatine in resting and exercised muscle of normal subjects by creatine supplementation. *Clin. Sci.* 83:367-374.

Harris, R.C., M. Viru, P.L. Greenhaff, and E. Hultman (1993). The effect of oral creatine supplementation on running performance during maximal short term exercise in man (abstract). *J. Physiol.* 467:74P.

Hatfield, F.C. (1987). *Ultimate Sports Nutrition.* Chicago: Contemporary Books, Inc.

Hay, J.G. (1985). *The Biomechanics of Sports* (3rd ed.). Englewood Cliffs, NJ: Prentice-Hall.

Heigenhauser, G.J.F., and N.L. Jones (1991). Bicarbonate loading. In: D.R. Lamb and M.H. Williams (eds.) *Perspectives in Exercise Science and Sports Medicine, Vol. 4: Ergogenics: Enhancement of Performance in Exercise and Sport.* Indianapolis, IN: Brown & Benchmark, pp. 183-203.

Hermansen, L. (1969). Anaerobic energy release. *Med. Sci. Sports* 1:32-38.

Hirvonen, J., H. Nummela, S. Rehunen, and M. Harkonen (1992). Fatigue and changes of ATP, creatine phosphate, and lactate during the 400-m sprint. *Can. J. Sport Sci.* 17:141-144.

Hirvonen, J., S. Rehunen, H. Rusko, and M. Harkonen (1987). Breakdown of high-energy phosphate compounds and lactate accumulation during short supramaximal exercise. *Eur. J. Appl. Physiol.* 56:253-259.

Hoffman, K. (1972). Stride length and frequency of female sprinters. *Track Tech.* 48:1522-1524.

Hultman, E., L.L. Spriet, and K. Soderlund (1987). Energy metabolism and fatigue in working muscle. In: D. Macleod, R. Maughan, M. Nimmo, T. Reilly, and C. Williams (eds.) *Exercise, Limitations and Adaptations.* London: E. & F.N. Spon, pp. 63-80.

Jacobs, I., M. Esbjoernsson, C. Sylven, I. Holm, and E. Jansson (1987). Sprint training effects on muscle myoglobin, enzymes, fibre types, and blood lactate. *Med. Sci. Sports Exerc.* 19:368-374.

Kindermann, W., J. Keul, and G. Huber (1977). Physical exercise after induced alkalosis (bicarbonate or tris-buffer). *Eur. J. Appl. Physiol.* 37:197-204.

Koceja, D.M., and G. Kamen (1988). Conditioned patellar tendon reflexes in sprint and endurance trained athletes. *Med. Sci. Sports Exerc.* 20:172-177.

Koshla, T. (1978). Standards of age, height and weight in Olympic running events for men. *Brit. J. Sports Med.* 12:97–101.

Koshla, T., and V.C. McBroome (1984). *The Physique of Female Olympic Finalists.* Cardiff, Wales: Welsh School of Medicine, pp. 1–23.

Kozlova, T. (1972). Sprinter Valery Borzov 'made not born.' *Track Field News* (April), 10.

Kraaijenhof, M. (1990). Trends in biomechanics and biochemistry of sprints methodology. *Track Field Quart. Rev.* 1:6–8.

Lacour, J.R., E. Bouvat, and J.C. Barthelemy (1990). Post competition blood lactate concentrations as indicators of anaerobic energy expenditure during 400-m and 800-m races. *Eur. J. Appl. Physiol.* 61:172–176.

Lakomy, H.K.A. (1986). Measurement of work and power output using friction-loaded cycle ergometers. *Ergonomics* 29:509–517.

Lakomy, H.K.A. (1987). The use of a non-motorized treadmill for analyzing sprint performance. *Ergonomics* 30:627–637.

Lambert, M.I., J.A. Hefer, R.P. Millar, and P.W. Macfarlane (1993). Failure of commercial oral amino acid supplements to increase serum growth hormone concentrations in male body builders. *Int. J. Sports Nutr.* 3:298–305.

Lemon, P.W.R., and D.N. Proctor (1991). Protein intake and athletic performance. *Sports Med.* 12:313–325.

Loader, W.R. (1960). *Testament of a Runner.* London: Heineman.

Lombardo, J.A., R.C. Hickson, and D.R. Lamb (1991). Anabolic/androgenic steroids and growth hormone. In: D.R. Lamb and M.H. Williams (eds.) *Perspectives in Exercise Science and Sports Medicine, Vol. 4: Ergogenics: Enhancement of Performance in Exercise and Sport.* Indianapolis, IN: Brown & Benchmark, pp. 249–278.

Mahler, P., C. Mora, G. Gremion, and A. Chantraine (1992). Isotonic muscle evaluation and sprint performance. *Excel* 8:139–145.

Matson, L.G., and Z.V. Tran (1993). Effect of sodium bicarbonate ingestion on anaerobic performance: a meta-analysis review. *Int. J. Sports Nutr.* 3:2–28.

Maughan, R.J., J.S. Watson, and J. Weir (1983). Relationship between muscle strength and muscle cross-sectional area in male sprinters and endurance runners. *Eur. J. Appl. Physiol.* 50:309–318.

McGilvery, R.W. (1975). The use of fuels for muscular work. In: H. Howald and J.R. Poortmans (eds.) *Metabolic Adaptation to Prolonged Physical Exercise.* Basel: Birkhauser Verlag, pp. 12–30.

McKenna, M.J., T.A. Schmidt, M. Hargreaves, L. Cameron, S.L. Skinner, and K. Kjeldsen (1993). Sprint training increases human skeletal muscle Na^+ $-K^+$ ATPase concentration and improves K^+ regulation. *J. Appl. Physiol.* 75:173–180.

Medbø, J.I., and I. Tabata (1993). Anaerobic energy release in working muscle during 30 s to 3 min exhausting bicycling. *J. Appl. Physiol.* 75:1654–1660.

Medbø, J.I., and S. Burgers (1990). Effect of training on the anaerobic capacity. *Med. Sci. Sports Exerc.* 22:501–507.

Medbø, J.I., A. Mohn, I. Tabata, R.M. Bahr, O. Vaage, and O.M. Sejersted (1988). Anaerobic capacity determined by maximal accumulated O_2 deficit. *J. Appl. Physiol.* 64:50–60.

Moravec, P., J. Ruzicka, P. Susanka, M. Dostal, M. Kodejs, and M. Norsek (1988). The 1987 International Athletic Foundation/IAAF scientific project report: time analysis of the 100 metres events at the II World Championships in Athletics. *New Studies Athletics* 3:61–96.

Neuman, G. (1988). Special performance capacity. In: A. Dirix, H.G. Knuttgen, and K. Tittel (eds.) *The Olympic Book of Sports Medicine.* Oxford: Blackwell Scientific Publications.

Nevill, M.E., L.H. Boobis, S. Brooks, and C. Williams (1989). Effect of training on muscle metabolism during treadmill sprinting. *J. Appl. Physiol.* 67:2376–2382.

Nevill, M.E., D.J. Holmyard, G.M. Hall, P. Allsop, A. van Oosterhout, and J.M. Burrin (1993). Growth hormone responses to treadmill sprinting in sprint-and endurance-trained male athletes (abstract). *J. Physiol.* 473:73P.

Olesen, H.L. (1992). Accumulated oxygen deficit increases with inclination of uphill running. *J. Appl. Physiol.* 73:1130–1134.

Pascoe, D.D., D.L. Costill, R.A. Robergs, J.A. Davis, W.J. Fink, and D.R. Pearson (1990). Effects of exercise mode on muscle glycogen restorage during repeated days of exercise. *Med. Sci. Sports Exerc.* 22:593–598.

Philips, W.N. (1991). *Anabolic Reference Guide* (5th ed.). Golden, CO: Mile High Publishing.

Quercetani, R.L. (1965). *A World History of Track and Field Athletica.* Oxford: Oxford University Press.

Radford, P.F. (1990). Sprinting. In: T. Reilly, N. Secher, P. Snell, and C. Williams (eds.) *Physiology of Sports.* London: E. & F.N. Spon, pp. 71–99.

Radford, P.F., and A.R.M. Upton (1976). Trends in speed of alternated movements during development and among elite sprinters. In: P.V. Komi (ed.) *Biomechanics.* Baltimore, MD: University Park Press, pp. 188–193.

Sadoyama, T., T. Masuda, H. Miyata, and S. Katsuta (1988). Fibre conduction velocity and fibre composition in human vastus lateralis. *Eur. J. Appl. Physiol.* 57:767–771.

Sahlin, K., and J. Henriksson (1984). Buffer capacity and lactate accumulation in skeletal muscle of trained and untrained men. *Acta Physiol. Scand.* 122:331–339.

Saltin, B. (1990). Anaerobic capacity: Past, present and prospective. In: A.W. Taylor, P.D. Gollnick, H.J.

Green, C.D. Ianuzzo, E.G. Noble, G. Metevier, and J.R. Sutton (eds.) *Biochemistry of Exercise, Vol. 21.* Champaign, IL: Human Kinetics, pp. 387–412.

Schlicht, W., W. Naretz, D. Witt, and H. Rieckert (1990). Ammonia and lactate: differential information on monitoring training load in sprint events. *Int. J. Sports Med.* 11 (suppl. 2):S85–S90.

Scott, C.B., F.R. Roby, T.G. Lohman, and J.C. Bunt (1991). The maximally accumulated oxygen deficit as an indicator of anaerobic performance. *Med. Sci. Sports Exerc.* 23:618–624.

Sharp, N.C.C. (1993). Immunological aspects of exercise, fitness and competition sport. In: D.A. Macleod, R.J. Maughan, C. Williams, C.R. Madeley, J.C.M. Sharp, and R.W. Nutton (eds.) *Intermittent High Intensity Exercise: Preparation, Stresses and Damage Limitation.* London: E. & F.N. Spon, pp. 201–213.

Sharp, R.L., D.L. Costill, W.J. Fink, and D.S. King (1986). Effects of eight weeks of bicycle ergometer sprint training on human muscle buffer capacity. *Int. J Sports Med.* 7:13–17.

Sherman, W.M., J.A. Doyle, D.R. Lamb, and R.H. Strauss (1993). Dietary carbohydrate, muscle glycogen, and exercise performance during 7 d of training. *Am. J. Clin. Nutr.* 57:27–31.

Sherman, W.M., and G.S. Wimer (1991). Insufficient dietary carbohydrate during training: does it impair athletic performance? *Int. J. Sports Nutr.* 1:28–44.

Short, S.H., and W.R. Short (1983). Four-year study of university athletes' dietary intake. *J. Am. Diet. Assoc.* 82:632–645.

Spriet, L.L., K. Soderlund, K. Bergstrom, and E. Hultman (1987). Anaerobic energy release in skeletal muscle during electrical stimulation in men. *J. Appl. Physiol.* 62:611–615.

Staron, R.S., R.S. Hikida, F.C. Hagerman, G.A. Dudley, and T.F. Murray (1984). Human skeletal muscle fibre type adaptability to various workloads. *J. Histochem. Cytochem.* 32:146–152.

Stone, M.H. (1993). Anabolic-androgenic steroid use by athletes. *Nat. Strength Cond. Assoc. J.* 15:10–27.

Tabatschnik, B. (1983). Looking for 100-m speed. *Mod. Athlete Coach* 9:14–16.

Tellez, T., and D. Doolittle (1984). Sprinting from start to finish. *Track Tech.* 88:2802–2805.

Temple, C. (1993). Tokyo world records forever tarnished. *The Times,* London, January 24, p. 10.

Tesch, P.A. (1992). Short and long term histochemical and biochemical adaptions in muscle. In: P.V. Komi (ed.) *Strength and Power in Sport.* Oxford: Blackwell Scientific Publications, pp. 239–248.

Tesch, P.A., and J. Karlsson (1985). Muscle fiber types and size in trained and untrained muscles of elite athletes. *J. Appl. Physiol.* 59:1716–1720.

Thorstensson, A., L. Larsson, P.A. Tesch, and J. Karlsson (1977). Muscle strength and fibre composition in elite athletes and sedentary men. *Med. Sci. Sports Exerc.* 9:26–30.

Tullson, P.C., and R.L. Terjung (1990). Adenine nucleotide degradation in striated muscle. *Int. J. Sports Med.* (suppl. 2):S47–S55.

Tvede, N., M. Kappel, J. Halkjaer-Kristensen, H. Galbo, and B.K. Pedersen (1993). The effect of light, moderate and severe bicycle exercise on lymphocyte subsets, natural and lymphokine activated killer cells, lymphocyte proliferative response and interleukin 2 production. *Int. J. Sports Med.* 14:275–282.

Van Der Beek, E.J. (1990). Vitamin supplementation and physical exercise performance. *J. Sports Sci.* 9:S77–89.

Vandewalle, H., G. Peres, and H. Monod (1987). Standard anaerobic exercise tests. *Sports Med.* 4:268–289.

Vollestad, N.K., I. Tabata, and J.I. Medbø (1992). Glycogen breakdown in different human muscle fire types during exhaustive exercise of short duration. *Acta Physiol. Scand.* 144:135–141.

Wilkes, D., N. Gledhill, and R. Smyth (1983). Effect of acute induced alkalosis on 800-m racing time. *Med. Sci. Sports Exerc.* 15:277–280.

Williams, C. (1993). Carbohydrate needs of elite athletes. In: A.P. Simopoulos and K. Pavlou (eds.) *Nutrition and Fitness for Athletes,* 71 New York: Karger, pp. 34–60.

Williams, M.H. (1989). *Beyond Training: How Athletes Enhance Performance Legally and Illegally.* Champaign, IL: Leisure Press.

Wootton, S.A., and C. Williams (1984). Influence of carbohydrate-status on performance during maximal exercise. *Int. J. Sports. Med.* 5:126–127.

3

Physiology and Nutrition for Competitive Swimming

JOHN P. TROUP, Ph.D.

DIETER STRASS, Ph.D.

TODD A. TRAPPE, M.S.

INTRODUCTION
CHARACTERISTICS OF ELITE SWIMMERS
    Body Composition and Anthropometry
    Flexibility
    Muscle: Strength and Power
    Fiber Typing and Performance
    Economy of Movement
    Anaerobic Power and Capacity
    Aerobic and Cardiopulmonary Capacities
LIMITATIONS TO SWIMMING TRAINING AND PERFORMANCE
    Limitations Imposed by Energy Metabolism
    Limitations Imposed by Disturbances in Acid-Base Balance
    Limitations Imposed by Cardiopulmonary Function
    Limitations Imposed by Body Fluid Homeostasis and Thermoregulation
HISTORICAL OVERVIEW OF TRAINING AND NUTRITION FOR SWIMMING
CURRENT CONCEPTS IN TRAINING AND NUTRITION FOR SWIMMING
    Traditional Practices
    Scientifically Based Swim Training
        Principle of Individualism
        Principle of Progressive Overload
        Principle of Training Specificity
        Training Intensity and Duration
        Recovery
    Specific Training Considerations
        Intensity vs. Volume
        Nutritional Concerns
    Monitoring Training
        Pace Prescription
        Predicting Race Performance

INTRODUCTION

Research in swimming is made difficult by the physical limitations that testing in water present to the investigator. However, the scope and impact of swimming research have grown over the last decade as new technologies have made evaluating swimming easier for the researcher. With the availability of swimming treadmills (Figure 3.1), computerized testing equipment, video technologies, and automated diagnostics, the amount and quality of research in swimming have increased substantially. These advances have contributed to greater knowledge about energy me-

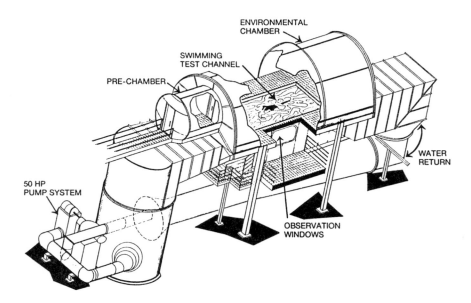

FIGURE 3-1. *Diagram of a swimming treadmill housed at the International Center for Aquatic Research, U.S. Olympic Training Center, Colorado Springs, Colorado. The treadmill allows for the testing and underwater observation of subjects swimming against a current of water, the velocity of which can be controlled. An environmental chamber surrounding the swimming treadmill allows for the manipulation of atmospheric pressure.*

tabolism, nutritional requirements, thermoregulation, and biomechanics of swimming (Cappaert et al. 1992; de Groot & van Ingen Schenau, 1989; Holmer, 1979). In addition, the relationships between swimming performance and anthropometric variables, muscle strength and power, training adaptations, and biomechanical technique have also been examined more closely (MacLaren et al., 1992; Ungerechts et al., 1988).

Some of the current interest in applied swimming research can be attributed to the declining rates of changes in swimming performances over the last 20 y. As the limits of swimming performance are approached, interest in science and its application increase so as to identify new and more effective approaches to training.

The purpose of this chapter is to review research in swimming conducted since 1980 with an emphasis upon the practical applications of that research. Readers are referred to Faulkner (1968) and Holmer (1979) for reviews of swimming research prior to 1980.

CHARACTERISTICS OF ELITE SWIMMERS

Body Composition and Anthropometry

One need only watch national and international caliber swimming competition to gain a quick idea of the physical morphology of elite swimmers. In general, successful swimmers tend to be lean and tall with long limbs, wide shoulders, and relatively large muscle masses, especially in their middle and upper bodies. Araujo (1978) and Ackland et al. (1991) reported that male swimmers are primarily of the ecto-mesomorphic somatotype and that females are endomesomorphic. Although elite swimming performance is not exclusive to this somatotype, it is more often than not the somatotype observed in the finalists of Olympic and national championships. For example, the average heights and weights of the male and female 1992 U.S. Olympic swimming team members were 75 inches (190.5 cm) and 192 pounds (87.1 kg) and 68 inches (172.7 cm) and 142 pounds (64.4 kg), respectively.

When swimmers are considered according to stroke, freestyle sprinters and backstrokers are found to be the tallest and heaviest, with the breaststrokers being shortest (Boulgakova, 1990). Similar observations were made by Spurgeon and Sargent (1978) on elite United States male swimmers (butterfly swimmers being the shortest) and on elite world female swimmers (Spurgeon & Giese, 1984). Khosla (1984) examined competitors from the 1976 Olympics and also reported taller and heavier swimmers in the sprint events, with the finalists being both taller and heavier than the non-finalists. Obvious gender differences exist, with males being taller, heavier, and having longer limbs than females. Interestingly, there appears to be a trend toward an increase in height without an increase in weight since the 1964 Tokyo Olympics (Lavoie & Montpetit, 1986). Grimston and Hay (1986) examined the effects of various anthropomorphic variables on swimming performance and concluded that these variables do not directly affect swimming speed, but they may affect stroke length and stroke frequency which, in turn, can affect swimming speed.

The lift and drag forces that are created as the hand and arm move through the water with each swimming stroke can be modeled in the laboratory. In a study by Troup (1992), four human arms were cast in plaster of Paris. These casts were then molded in rubber and attached to an apparatus in the swimming flume that measured the drag force in the direction of the water flow and the lift force in the side-to-side direction. The results indicated that the resultant propulsive force increased with the surface area of the hand. Thus, all things being equal, swimmers with large hands should be faster swimmers. Also, Clarys (1986) studied the differences in body dimensions between elite and sub-elite swimmers and evaluated how these differences related to performance. He concluded that the body configuration of elite swimmers allowed a more effective application of lift force during swimming, but did not reduce drag.

The percent body fat of elite male and female swimmers is lower than that seen for the average population (approximately 15–20% body fat for males, 20–25% body fat for females). For example, the average body fat for the 1992 United States Olympic Swimming Team members was 9.4% (males) and 15.9% (females). However, because there is a rather large range in body fat in the most successful swimmers, a low percent body fat appears to have little effect on swimming performance. While there may be an ideal range of body fat for swimmers, there is no scientific support for the use of a single ideal value.

Flexibility

It has been suggested that increased joint flexibility enables the swimmer to achieve a greater range of motion during the arm stroke. Kavouras (1993) has shown that elite swimmers are more flexible around the shoulders and ankles than their non-elite counterparts; this relationship is true for age-group as well as Olympic competitors. Flexibility is influenced by the functional anatomy (tendons, ligaments, etc.) around a single or composite joint and by the size of the surrounding musculature.

Flexibility varies with gender and among swimmers of different stroke specialties (Kavouras, 1993). Females tend to be more flexible than males of the same age and ability; breaststrokers have more flexible ankles (inversion and eversion) as well as greater lateral rotation at the hip compared to swimmers of other strokes, and butterfly swimmers have greater back (trunk extension) and shoulder (horizontal extension and flexion) flexibility (Kavouras, 1993).

Muscle Strength and Power

Strength training is incorporated into almost all of the training programs for elite swimmers. It can be argued that strength training may be the most important factor in enhancing swimming performance in the sprint events (Strass, 1988). The availability and use of dry-land testing devices that mimic the swimming stroke allow the measurement of muscle strength and power that is more specific to the movements common in competitive swimming. Using such a device (Swim Bench®) to measure the upper-body muscular power of competitive swimmers, Costill et al. (1980) and Sharp et al. (1982) demonstrated that swimming is a sport in which the generation of adequate power can be a decisive factor in performance. Sharp et al. (1982) reported a significant correlation ($r = 0.94$) between the power-per-arm-pull on the Swim Bench® and the time for a 25-y freestyle swim in a group of non-elite swimmers; the relationship between arm power and swim time became less important among national and international level swimmers ($r = 0.62$). This suggests that a certain amount of muscle power is important to the developing swimmer, perhaps to compensate for relatively poor mechanical efficiency. For highly skilled swimmers already capable of generating adequate power, further improvement in power appears to be a less important factor in determining swim performance. Rather, the ability to maintain a high percentage of peak power throughout the swimming event may be a more valuable attribute. This capacity is related to the swimmer's fitness, swimming technique, and ability to maintain mechanical (propelling) efficiency (Cappaert, 1991a).

Propelling efficiency is determined by the application of sufficient power throughout the stroke pattern, in combination with proper swimming mechanics (Cappaert et al. 1992; Toussaint et al., 1988). The effective application of power is more critical to swimming performance than the ability to generate even greater forces (Toussaint & Beek, 1990). Once a swimmer is capable of generating and maintaining a certain power output, a change in mechanical efficiency is likely to be the primary determinant of changes in swimming performance (Cappaert et al., 1992).

Power generation during sprint swimming depends on the maximal force and velocity produced by the muscle's contractile elements (Strass, 1988) and upon the muscle's capacity for generating an adequate supply of ATP to meet the needs of the contractile elements. Muscles with a large cross-sectional area can generate large forces, and longer muscles have greater potential for achieving rapid shortening velocity (Huijing, 1992). Thus, from a theoretical standpoint, swimmers with long arms and legs who are heavily muscled should have an advantage over their shorter, more ectomorphic counterparts.

Muscle strength and resultant power production are in large part functions of the recruitment and discharge frequency of motor units and of the muscle cross-sectional area. Longitudinal studies (MacDougall, 1986; Schmidtbleicher, 1988) show clear evidence that strength training characterized by a large number of sets and repetitions with submaximal loads (60 to 80% of maximal voluntary contraction) is followed by an increase in muscle cross-sectional area (hypertrophy) and in maximal strength. On the other hand, neural changes from a strength-training program characterized by near maximal loads and low repetitions are achieved by shortening the time for the recruitment of motor units and by increasing the tolerance of the motoneurons to elevated innervation frequency (Häkkinen & Komi 1983; Sale, 1986; Schmidtbleicher & Buehrle 1987). This training method also produced improvements in the rate of force development (Schmidtbleicher, 1988; Strass, 1988). Studies using electromyographic (EMG) techniques have provided new insight into the characteristics of fiber recruitment during exercise (Häkkinen, 1986; Strass, 1991).

This information is of practical importance when considering the specific muscle function requirements of swimming races. During distance competition (800-m, 1500-m), muscle force production during each stroke is comparatively low, and fatigue-resistant Type I fibers are preferentially activated. For the generation of submaximal forces during the 200-m and 400-m races, Type I and IIA fibers are likely to be recruited. The Type IIA fibers produce considerably more force than Type I fibers, but they fatigue sooner (Burke, 1981). Type I, IIA, and IIB (the "fastest" muscle fiber type) are all recruited in short-duration, high-intensity swimming events (50-m and 100-m), in which maximal or near-maximal forces are required. Type IIB fibers produce large forces very quickly, but they are fatigue sensitive (Burke, 1981). Fatigue of type IIB fibers may well limit performance during sprint swimming.

Fiber Typing and Performance

Studies examining muscle fiber types in swimmers have reported varying results; fiber type percentages ranging from 30–70% Type I fibers have been reported in competitive swimmers. This rather large range may be due to the methods and sampling patterns used in collecting the biopsies, the inherent variations among swimmers, and the actual muscles biopsied. Gollnick et al. (1972) found 25% Type II and 75% Type I fibers in the deltoid muscles of highly trained competitive swimmers. Lavoie et al. (1981) reported 50% Type I fibers in the triceps brachii of elite Canadian swimmers. Costill et al. (1985) found 68% Type I fibers in the deltoid muscles of elite collegiate (NCAA, Division I) swimmers. Prins (1981) reported that a former Olympic 100-m freestyle champion and world record holder had 60% Type II fibers (m. vastus lateralis). Nygaard and Nielsen (1978) distinguished between intermediate fibers (I, IIA, IIB) and reported 40% Type I, 41% Type IIA, and 19% Type IIB in the deltoid muscles of competitive swimmers, which closely agrees with the 60% Type II fibers of sprint swimmers reported by Costill (1978). Lavoie et al. (1981) reported that six months of swim training was associated with enlarged fiber areas in both slow (Type I) and fast (Type II) fibers of the triceps brachii muscle. Troup (unpublished data, 1991) found 72% Type II fibers in the deltoid muscle of a world-record holder in the 400-m freestyle. Based upon the seemingly large variation in muscle fiber types among successful competitive swimmers, it is clear that muscle fiber type alone does not provide a good method of predicting swimming performance.

Economy of Movement

Swimming economy is defined as the oxygen uptake required by a swimmer to sustain a given velocity of swimming (Costill et al., 1992). If oxygen uptake values are plotted against swimming speed, a best-fit straight line can be drawn through these points, and swimming economy can be extrapolated to intensities that exceed the $\dot{V}O_2$max (Toussaint, 1988). Using this method, it has been shown that elite swimmers are much more economical than non-elite swimmers (Van Handel et al., 1988). Compared to sub-elite swimmers, elite and highly trained swimmers use less oxygen at any given swimming velocity.

Changes in swimming technique have a major impact upon swimming economy; as swimming technique becomes more efficient, the energy cost of maintaining a given swimming velocity falls. Thus, improvements in stroke mechanics reduce the energy demands for a given swimming speed. This results in a "flatter" economy profile that characterizes elite versus sub-elite swimmers.

Anaerobic Power and Capacity

More than 80% of competitive swimming races cover 200 m or less (about 130 s or less), a fact that underscores the importance of anaerobic energy production. Data describing the anaerobic characteristics of swimmers are not easy to generate, but some tests have been developed (Medbø et al., 1988; Rohrs et al., 1990). These include tests of oxygen deficit, oxygen debt, post-exercise blood lactate concentration, tethered-swimming tests, modified Wingate tests, and Swim Bench® tests.

Oxygen-deficit testing has demonstrated that elite swimmers have larger anaerobic capacities and rely more upon anaerobic energy production during high-intensity exercise, as compared to their sub-elite counterparts (Medbø & Burgers, 1990; Troup et al., 1991b). Well-trained elite swimmers derive more energy from anaerobic sources to meet the energy demands of a given swimming velocity than do their sub-elite counterparts; this may be another reason why the slope of the swimming-economy profile is less steep for elite than for sub-elite swimmers.

Aerobic and Cardiopulmonary Capacities

Swimmers have large cardiopulmonary and aerobic capacities (Holmer, 1979). Aerobic capacity ($\dot{V}O_2$max) during swimming can be measured in swimming pools, with the subject gradually increasing swimming velocity, and in swimming flumes where the speed of the water can be increased as the swimmer attempts to swim in place. In swimming research, maximal oxygen uptake is often expressed in absolute terms (L/min) because of the drastic reduction in body weight accompanying immersion in water. Hermansen and Karlsson (1967) tested nine elite male swimmers with an average $\dot{V}O_2$max of 5.16 L/min (range 4.64–5.81), and Holmer et al. (1974a) studied 12 elite male swimmers and reported that $\dot{V}O_2$max averaged 5.05 L/min (range 4.04–5.93). In the same study (Holmer et al., 1974a), 11 elite female swimmers achieved an average $\dot{V}O_2$max of 3.42 L/min (range 2.94–3.73). Studies of elite swimmers by Montpetit et al. (1987) and by Van Handel et al. (1988) showed poor correlations between training-induced changes in $\dot{V}O_2$max and changes in swimming performance. Perhaps these low correlations can be attributed to the extensive reliance on anaerobic energy production in most swimming events.

LIMITATIONS TO SWIMMING TRAINING AND PERFORMANCE

As in many other sports, maximal swimming performance can be limited by a number of factors, including those related to energy metabolism and acid-base balance. The aquatic environment also presents a unique set of challenges to both the coach and the sport scientist, in part because some of the physiological responses to exercise in water differ from those on land. In particular, cardiovascular responses, body fluid balance, and thermoregulation are uniquely affected when humans exercise in water.

Limitations Imposed by Energy Metabolism

Intramuscular adenosine triphosphate (ATP), phosphocreatine (PCr), and glycogen stores are the main fuel sources during high-intensity exercise (Bergström & Hultman, 1972). The majority of the energy for all competitive swimming events (the longest event being the 1500-m freestyle, lasting about 15 min) is likely derived from fuel stored in the muscle. Based primarily upon biopsy studies of the vastus lateralis muscle during cycling, it seems probable that the amount of glycogen that is normally stored in skeletal muscle is more than adequate to meet the demands of competitive swimming events; only a small fraction of a muscle's stored glycogen is used (Saltin, 1973). Problems or limitations in performance may arise, however, when pre-exercise glycogen levels are severely depleted following intense training.

Swimming performance can be limited by many of the same factors that apparently limit performance in other sports: 1) a reduction of intramuscular ATP and PCr stores, 2) limitations in the rate of energy production and utilization (Medbø & Burgers, 1990), and 3) a disturbance of muscle function related to changes in intramuscular pH (Gullstrand & Lawrence, 1987; Olbrecht et al., 1992). The rate at which ATP is produced is related to the flux of substrate (carbohydrates and fatty acids) through the metabolic pathways as regulated by enzymatic activity (Newsholme, 1988). To this end, the activities of important glycolytic enzymes (e.g., phosphofructokinase) are relatively great in swimmers, as well as in sprint-trained athletes of other sports (Costill et al., 1992).

Limitations Imposed By Disturbances in Acid-Base Balance

The alterations in intramuscular pH that likely occur during competitive swimming have not been extensively investigated. Most studies (Mader et al., 1980; Madsen & Olbrecht, 1983; Olbrecht et al., 1988) have focused on blood lactate levels as an indirect reflection of acid-base status. Costill et al. (1984) reported that decreased plasma pH during cycle ergometry of similar duration and intensity to most swimming events, negatively affected performance. This suggests that acid-base balance is potentially an important limiting factor for metabolism in swimming performance, particularly in events lasting between 1–3 min. Sharp et al. (1983) observed that sprint-trained cyclists have larger bicarbonate buffer capacities than untrained subjects. Thus, an improved capacity to buffer metabolic acids may allow the trained swimmer to sustain high-intensity swimming for a longer period of time before acidosis becomes limiting.

Limitations Imposed by Cardiopulmonary Function

Water immersion is accompanied by an increase in hydrostatic pressure (the weight of the water acting on the surface of the body). In addition, the supine body posture, the reduction in gravitational effects, and the restrictions placed on breathing by the stroking pattern result in cardiovascular and respiratory adjustments unique to swimming.

The supine position (in or out of the water) results in an increase in venous filling of the heart (greater end-diastolic volume), which allows for a lower heart rate at a given cardiac output (Arborelius et al., 1972; Lange et al., 1974). For a given submaximal $\dot{V}O_2$, heart rate is usually lower while swimming than while running or cycling on land (Magel, 1971; McArdle et al., 1971). Holmer et al. (1974b) reported an exception to this principle; they found similar heart rates at a given $\dot{V}O_2$ during swimming and running.

Respiratory volume and frequency in swimming are, in part, determined by the limitations imposed by the swimming stroke. In an effort to help swimmers better cope with these demands, many coaches employ "hypoxic" training. Hypoxic swimming involves taking fewer breaths than normal (Counsilman, 1975). For example, instead of breathing every stroke cycle, breathing might occur every second or third stroke cycle. In theory, the decrease in frequency of ventilation causes a greater extraction of O_2 by the exercising muscles and increases the venous PCO_2 (Craig, 1979). Oddly, Gullstrand and Holmer (1980) found lower heart rates and blood lactate values during 100-m and 200-m bouts of interval training when hypoxic breathing patterns were compared to normal breathing, whereas Counsilman (1975) found an increase in heart rate during hypoxic training. Considering that little is known about the potential benefits and risks (increases in PCO_2 have been related to complaints of headache and loss of consciousness; Craig, 1976) of hypoxic training, more research is needed.

Limitations Imposed By Body Fluid Homeostasis and Thermoregulation

The supine body position and the increase in hydrostatic pressure that accompany swimming cause a redistribution of fluids among the body's fluid compartments. The depth of immersion also influences fluid shifts by changing the hydrostatic pressure, but immersion depth is basically constant in competitive swimming. The temperature of the water also obviously affects both body fluid balance and heat exchange.

Fluid is redistributed during water immersion mainly due to the buoyancy effect of water displacement; e.g., a 70 kg swimmer will weigh only about 10 kg or less in the water. The buoyancy effect is most pronounced in the legs. Thus, when a person stands on land, the legs act as vascular columns, and the pressure created by this column of blood causes fluid to pass out of the vasculature and into the interstitial and intracellular fluid compartments. Moving from standing on land to supine immersion in the water alleviates some of this pressure (McCally, 1965). Consequently, fluid flows from the extravascular spaces into the vasculature, causing a hemodilution (Epstein, 1978; Khosla & DuBois, 1979). This increase in blood volume triggers a renal diuresis and subsequent hemoconcentration (Boening et al., 1972; Khosla & DuBois, 1979, 1981; McCally, 1965; Vogt & Johnson, 1965). This is the reason most swimmers feel an urge to urinate not long after entering the water. A few studies have examined the effects on body fluid homeostasis that are superimposed by exercise in the water (Guezennec et al., 1986; McMurray, 1983; Nielsen et al., 1984), but have failed to use intensities and/or water temperatures normally seen in competitive swimming.

Temperature regulation during water immersion and swimming has received much greater attention (Craig & Dvorak, 1968; Galbo et al., 1979; Hayward et al., 1977; McArdle et al., 1976; McMurray & Horvath, 1979; Nadel, 1977; Nadel et al., 1974; Nielsen, 1976). However, very little of the research has involved swimming intensities commonly elicited in training and competition. Nevertheless, the results of these studies do have practical implications for the long-distance (marathon and channel) swimmer and provide a fundamental basis for understanding temperature control in water.

In air, the primary mode of heat loss during exercise is provided by the evaporation of sweat. In swimming, even though metabolic rates are similar to those during running or cycling, evaporation of sweat is prevented by the surrounding water; convection and conduction are the major means for heat loss. Virtually all swimming competitions are governed by FINA (Fédération International Natation Association) regulations that recommend that the water temperature fall within a "competitive" range of 25–27° C. Swim training presents more of a potential hyperthermic challenge than does swimming competition because training is conducted at high intensities (high heat production) for long, mostly continuous periods. However, research regarding the thermoregulatory response to swim training is very limited. Upon entering the water, the skin temperature quickly reaches equilibrium with the water temperature (Nadel et al., 1974). If the water temperature is below 33–34° C (thermoneutrality) and the swimmers are performing little or no exercise, hypothermia will occur after prolonged immersion (Holmer & Bergh, 1974; Nadel et al., 1974). In the only description of core-temperature changes during swim training, Barzdukas et al. (1993) reported that core temperature is significantly elevated during high-volume training (high-volume refers to the distances swum during training on a daily or weekly basis). An increase in core temperature of 1–2° C was recorded during a 2 h training session of 8,000–10,000 m.

HISTORICAL OVERVIEW OF TRAINING AND NUTRITION FOR SWIMMING

Organized swimming competition preceded organized training programs for swimmers. Competitive swimming began in the late 19th century, and the first Olympic competition took place in 1896. In the early 20th century, swimming competitions were completed by "skilled" swimmers, and training was not systematically used in preparation for these events.

With the introduction of interval training in the 1950s, the volume and duration of swim training gradually increased. Training volumes ranging from 1000 m to 3000 m per training session became common. Many of the ideas developed about swim training in the 1960s were derived from research on running (Wilt, 1964). With the lack of specific training studies available in swimming, coaches designed training programs by mixing some fundamental principles of run training with a large portion of empirical observation and experience. During the 1960s, the number of organized competitive swimming programs grew, and training volume continued to increase; at about the same time, strength training began to be incorporated as a supplement to swimming workouts. The marked increase in training volume since 1960 is illustrated in Figure 3.2. Because greater distances were swum per hour, the average swimming speed and intensity must have also increased. These increases in volume and intensity were associated with improved swimming performance, as exemplified in Figure 3.3. Peak training volumes of approximately 15,000–20,000 m/d were reached in the late 1970s, and this increase appears to have contributed to improvements in performance, probably as a combined result of improvements in both swimming skill and fitness.

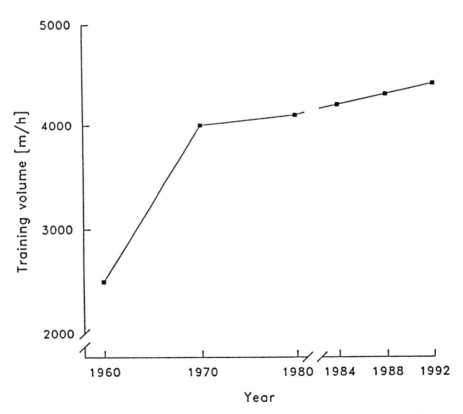

FIGURE 3-2. *Schematic of the yearly progression of maximal swimming distances (meters) attainable in one hour of training.*

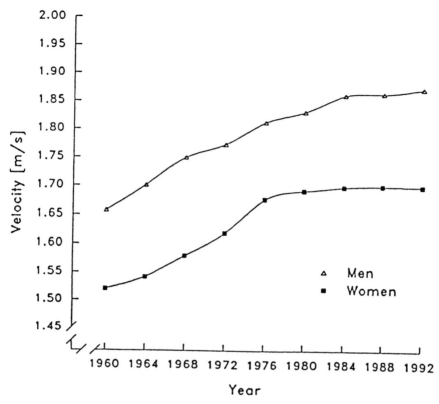

FIGURE 3-3. *Quadrennial progression of 200-m freestyle Olympic gold medal times expressed as swimming velocity (m/s).*

By studying how performances in competitive swimming events have changed over time, it is possible to gain some insight into how changes in training techniques may have influenced performance (Costill et al., 1979). This can be determined by observing the percent changes in maximal swimming velocity (% $\dot{V}$max) for freestyle swimming events from 50-m (assumed to represent peak swimming velocity) to 1500-m (approximately 85% of peak swimming velocity). Data from the 1960, 1978, and 1992 Olympic games illustrate that % $\dot{V}$max improved only slightly for distances from 400–1500 m. Greater improvements in % $\dot{V}$max were observed in the 50-m and 100-m events. This suggests that power-oriented swim training was likely emphasized more than distance swimming. Additionally, improved techniques in each of the four swimming strokes and in the start, turn, and finish phases of swimming events also seem likely to have contributed to the observed performance improvements.

Nutritional survey studies from the mid-1980's (Van Handel et al.,

1985) reported that many elite U.S. swimmers were not ingesting sufficient calories, were more concerned about losing weight than about the nutritional value of their diets, and did not consume fluids during workouts. At the same time, measurements of body fat became an obsession in many swimming programs as a method of applying science in training.

CURRENT CONCEPTS IN TRAINING AND NUTRITION FOR SWIMMING

Traditional Practices

Most swim training programs are based upon the training philosophies and practices employed by successful coaches, mixed with personal and anecdotal experience. Design of a training program employing this approach typically involves determining how training volume (distance to be covered) and training intensity should be matched. Analysis of the training sessions of swimmers reveals that 40–50% of the training session is typically completed at intensities less than 80% $\dot{V}O_2$max. Another 40–60% of swimming is performed at 80–100% $\dot{V}O_2$max, and less than 5% of the training is accomplished at intensities above 100% $\dot{V}O_2$max. This distribution varies, depending upon the time of the training season and the event specialty of the swimmer. Nevertheless, very little swimming (typically less than 5% of total training distance) appears to be completed at event-specific training paces.

Scientifically Based Swim Training

Many current training programs require the coach to: 1) identify the physiological, muscle strength and power, flexibility, and technique requirements of the event; 2) design specific and individualized training bouts that reflect the physiological demands of the event; and 3) design training programs that employ different types and combinations of training. Based upon this fundamental assessment, the coach can design specific workouts by addressing the following issues:

1. What is the workout bout designed to accomplish (e.g., endurance, strength, speed, technique, etc.)?
2. What training intensities are needed to stimulate the physiological and biochemical changes required for success in the event?
3. How much recovery time between training sets, repeats, and workouts is required?
4. What is the total amount of work (meters/workout) needed to bring about the physiological and biochemical changes required for success in the event?

The coach's ability to address each of these questions in designing the training program is a critical factor in the eventual success of his or her swimmers. In designing a training program based upon the above considerations, a coach must contemplate many factors, including the time of the training season and the individual's capacity for training.

Principle of Individualism. This principle may be the most important concept in training program design, but one that is arguably the most often overlooked in swimming. The individual's physical capacities, learning characteristics, communication skills, motivations, and training response must be known by the coach. Based on these individual differences, training can be made specific for the competitive athlete. An individual training plan must take into account the following: 1) developmental stage, 2) training and competitive experience, 3) physical capacity, 4) the response to training loads of different intensity and volume, 5) gender differences, and 6) emotional status and maturity (Pfeiffer, 1991).

Principle of Progressive Overload. Training intensity and duration should gradually be increased to allow the muscles and other organ systems to systematically adapt to the physiological demands of training. Progressive overload can be achieved in three different ways: 1) gradual increase in training volume, 2) gradual increase in training intensity, and/ or 3) gradual decrease in the rest interval for a given bout of interval training.

Principle of Training Specificity. The physiological demands of some portion of the training program must reflect the specific physiological requirements of the swimmer's primary events. The length of time that a specific type of training is incorporated into a training program depends upon the swimmer's response to the training stimulus. The reader may wish to consult textbooks that describe recommended training regimens for producing optimal adaptations of aerobic power, anaerobic power, and muscle strength and power production (Brooks & Fahey, 1984; McArdle et al., 1991; Wilmore & Costill, 1988). Additional information is provided below under Training Modes.

Training Intensity and Duration. Training intensity can be based upon heart rate response (Bompa, 1983; Treffene, 1983), $\%\dot{V}O_2$max (Pfeiffer, 1991), lactate response (Olbrecht et al., 1988; Mader et al., 1980; Stegmann & Kindermann, 1982), or $\%\dot{V}$max values (Bompa, 1983). Table 3.1 contains simple guidelines for helping coaches design training programs in which the intensity and duration of swim sets can be varied according to the physiological objectives of the training session.

Recovery. The amount of recovery needed during interval training is dependent upon the duration of the individual swim and the intensity of the effort. In general, the higher the intensity of the swim, the longer will be the rest. The longer the distance of the swim, the lower the intensity, and the shorter the recovery period. Recent studies (Beltz et al., 1988; Troup et al., 1991a) have provided guidelines for selecting appropriate recovery intervals when using interval training.

TABLE 3-1. *Categories of swim training*

	TYPE OF TRAINING					
	Aerobic				Anaerobic	
	warm-up & recovery	*base training*	*endurance*	*aerobic capacity*	*400-m pace*	*sprint*
Distance of training set (y or m)	500–2000	500–4000	800–4000	500–2000	200–1200	50–500
Total time of training set (min)	5–30	15–60	10–60	5–20	5–15	5–10

Specific Training Considerations

Intensity versus Volume. In both the scientific and coaching communities, there has been debate as to the optimal combination of intensity and duration of training that will best develop peak performance (Costill et al., 1992). Most competitive swimming events rely upon rapid glycolytic flux to produce ATP, and prolonged (high-volume) training may not provide the stimulus needed to provoke such a rapid generation of ATP. Consistent with this hypothesis, Fitts et al. (1989) presented data on the contractility of single human muscle fibers following a period of increased training volume during swimming. They showed a decrease in the maximal shortening velocity of the fast twitch fibers following endurance-oriented swim training. These results suggest that too much emphasis on endurance training may impair a swimmer's potential for high-power swim performance.

Although the training intensity should reflect the specificity needed in training for specific swimming events, emphasis upon training intensity alone neglects other aspects of the developmental process needed in training. Similarly, concentrating solely upon the distance covered in each training session does not adequately address the specific demands of each event. Costill et al. (1992) demonstrated that increases in training distance beyond a certain point resulted in no further improvement in endurance capacity (i.e., $\dot{V}O_2$max). Based on the changes seen in swimming economy, along with survey information from coaches about the training response of swimmers, it appears as though the benefits of the extra training distance are something other than the potentially small increases in maximal aerobic power.

While there is no substitute for the specificity of training achieved with high-intensity training, most coaches would agree that longer-distance training prepares swimmers for the physical rigors of intense training. In fact, this has been an accepted concept in training among swimming coaches in the U.S. and other countries (Maglischo, 1982; Wilt, 1964). The tangential benefits of long distance training can be seen by examining the changes that occur in swimming economy following such training (Van Handel et al., 1988). Physiological adaptations to distance swim training result in a right and downward shift in the curve relating energy costs to swimming velocity. Oxygen-deficit test results (Hermansen, 1969; Medbø & Burgers, 1990) have illustrated that the anaerobic energy demands for high power production also decrease with training as the aerobic contribution increases. This suggests that endurance training may benefit both distance and sprint athletes prior to the start of their event-specific training. After a certain point in training, however, endurance capacity will be slow to improve, thus providing no further fitness-related benefit to increasing training volume (Costill et al., 1992).

Nutritional Concerns. There is a dearth of evidence about the effects of dietary manipulation on swimming performance, so dietary recommendations must be derived largely from experiments on cyclists and runners. Thus, with the exception of prolonged swims (Ironman triathlons, channel swims, etc.), it is unlikely that carbohydrate feedings shortly before and/or during competitive swimming events will be beneficial to performance (see Maughan, 1991, and Sherman, 1990, for review).

However, it seems logical that daily diets containing large proportions of carbohydrate could be advantageous to swimmers during training, when it is common for elite swimmers to swim in excess of 4 h/d. Considering the large energy expenditures associated with swim training, it is obvious that inadequate ingestion of carbohydrate can potentially impact muscle and liver glycogen stores, reducing the swimmer's capacity for training and competitive performance. For example, based primarily on studies of cyclists, it seems likely that a regimen of reduced training and increased carbohydrate intake for 5–6 d before competition would restore glycogen levels to supranormal levels (Sherman, 1981).

Likewise, it seems reasonable to suspect that a habitual high-carbohydrate diet might improve both the volume of swim training that could be endured on a daily basis and the intensity of that training. This notion is supported by the data of Costill et al. (1988), who showed that four swimmers in a group of 12 had relatively low daily carbohydrate intakes (396 g/d) compared to the other eight (612 g/d), and only the four with low carbohydrate intakes were unable to maintain increased training loads.

In contrast, the results of an experiment on swimmers who consumed 80% versus 43% carbohydrate diets for 9 d each were not consistent with the notion that high-carbohydrate diets are advantageous during swim training (Lamb et al., 1990). In this study, there were no apparent effects of diet during training on interval swim times, heart rates, or ratings of perceived exertion. Because the swimmers in the study by Lamb et al. (1990) consumed an average of 4675 kcal (19.6 MJ), even the 43% carbohydrate diet provided 502 g of carbohydrate on a daily basis (versus 935 g for the 80% carbohydrate diet). Thus, 502 g of carbohydrate may have been sufficient to adequately replenish glycogen stores (Costill et al., 1981). It is almost certain that a high-carbohydrate diet is advantageous to endurance performance when compared to a *very low* carbohydrate diet (Bergström & Hultman, 1972), and long-term high carbohydrate diets do enhance muscle glycogen stores when compared to either *low* or *moderate* carbohydrate diets (Simonsen et al., 1991). Still, there is insufficient evidence to conclude with confidence that exercise performance is enhanced by a long-term, high-carbohydrate diet versus a moderate carbohydrate diet (Sherman & Wimer, 1991). Nevertheless, there is no substantial evidence that a high-carbohydrate diet impairs performance, and such a diet is known to be associated with a decreased risk for a cardiovascular disease. Consequently, it is prudent to continue advising swimmers and other athletes—in addition to sedentary individuals—to eat diets containing at least 60% of total energy as carbohydrate.

The dietary protein requirements of athletes have been characterized, and it has been suggested that exercise training can increase the dietary protein requirement above that needed by non-athletes (Lemon & Proctor, 1991). However, nearly all athletes, swimmers presumably included, consume more than enough of the proteins recommended for athletes in their regular diets (Butterfield, 1991).

Monitoring Training

By using tests to evaluate actual swim performance during training, it is possible to determine whether or not training has been effective in improving performance capacity. A few of these tests are described below.

Pace Prescription. Perhaps the most commonly employed determinant of swimming pace during training is exercise heart rate. However, such recommendations are often based upon the coach's experience, rather than results of well-controlled testing. It has been suggested that paces for endurance training can be determined from a single 30-min swim or a 2 × 400-m swim test (Madsen & Lohberg, 1987; Olbrecht et al., 1985). The intent of these tests is for the swimmer to swim a fast but constant pace for the entire distance. The average 100-m pace can then be determined from the 30-min test and used to help design bouts of interval training (Madsen & Olbrecht, 1983; Olbrecht et al., 1988). Coincidentally, the blood lactate values at these swimming paces average about 4 mM. Olbrecht et al. (1985) found that the swimming velocity associated with a blood lactate level of 4 mM, extrapolated from the lactate data generated from 2 × 400-m swims, correlated highly ($r = 0.97$) with the swim speed derived from the 30-min swim.

Predicting Race Performance. Maximal swimming sets have been used in order to predict race performance. These include sets such as 6 × 50-m on 3 min, 5 × 100-m on 5 min, and 6 × 200-m on 8 min. By doubling the average time for each swim in a set, the performance at the next-higher distance can be predicted. For example, 100-m time should be twice the average time for a 50-m swim in the 6 × 50-m set. A correlation coefficient ($r = 0.98$) between the predicted time and the actual race time was reported. Additional research is needed to help identify similar, scientifically valid test procedures that can be easily employed by the coach for the purposes of predicting race performance and assessing training response.

MEDICAL CONSIDERATIONS

The majority of the medical problems encountered in swimming are joint injuries, most often to the shoulder and knee, and certain infections that accompany chronic immersion of the body in water (Costill et al., 1992).

Musculoskeletal Injuries

Two of the most common types of injuries in swimming are overuse injuries of the shoulder and knee joints. These injuries may stem simply from overuse due to the long daily training sessions conducted year-round, from biomechanical deficiencies in swimming technique, or from a combination of both. Swimmers in high-volume training programs may take as many as one-million arm strokes per year while training. The repetitive stress from this many strokes, particularly in conjunction with a biomechanical deficiency, predisposes swimmers to shoulder injuries. The relative instability of the shoulder joint is also thought to be a causative factor (Richardson et al., 1980). Weaknesses in the rotator-cuff muscles can destabilize the joint, and subsequent chronic irritation of the tendons, ligaments, and bursae of the joint leads to inflammation and pain (McMaster 1986a, 1986b; Merino & Llobet, 1978). Problems of this nature usually surface many years into the swimmer's career, but have also been seen in comparatively young age-group swimmers (Dominquez, 1978b; McMaster et al., 1989). Another predisposing factor to shoulder injury may be occlusion of the vasculature supplying the shoulder joint consequent to repeated rotation of the humerus during the swimming stroke (Ciullo, 1986).

Implementation of a few simple shoulder-strengthening exercises and shoulder-flexibility exercises may reduce the risk of shoulder injuries. After the injury has occurred, application of cold packs to reduce inflammation, anti-inflammatory medication, and rest are the three standard prescriptions for relief of the injured shoulder (Cofield & Simonet, 1984). In some extreme cases, surgery is needed (Dominquez, 1978a; 1980).

Injuries to the knee are common in breaststroke swimmers (Kennedy & Hawkins, 1974; Rovere & Nichols, 1985; Stulberg et al., 1980). The mechanical stresses placed upon the knee during the breaststroke kick are quite unorthodox in comparison to the normal structure and function of the knee joint (Richardson, 1986; Vizsolyi et al., 1987). The breaststroke kick places a large amount of strain on the medial collateral ligament; this strain often accounts for knee injuries (Richardson, 1986). Swimmers specializing in the other strokes are not immune from knee problems; the kicks used in the other competitive strokes, as well as the involvement of the knee joint in swimming starts and turns, place a large compressive force on the kneecap (Richardson, 1986).

"Swimmer's Ear"

Clinically termed *otitis externa*, inflammation of the external ear canal is often called "swimmer's ear" due to its prevalence in the swimming population, especially in younger swimmers (Fabiani et al., 1982; Roydhouse, 1978). The external ear canal is normally coated with a waxy substance that protects the ear from foreign particles and bacteria. This waxy substance is reduced or eliminated in swimmers after hours of exposure to the water (Strauss & Cantrell, 1979). Swimmers then are susceptible to various infections of the ear, which can become painful if left untreated. Various over-the-counter ear drops are useful in eliminating the infection. Drops to dry the ear canal after exposure to the water, are also effective in preventing ear infections.

Infections of the middle ear (*otitis media*) also occur in competitive swimmers, but to a lesser extent than do infections of the external ear canal. Symptoms commonly encountered are fever, hearing loss, and loss of balance. Infections of the middle ear can be treated quite effectively by a physician and should not be taken lightly (Strauss & Cantrell, 1979). Most infections of the ear can be prevented simply by proper drying and cleaning of the ear after prolonged water immersion, as well as the use of ear plugs and/or a swimming cap during training sessions.

Exercise-Induced Asthma

Some nine million Americans, including three to four million children and young adults, have some form of asthma. It is estimated that 60–90% of these nine million people are susceptible to exercise-induced asthma (bronchoconstriction). Swimming is one exercise that often causes little or no bronchoconstriction in asthmatic patients (Fitch & Morton, 1971); in fact, Fitch (1975) reported that at each of the Olympiads from 1956 to 1972 (and in 1984), there was a gold medalist in swimming who had asthma. The exact mechanisms for exercise-induced asthma are not known (Fitch, 1975; Fitch & Morton, 1971; Inbar et al., 1980; Regianni et al., 1988). Explanations for the differences in how asthmatics respond to different exercise modes (i.e., swimming, cycling, running) have included increased humidity of the air above the water, the effects of horizontal posture and water immersion, the absence of pollen over the water, and the relative hypoventilation that may occur during swimming.

Other Considerations

Irritation and reddening of the eyes or blurring of vision are sometimes encountered in swimmers, but these problems have mostly been eliminated in recent years with the use of swimming goggles. A high incidence of low back pain in competitive swimmers has also been noted by some investigators (Mutoh, 1978; 1983). Finally, abnormalities in spinal curvatures may occur in some swimmers (Iwanowski, 1983).

SUGGESTED DIRECTIONS FOR FUTURE RESEARCH ON SWIMMING

Over the last decade, the rate of improvement in swimming performance has declined. From a scientific standpoint, continued improvements in performance will likely result from a better understanding of the physiological and biochemical factors that serve to limit the human capacity for high-intensity exercise. A keener understanding regarding how physical characteristics such as muscle strength and power, flexibility, and anaerobic capacity interact with stroke biomechanics to determine a person's potential for success in competitive swimming is also required. Better scientific insights regarding the relationship among exercise intensity, duration, and recovery will help coaches design and implement interval-training programs. Basic research in muscle energy metabolism and its relation to swimming should be continued to better understand the biochemical and physiological responses to swimming racing and training. More studies are needed to help identify the manner in which swimmers adapt to various training regimens, and to develop practical means by which the coach can assess how the swimmers are responding to training. A more complete understanding of how individual swimmers respond to training and how training can be made most effective also requires further investigation in both the laboratory and the pool.

SUMMARY

A greater scientific understanding of the physiology, biochemistry, and biomechanics of swimming will undoubtedly continue to provide information that will prove of practical value to the swimming coach. In many respects, swimming science is still in its infancy, with many questions of scientific and practical interest remaining to be addressed. As more sophisticated technology becomes available, researchers will be able to overcome some of the limitations to research imposed by the aquatic environment, and the quality and quantity of swimming research will increase. The existing state of the science in swimming already provides many insights that can help coaches design and implement effective training programs for swimmers of all levels. The enormous amount of experience represented in the coaching community represents a wealth of information and ideas for sports scientists to pursue in the quest to forge an effective link between the laboratory and the swimming pool.

ACKNOWLEDGEMENTS

We thank Stavros Kavouras and Kay Prater for review and preparation of the manuscript.

BIBLIOGRAPHY

Ackland, T.R., J.C. Mazza, L. Carter, and W.D. Ross (1991). A survey of physique of world champion aquatic athletes. *Sports Coach* 14:10–11.

Araujo, C.G.S. (1978). Somatotyping of Top Swimmers by the Heath-Carter Method. In: B. Eriksson and B. Furberg (eds.) *Swimming Medicine* IV, Baltimore: University Park Press, pp. 188–199.

Arborelius, M., Jr., U.I. Balldin, B. Lilja, and C.E.G. Lundgren (1972). Hemodynamic changes in man during immersion with the head above water. *Aerospace Med.* 43:592–598.

Arredondo, S.M., S. Spry, S. Takahashi, G. Langhans, L.J. D'Acquisto, and J.P. Troup (1990). Performance related differences in oxygen uptake, velocity and blood lactate at lactate threshold (abstract). *Med. Sci. Sports Exerc.* 22:S124.

Barzdukas, A.P., T.A. Trappe, A.C. Jozsi, S.G. Gregg, and J.P. Troup (1993). The effects of hydrating on thermal load and plasma volume during high intensity swimming training. *Med. Sci. Sports Exerc.* 25: S20.

Beltz, J.D., D.L. Costill, R. Thomas, W.J. Fink, and J.P. Kirwan (1988). Energy demands of interval training for competitive swimming. *J. Swim. Res.* 4:5–9.

Bergström, J., and E. Hultman (1972). Nutrition for maximal sports performance. *J. Am. Med. Assoc.* 221:999–1006.

Berning, J.R. (1992). The Effect of Carbohydrate Feedings on Four-Hour Swimmers. In: J. P. Troup (ed.) *International Center for Aquatic Research Annual.* Colorado Springs: U.S. Swimming Press, pp. 145–149.

Boening, D., H.-V. Ulmer, U. Meier, W. Skipka, and J. Stegemann (1972). Effects of a multi-hour immersion on trained and untrained subjects: I. Renal function and plasma volume. *Aerospace Med.* 43:300–305.

Bompa, T.O. (1983). *Theory and Methodology of Training: The Key to Athletic Performance.* Dubuque: Kendall/Hunt.

Bone, M., S.M. Arredondo, J.M. Cappaert, A. Barzdukas, L. D'Acquisto, A.P. Hollander, and J.P. Troup (1991). Validation of dryland swimming-specific measurement of anaerobic power. *J. Sports Sci.* 9:79–80.

Boulgakova, N. (1990). *Selection Et Preparation Des Jeunes Nageus.* Paris: Vigot.

Brooks, G.A., and T.D. Fahey (1984). *Exercise Physiology: Human Bioenergetics and its Applications.* New York: Wiley.

Burke, R.E. (1981) Motor units: anatomy, physiology, and functional organization. In: V.B. Brooks (ed) *Handbook of Physiology.* Section I, The Nervous System II, Washington: American Physiological Society, pp. 345–422.

Butterfield, G. (1991). Amino acids and high protein diets. In: D.R. Lamb, and M.H. Williams (eds.) *Perspectives in Exercise Science and Sports Medicine, Vol. 4: Ergogenics—Enhancement of Exercise and Sports Performance.* Indianapolis, IN: Benchmark Press, pp. 87–122.

Cappaert, J.M., M. Bone, and J.P. Troup (1992). Intensity and performance related differences in propelling and mechanical efficiencies. In: D. Mac Laren, T. Reilly, and A. Lees (eds.). *Swimming Science VI.* London: E. & F.N. Spon, pp. 53–56.

Cappaert, J.M. (1991a). The Importance of Propelling and Mechanical Efficiencies. In: J.P. Troup (ed.) *International Center for Aquatic Research Annual.* Colorado Springs: U.S. Swimming Press, pp. 75–80.

Cappaert, J.M. (1991b). *FINA World Championship Report.* Lausanne: FINA.

Ciullo, C.V. (1986). Swimmer's shoulder. *Clin. Sports Med.* 5:115–137.

Clarys, J.P. (1986). Human body dimensions and applied hydrodynamics: selection criteria for top swimmers. *SNIPES Journal,* 23:32–41.

Cofield, R.H., and W.T. Simonet (1984). The shoulder in sports. *Mayo Clinic Proceedings* 59:157–164.

Costill, D.L. (1978). Adaptations in skeletal muscle during training for sprint and endurance swimming. In: B.O. Eriksson & B. Furberg (eds.) *Swimming Medicine IV.* Baltimore: University Park Press, pp. 233–248.

Costill, D.L., and J. Miller (1980). Nutrition for endurance sport: carbohydrate and fluid balance. *Int. J. Sports Med.* 1:2–14.

Costill, D.L., E. Coyle, W. Fink, G. Lesmes, and F. Witzmann (1979). Adaptations in skeletal muscle following strength training. *J. Appl. Physiol.* 46:96–99.

Costill, D.L., R. Sharp, and J.P. Troup (1980). Muscle strength: Contributions to sprint swimming. *Swimming World* 21:29–34.

Costill, D.L., F. Verstappen, H. Kuipers, E. Janssen, and W. Fink (1984). Acid-base balance during repeated bouts of exercise: Influence of HCO3. *Int. J. Sports Med.* 5:228–231.

Costill, D.L., W.J. Fink, M. Hargreaves, D.S. King, R. Thomas, and R. Fielding (1985). Metabolic characteristics of skeletal muscle during detraining from competitive swimming. *Med. Sci. Sports Exerc.* 17:339–343.

Costill, D.L., M.G. Flynn, J.P. Kirwan, J.A. Houmard, J.B. Mitchell, R. Thomas, S.H. Park. (1988). The effects of repeated days of intensified training on muscle glycogen and swimming performance. *Med. Sci. Sports Exerc.* 20:249–254.

Costill, D.L., E.W. Maglischo, and A.B. Richardson. (1992). *Swimming.* London: Blackwell Scientific.

Costill, D.L., W.M. Sherman, W.J. Fink, C. Maresh, M. Witten, and J.M. Miller (1981). The role of dietary carbohydrates in muscle glycogen resynthesis after strenuous running. *Am. J. Clin. Nutr.* 34:1831–1836.

Counsilman, J.E. (1975). Hypoxic and other methods of training evaluated. *Swim. Tech.* 12:19–26.

Craig, A.B. (1976). Summary of 58 cases of consciousness underwater during swimming. *Med. Sci. Sports* 8:171–175.

Craig, A.B. (1979). The fallacies of hypoxic training in swimmers. In: J. Terauds and W. Bedingfield (eds.) *Swimming III.* Baltimore: University Park Press, pp. 235–239.

Craig, A.B., and M. Dvorak (1968). Thermal regulation of man exercising during water immersion. *J. Appl. Physiol.* 25:28–35.

Craig, A.B. and D.R. Pendergast (1979). Relationships of stroke rate, distance per stroke, and velocity in competitive swimming. *Med. Sci. Sports Exerc.* 11: 278–283.

Craig, A.B., P.L. Skehan, J.A. Pawelezyk, and W.L. Boomer (1985). Velocity, stroke rate, and distance per stroke during elite swimming competition. *Med. Sci. Sports Exerc.* 17:625–634.

de Groot, G., and G.J. van Ingen Schenau (1988). Fundamental mechanics applied to swimming: technique and propelling efficiency. In: B. E. Ungerechts, K. Wilke, and K. Reischle (eds.) *Swimming Science V.* Champaign, IL: Human Kinetics, pp. 17–29.

Dominquez, R.H. (1978a). Coracoacromial ligament resection for severe swimmer's shoulder. In: B. Eriksson and B. Furgerg (eds.) *Swimming Medicine IV.* Baltimore: University Park Press, pp. 110–114.

Dominquez, R.H. (1978b). Shoulder pain in age group swimmers. In: Eriksson, B. and B. Furgerg (eds.) *Swimming Medicine IV.* Baltimore: University Park Press, pp. 105–109.

Dominquez, R.H. (1980). Shoulder pain in swimmers: Even though more swimmers are seeing physicians for shoulder pain, fewer need to be considered for surgery. *Phys. Sportsmed.* 8:35–42.

Epstein, M. (1978). Renal effects of head-out water immersion in man: implications for an understanding of volume homeostasis. *Physiol. Rev.* 58:529–581.

Fabiani, M., P. Bolasco, and M. Barbara (1982). Incidence of otorhinolaryngological diseases in water sports. *J. Sports Med. Phys. Fit.* 22:108–112.

Faulkner, J.A. (1968). Physiology of swimming and diving. In: H.B. Falls (ed.) *Exercise Physiology.* New York: Academic Press, pp. 415–446.

Fitch, K.D. (1975). Exercise-induced asthma and competitive athletics. *Pediatrics* 56:942–943.

Fitch, K.D., and A.R. Morton (1971). Specificity of exercise in exercise-induced asthma. *Brit. Med. J.* 4:577–581.

Fitts, R.H., D.L. Costill, and P.R. Gardetto (1989). Effect of swim exercise training on human muscle fiber function. *J. Appl. Physiol.* 66:465–475.

Galbø, H., M.E. Houston, N.J. Christensen, J.J. Holst, B. Nielsen, E. Nygaard, and J. Suzuki (1979). *Acta Physiol. Scand.* 105:326–337.

Gollnick, P.D., R.B. Armstrong, C.W. Sawbert, K. Piehl, and B. Saltin (1972). Enzyme activity and fibre composition in skeletal muscle of trained and untrained men. *J. Appl. Physiol.* 3:312–319.

Grimston, S.K., and J.G. Hay (1986). Relationships among anthropometric and stroking characteristics of college swimmers. *Med. Sci. Sports Exerc.* 30:60–68.

Guezennec, C.Y, G. Defer, G. Gazorla, C. Sabathier, and F. Lhoste (1986). Plasma renin activity, aldosterone and catecholamine levels when swimming and running. *Eur. J. Appl. Physiol.* 54:632–637.

Gullstrand, L., and I. Holmer (1980). Physiological responses to swimming with controlled frequency of breathing. *Scand. J. Sports Science* 2:1–6.

Gullstrand, L., and S. Lawrence (1987). Heart rate and blood lactate response to short intermittent work at race pace in highly trained swimmers. *Aust. J. Sci. Med. Sport* 19:10–14.

Häkkinen, K. (1986). Training and detraining adaptations in electromyography. Muscle fibre and force production characteristics of human leg extensor muscle with special reference to prolonged heavy resistance and explosive type strength training. *Studies in Sport, Physical Education and Health No. 20.* University of Jyvaeskylae, Jyvaeskylae.

Häkkinen, K. and P.V. Komi (1983). Changes in neuromuscular performance in voluntary and reflex contraction during strength training in man. *Int. J. Sports Med.* 4:282–288.

Hayward, J.S., J.D. Eckerson, and M.L. Collis (1977). Thermoregulatory heat production in man: prediction equation based on skin and core temperatures. *J. Appl. Physiol.* 42:377–384.

Hermansen, L. (1969). Anaerobic energy release. *Med. Sci. Sport* 1:32–38.

Hermansen, L. and J. Karlsson (1967). The results from the physiological investigation of our elite swimmers. *Simsport.* 22:19–27.

Holmer, I. (1979). Physiology of swimming man. Exerc. Sports Sci. Rev. 7:87–124.

Holmer, I. and U. Bergh (1974). Metabolic and thermal responses to swimming in water at varying temperatures. *J. Appl. Physiol.* 37:702–705.

Holmer, I., A. Lundin, and B.O. Eriksson (1974a). Maximum oxygen uptake during swimming and running by elite swimmers. *J. Appl. Physiol.* 36:711–714.

Holmer, I., E.E. Stein, B. Saltin, B. Ekblom, and P.O. Astrand (1974b). Hemodynamic and respiratory responses compared in swimming and running. J. Appl. Physiol. 37:49–54.

Huijing, P.A. (1992). Mechanical Muscle Models. In: P.V. Komi (ed.) *Strength and Power in Sports.* London: Blackwell Scientific, pp. 151–168.

Inbar, O., R. Dotan, R.A. Dlin, I. Neuman, and O. Bar-Or (1980). Breathing dry or humid air and exercise-induced asthma during swimming. *Eur. J. Appl. Physiol.* 44:43–50.

Ivy, J. L., A.L. Katz, C.L. Cutler, W.M. Sherman, and E.F. Coyle (1986). Muscle glycogen utilization during prolonged strenuous exercise when fed carbohydrate. *J. Appl. Physiol.* 65(4):1703–1709.

Iwanowski, W. (1983). Spherosomatometric method for analysis of anteroposterior spine curvatures in swimmers. In: L. Lewillie and J.P. Clarys (eds.) *Swimming II.* Baltimore: University Park Press, pp. 316–320.

Kavouras, S.A. (1992). *Developmental Stages of Competive Swimmers: 1991 United States Swimming Camp Report.* Colorado Springs: U.S. Swimming Press.

Kavouras, S.A. (1993). *Growth, Maturation and Performance Evaluation of Elite Age Group Swimmers: 1992 United States Swimming Camp Report.* Colorado Springs: U.S. Swimming Press.

Kennedy, J.C., and R. Hawkins (1974). Breaststroker's knee. *Phys. Sportsmed.* 2(1):33–35.

Khosla, S.S., and A.B. DuBois (1979). Fluid shifts during initial phase of immersion diuresis in man. *J. Appl. Physiol.* 46:703–708.

Khosla, S.S. and A.B. Dubois (1981). Osmoregulation and interstitial fluid pressure changes in humans during water immersion. *J. Appl. Physiol.* 51:686–692.

Khosla, T. (1984). Physique of female swimmers and divers from the 1976 Montreal Olympics. *J. Am. Med. Assoc.* 252:536–537.

Lamb, D.R., K.F. Rinehardt, R.L. Bartels, W.M. Sherman, and J.T. Snook (1990). Dietary carbohydrate and intensity of interval swim training. *Am. J. Clin. Nutr.* 52:1058–1063.

Lange, L., S. Lange, M. Echt, and F. Gauer (1974). Heart volume in relation to body posture and immersion in a thermo-neutral bath. *Pfluegers Archiv.* 352:219–226.

Lavoie, J.M. and R.R. Montpetit (1986). Applied physiology of swimming. *Sports Med.* 3:165–189.

Lavoie, J.M., A.W. Taylor, and R.R. Montpetit (1981). Histochemical and biochemical profile of elite swimmers before and after six month training period. In: J. Poortmans and G. Nisert (eds.) *Biochemistry of Exercise.* Baltimore: University Park Press, pp. 259–266.

Lemon, P.W.R., and D.N. Proctor (1991). Protein intake and athletic performance. *Sports Med.* 12:313–325.

MacDougall, J. (1986). Morphological changes in human skeletal muscle following strength training and immobilization. In: L. Jones, N. Mc Cartney, and A. McComas (eds.) *Human Muscle Power.* Champaign, Ill: Human Kinetics Publishers, pp. 269–284.

Mac Laren, D., T. Reilly, and A. Lees (1992). Biomechanics and Medicine in Swimming. *Swimming Science VI.* London: E. & F.N. Spon.

Mader, A., Ø. Madsen, and W. Hollmann (1980). The evaluation of the anaerobic energy supply with regard to the performances in training and competition in swimming. *Leistungssport,* 10:263–279, 408–418.

Madsen, Ø., and M. Lohberg (1987). The lowdown on lactates. Swim Tech. May-June:21–26.

Madsen, Ø., and J. Olbrecht (1983). Specifics of aerobic training. In: R.M. Ousley (ed.) *Annual of American Swimming Coaches Association.* Ft. Lauderdale, FL: ASCA Press, pp. 15–33.

Magel, J.R. (1971). Comparison of the physiologic response to varying intensities of submaximal work in tethered swimming and treadmill running. *J. Sports Med. Phys. Fit.* 11:203–312.

Maglischo, E.W. (1982). *Swimming Faster.* Palo Alto: Mayfield Publishing Company.

Malina, R.M., and C. Bouchard (1988). *Growth, Maturation, and Physical Activity.* Champaign, IL: Human Kinetics.

Maughan, R. (1991). Carbohydrate-electrolyte solutions during prolonged exercise. In: D.R. Lamb and M.H. Williams (eds.) *Perspectives in Exercise Science and Sports Medicine, Vol. 4: Ergogenics—Enhancement of Performance in Exercise and Sport.* Indianapolis: Benchmark Press, pp. 36–86.

McArdle, W.D., R.M. Glaser, and J.R. Magel (1971). Metabolic and cardiorespiratory response during free swimming and treadmill walking. *J. Appl. Physiol.* 30:733–738.

McArdle, W.D., J.R. Magel, G.R. Lesmes, and B. Pechar (1976). Metabolic and cardiovascular adjustment to work in air and water at 18, 25 and 33 degrees C. *J. Appl. Physiol.* 40:85–90.

McArdle, W.D., F.I. Katch, and V.L. Katch (1991). *Exercise Physiology: Energy, Nutrition, and Human Performance.* Malvern, PA: Lea & Febiger.

McCally, M. (1965). *Body fluid volumes and renal response of human subjects to water immersion.* AMRL-TR-65-115, Aerospace Medical Research Laboratories, Wright-Patterson Air Force Base.

McMaster, W.C. (1986a). Anterior glenoid labrum damage: a painful lesion in swimmers. *Am. J. Sports Med.* 14:383–387.

McMaster, W.C. (1986b). Painful shoulder in swimmers: a diagnostic challenge. *Phys. Sportsmed.* 14:108–112.

McMaster, W.C., J.P. Troup, and S. Arredondo (1989). Incidence of shoulder problems in developing elite swimmers. *J. Swim. Res.* 5:11–16.

McMurray, R.G. (1983). Plasma Volume Changes During Submaximal Swimming. *Eur. J. Appl. Physiol.* 51:347–356.

McMurray, R.G. and S.M. Horvath (1979). Thermoregulation in swimmers and runners. *J. Appl. Physiol.* 46:1086–1092.

Medbø, J. I. and S. Burgers (1990). Effect of training on the anaerobic capacity. *Med. Sci. Sports Exerc.* 22:501–507.

Medbø, J.I., A.-C. Mohn, I. Tabata, R. Bahr, and O. Vaage, O. M. Sejersted (1988). Anaerobic capacity determined by maximal accumulated O_2 deficit. *J. Appl. Physiol.* 64:50–60.

Merino, J.A., and M. Llobet (1978). Insertion Tendinitis Among Swimmers. In: B. Eriksson and B. Furger (eds.) *Swimming Medicine IV.* Baltimore: University Park Press, pp. 101–104.

Montpetit, R., A. Duvallet, G. Cazorla, and H. Smith (1987). The Relative Stability of Maximal Aerobic Power in Elite Swimmers and its Relation to Training Performance. *J. Swim. Res.* 3:15–18.

Mutoh, Y. (1978). Low back pain in butterfliers. In: B. Ericksson and B. Furberg (eds.). *Swimming Medicine IV.* Baltimore: University Park Press, pp. 115–123.

Mutoh, Y. (1983). Mechanism and prevention of swimming injury. *Jap. J. Sports Sci.* 2: 527–544.

Nadel, E.R. (1977). Thermal and Energetic Exchanges During Swimming. In: E.R. Nadel (ed.) *Problems with Temperature Regulation During Exercise.* New York: Academic Press, pp. 91–119.

Nadel, E.R., I. Holmer, U. Bergh, P.-O. Astrand, and J. A. J. Stolwijk (1974). Energy exchanges of swimming man. *J. Appl. Physiol.* 36:465– 471.

Newsholme, E.A. (1988). Basic Aspects of Metabolic Regulation and Their Application to Provision of Energy in Exercise. In: M. Hebbelinck and R. J. Shephard (eds.) *Principles of Exercise Biochemistry.* Basel: Karger, pp. 40–77.

Nielsen, B., G. Sjøgaard, F. Bonde-Petersen (1984). Cardiovascular, hormonal and body fluid changes during prolonged exercise. *Eur. J. Appl. Physiol.* 53:63–70.

Nielsen, B. (1976). Temperature regulation during exercise in water and air. *Acta Physiol. Scand.* 98:500–508.

Nygaard, E. and E. Nielsen (1978). Skeletal muscle fibre capillarisation with extreme endurance training in man. In: B. Eriksson and B. Furberg (eds.) *Swimming Medicine IV.* Baltimore: University Park Press, pp. 282–293.

Olbrecht, J., Ø. Madsen, A. Mader, H. Liesen, and W. Hollmann (1985). Relationship between swimming velocity and lactic concentration during continuous and intermittent training exercise. *Int. J. Sports Med.* 6:74–77.

Olbrecht, J., A. Mader, H. Heck, and W. Hollman (1992). Importance of a calculation scheme to support the interpretation of lactate tests. In: D. Mac Laren, T. Reilly, and A. Lees (eds.) *Swimming Science VI.* London: E & FN SPON, pp. 243–249.

Olbrecht, J., A. Mader, A. Madsen, H. Liesen, and W. Hollman (1988). The Relationship of Lactic Acid to Long-Distance Swimming and the 2 × 400-m "2-Speed Test" and the Implications for Adjusting Training Intensities. In: B.E. Ungerechts, K. Wilke, and K. Reischle (eds.) *Swimming Science V.* Champaign: Human Kinetics, pp. 261–267.

Pfeiffer, H. (1991). *Schwimmen.* Berlin: Sportverlag.

Prins, J. (1981). Muscles and their function. In: E.R. Flavell (ed.) *Biokinetics Strength Training,* Albany, CA: Isokinetics Inc., pp. 72–77.

Reggiani, E., L. Marugo, A. Delpino, G. Piastar, G. Chiodini (1988). A comparison of various exercise challenge tests on airway reactivity in atopical swimmers. *J. Sports Med. Physic. Fitness* 28:394–401.

Richardson, A.B. (1986). The biomechanics of swimming: the shoulder and knee. In: J.V. Ciullo (ed.) *Clinics in Sports Medicine: Swimming.* Philadelphia: W.B. Saunders, pp. 103–114.

Richardson, A.B., F.W. Jobe, and H.R. Collins (1980). The shoulder in competitive swimming. *Am. J. Sports Med.* 8:159–163.

Rohrs, D.M., J.L. Mayhew, C. Arabas, and M. Shelton (1990). The relationship between seven anaerobic tests and swim performance. *J. Swim. Res.* 6:15–19.

Rovere, G.D., and A.W. Nichols (1985). Frequency, associated factors and treatment of breaststroker's knee in competitive swimmers. *Am. J. Sports Med.* 13:95–98.

Roydhouse, N. (1978). Earaches and adolescent swimmers. In: B. Eriksson and B. Furberg (eds.) *Swimming Medicine IV.* Baltimore: University Park Press, pp. 79–84.

Sale, D. (1986). Neural adaptation in strength and power training. In: L. Jones, N. McCartney, and A. McComas (eds.) *Human Muscle Power.* Champaign, Ill: Human Kinetics Publishers, pp. 289–304.

Saltin, B. (1973). Metabolic fundamentals in exercise. *Med. Sci. Sports* 5:137–146.

Schmidtbleicher, D. (1988). Muscular mechanics and neuromuscular control. In: B.E. Ungerechts, K. Wilke, and K. Reischle (eds.) *Swimming Science V*. Champaign, IL: Human Kinetics, pp. 131–148.

Schmidtbleicher, D. and M. Buehrle (1987). Neuronal adaptations and increase of cross-sectional area studying different strength training methods. In: B. Jonsson (ed.) *Biomechanics X-B*. Champaign, IL: Human Kinetics, pp. 615–620.

Sharp, R.L., L.E. Armstrong, D.S. King, and D.L. Costill (1983). Buffer capacity of blood in trained and untrained males. In: H.G. Knuttgen, J.A. Vogel, J. Poortmans (eds.) *Biochemistry of Exercise*. Champaign: Human Kinetics, pp. 595–599.

Sharp, R.L., J.P. Troup, and D.L. Costill (1982). The relationship between power and sprint freestyle swimming. *Med. Sci. Sports Exerc.* 14:53–36.

Sherman, W.M. (1990). Carbohydrate feedings before and after exercise. In: D.R. Lamb and M.H. Williams (eds.) *Perspectives in Exercise Science and Sports Medicine, Vol. 4: Ergogenics—Enhancement of Performance in Exercise and Sport*. Indianapolis: Benchmark Press, pp. 1–34.

Sherman, W.M., D.L. Costill, W.J. Fink, and J.M. Miller (1981). Effect of exercise-diet manipulation in muscle glycogen and its subsequent utilization during performance. *Int. J. Sports Med.* 2:114–118.

Sherman, W.M., and G.S. Wimer (1991). Insufficient dietary carbohydrate during training: Does it impair athletic performance? *Int. J. Sports Nutr.* 1:28–44.

Simonsen, J.C., W.M. Sherman, D.R. Lamb, A.R. Dernbach, J.A. Doyle, and R. Strauss (1991). Dietary carbohydrate, muscle glycogen, and power output during rowing training. *J. Appl. Physiol.* 70:1500–1505.

Spurgeon, J.H. and A.G. Sargent (1978). Measures of physique and nutrition on outstanding male swimmers. *Swim. Tech.* 15:26–32.

Spurgeon, J.H. and W.K. Giese (1984). Physique of world class female swimmers. *Scand. J. Sports Sci.* 6:11–14.

Stegmann, H., and W. Kindermann (1982). Comparison of prolonged exercise tests at the individual anaerobic threshold of 4 mmol/L lactate. *Int. J. Sports Med.* 3:105–110.

Strass, D. (1988). Effects of maximal strength training on sprint performance of competitive swimmers. In: B.E. Ungerechts, K. Wilke, and K. Reischle (eds.) *Swimming Science V*. Champaign, IL: Human Kinetics, pp. 149–156.

Strass, D. (1991). Electromyographic evaluation of selected arm and shoulder muscles of sprint swimmers in different technical positions. *J. Sports Sci.* 9:105–106.

Strauss, M.B., and R.W. Cantrell (1979). Swimmer's ear. Ear canal infections may be minor in terms of severity, but their frequency qualifies them as significant diving and swimming medi ·al problems. *Phys. Sportsmed.* 7:103–105.

Stulberg, S.D., K. Shulman, S. Stuart, and P. Culp (1980). Breaststroker's knee: pathology, etiology, and treatment. *Am. J. Sports Med.* 8:164–171.

Toussaint, H.M. (1988). *Mechanics and energetics of swimming*. Dissertation, Vrije Universiteit Amsterdam.

Toussaint, H.M., and P. Beek (1990). Biomechanics of competitive front crawl swimming. *Sports Med.* 89:8–24.

Toussaint, H., M.A. Beelen, A. Rodenburg, A.J. Sargeant, G. de Groot, A.P. Hollander, and G.J. van Ingen Schenau (1988). Propelling efficiency of front crawl swimming. *J. Appl. Physiol.* 65:2506–2512.

Trappe, S.W. (1991). *Anaerobic contributions: Physiological and biochemical perspectives of elite sprint and endurance trained cyclists*. MS Thesis. University of Colorado, Boulder, CO.

Treffene, R. (1983). Heart rate measurement technique in swimming performance prediction. In: A.P. Hollander, P.R. Huijing and G. de Groot (eds.) *Biomechanics and Medicine in Swimming*. Champaign, IL: Human Kinetics, pp. 339–344.

Troup, J.P. (1992). *International Center for Aquatic Research Annual, 1991–92*, Colorado Springs, CO: U.S. Swimming Press.

Troup, J.P., and J. Daniels (1986). Swimming Economy: An Overview. *J. Swim. Res.* 2:1–7.

Troup, J.P., S. Trappe, G. Crickard, L. J. D'Acquisto, and A.P. Barzdukas (1991a). Aerobic-anaerobic contributions during various interval training distances at common work:rest ratios (abstract). *J. Sports Sci.* 9:108.

Troup, J.P., A.P. Hollander, M. Bone, S. Trappe, and A.P. Barzdukas (1991b). Performance-related differences in the anaerobic contribution of competitive freestyle swimmers (abstract). *J. Sports. Sci.* 9:106–107.

Ungerechts, B., K. Wilke, and K. Reischle (1988). *Swimming Science V*. Champaign, IL: Human Kinetics.

Van Handel, P.J., A. Katz, J.P. Troup, and P.W. Bradley (1988). Aerobic economy and competitive swim performance of U.S. elite swimmers. In: B.E. Ungerechts, K. Wilke, and K. Reischle (eds.) *Swimming Science V*. Champaign, IL: Human Kinetics, pp. 219–227.

Van Handel, P.J., K.M. Cella, P.W. Bradley, and J.P. Troup (1985). Nutritional status of the elite swimmer. *J. Swim. Res.* 1:27–31.

Vizsolyi, P., J. Taunton, G. Robertson, L. Filsinger, H.S. Shannon, D. Whittingham, and M. Gleave (1987). Breaststroker's knee: an analysis of epidemiological and biomechanical factors. *Am. J. Sports Med.* 15:63–71.

Vogt, F.B., and P.C. Johnson (1965). Study of the effect of water immersion on healthy adult male subjects: plasma volume and fluid–electrolyte changes. Aerospace Med. 36:447–451.

Wakayoshi, K., T. Nomura, G. Takahashi, Y. Mutoh, and M. Miyashita. (1992). Analysis of swimming races in the 1989 Pan Pacific swimming championships and 1988 Japanese Olympic trials. In: D. Mac Laren, T. Reilly, and A. Lees (eds.) *Biomechanics and Medicine in Swimming.* Swimming Science VI. London: E. & F.N. Spon, pp. 135–141.

Wilmore, J.H., and D.L. Costill (1988). *Training for Sport and Activity: The Physiological Basis of the Conditioning Process.* Dubuque, IA: W.C. Brown.

Wilt, F. (1964). *Run Run Run.* Los Altos, CA: Tafnews Press.

DISCUSSION

GREGG: Please address the following questions: 1) Does body composition affect swimming performance? 2) Is the large volume of training currently in vogue important for physiological improvement or for technique improvement? 3) Are the remarkably high swim training intensities of 90–100% $\dot{V}O_2$max that have been reported flawed by a methodological error in the assessment of $\dot{V}O_2$max?

TROUP: There is a wide range of % body fats in elite swimmers. For example, our 1984 and subsequent Olympic women's team members ranged from 10–23% body fat. All those women swam fast. My guess is that a body composition in the range of 10–23% body fat will not provide any noticeable advantage to swim performance. There may be a disadvantage if body fat is greater than 23%, because it may create more drag. Eating disorders, particularly in women, may be caused by coaches who attempt to get swimmers to reduce body fat to extremely low levels. I do not believe that body composition contributes much to swim performance as long as body fat is within reasonable limits.

The volume of training required for optimal development of swim performance is controversial. One school believes that only high-intensity speed training should be done, but most of the coaching community subscribes to the need for high-volume training, i.e., a minimum of about 15,000 m/d or 6 h of training per day. Presumably, high-volume training improves swimming economy, at least partly by improving technique. I think that both the volume and intensity of training are important.

I am confident that elite swimmers do, in fact, train largely at 90–100% $\dot{V}O_2$max. Heart rates are in the range of 170–180 during the course of those workouts. The reason that swimmers can train this intensely is probably a function of the fact that they primarily swim alternating exercise-rest intervals rather than continuously at one pace.

KNUTTGEN: In relation to body composition, how important is buoyancy in elite swimmers?

TROUP: By allowing the swimmer to ride higher in the water, increased buoyancy may reduce drag to a certain extent and thus provide an advantage, especially in long distance swimming. Our elite distance swimmers tend to have a greater % fat than do the sprinters and they may be more buoyant.

KANTER: Body composition of elite swimmers tends to be higher in fat than that of elite runners and cyclists, who also do large volumes of training. Does this, in part, have to do with the fact that cooling is more effective in water and, consequently, it is easier to maintain a lower metabolic rate?

TROUP: I do not know if cooling is necessarily more effective in water.

NADEL: Heat transfer from the skin would be much more rapid per unit of temperature difference between skin and water versus skin and air because of the high heat transfer characteristics of water. But the cooling characteristics of the body are related not only to the skin-to-water temperature difference, but also to the body's resistances to heat transfer, i.e., the insulative layer of body fat and the variable circulation of blood to the periphery.

KANTER: Does the extra layer of fat make you a better swimmer or is it that you will retain the extra layer of fat if you swim because of some physiological adaptation resulting from swim training?

TROUP: I do not know.

GREGG: One of the comments that we hear from the public and coaches is that swimming is a bad sport to use to reduce body fat. If we could measure energy expenditure during 2 h of swimming versus cycling or running, would we see similar values for all three sports? If there is a difference, that might explain differences in body composition among swimmers and other endurance athletes.

BAR-OR: Perhaps a greater fat percentage is advantageous for swimmers because it provides a hydrodynamic advantage by causing a rounding of shoulders and other body parts. Maybe rounded edges give the swimmer a biomechanical edge.

TROUP: What you suggest may have merit. However, one must also consider how the extra body fat is distributed. For example, a beneficial effect of more rounding of the shoulders may be offset by the adverse effect of extra fat on increasing drag for the legs and trunk.

MAUGHAN: Maybe we can learn from some of the other sports. Distance runners have lower body fat than cyclists. Distance runners have to support their body weight during training and competition but cyclists do not. Race walkers have a higher body fat than the distance runners because the walkers have less oscillation of the center of gravity than do runners. Perhaps the requirement to move the body mass against gravity is the most important factor affecting body composition of various sport competitors.

BURKE: We need to consider age when addressing this body composition issue. It seems to me that most of the studies on swimmers use very young subjects, whereas runners and cyclists studied tend to be older than 25.

BAR-OR: As discussed by Ethan Nadel, immersion in cool water, which has a very high thermoconductivity, can lead to rapid heat transfer and body cooling. In addition to insulation by the subcutaneous layer of fat and to changes in peripheral blood flow, the ratio of body surface area to body mass also affects the rate of heat loss while immersed in cool water. This factor is particularly important for young age-group swimmers, whose surface area to mass ratio is greater than that for adults. The smaller the child, the greater the likelihood of excessive heat loss. Coaches of young swimmers must be aware of this phenomenon.

Another age group consideration is that prepubescent children are characterized by a much lower anaerobic power than are adults and may, therefore, perform relatively better at longer, more aerobic distances.

Finally, with respect to swimming and asthma, Inbar et al. showed in 1992 that the prone position does not give any advantage as far as bronchoconstriction in asthmatics. In other words, there is no support for the notion that the horizontal posture in swimming contributes to the apparent value of swimming for asthmatics.

NADEL: Body cooling might not affect performance in a very short event, but cooling may well affect the ability to train in the water for several hours. Cooling certainly could affect performance in events longer than 5–10 min. In the late 1970s, Bergh and Holmér reported that $\dot{V}O_2$ max after immersion was lower when the body temperature was lower and higher when the temperature was higher. This indeed will affect performance. Is there recent information in this area?

TROUP: Steve Gregg and some members of our group recorded plasma volume changes and core temperature changes during a training session, but I am unaware of other recent studies. I agree that heat loss is an important consideration for training sessions and during competitive distance swimming. Long distance races can last 5–6 h. Most of the distance competitions are held in North America, particularly in Canada, where the water temperatures range from 18–22° C. As it turns out, most successful open water swimmers have a relatively high percentage of body fat.

KNUTTGEN: Given that stroke length seems to be important to swimming success, do you think the ratio of the swimmer's arm length to body height might be a predictive factor for swimming success? It seems to me that many of the elite American women swimmers seem to be fairly small individuals. How does this all tie together?

TROUP: Distance covered per stroke may be related to endurance conditioning, and actual stroke length may be a function of muscle strength and power. Matt Bionde, who is very tall and has very long arms, has a moderate stroke length and distance per stroke. Janet Evans, who is half his size and has shorter arms, makes up for a shorter stroke length by having a much higher stroke frequency. The product of those components determines swimming velocity. I do not think we know whether stroke length or stroke frequency is more important.

HAGERMAN: Have you measured the length and width of swimmers' feet? If so, were there any correlations with performance?

TROUP: Last summer we began collecting data on length and width of swimmers' feet, but these studies are not complete. It has been estimated by Counsilman and others that the feet in freestyle contribute 10–20% of propulsion. I have heard higher or lower values presented by other biomechanists.

BAR-OR: You have chosen to use the oxygen deficit as an index of anaerobic performance, but isn't anaerobic performance localized to specific muscles performing the activity rather than generalized to the whole body? For example, the anaerobic performance of the swimmer's arms could be quite different from that of the legs. Is there any information on the anaerobic performance of specific limbs of swimmers?

TROUP: Hollander studied oxygen deficit in freestylers versus breaststrokers and found that it was greater in the breaststrokers, but that is the closest people have gotten to addressing your question.

KRAEMER: It seems to me that most resistance training programs used by swimmers either use a very low volume of training or the exercise choice is so specific that it limits power development capabilities. More research is needed on resistance training for swimmers.

COYLE: John, you suggest that swimming economy improves with training and that one of the justifications for prolonged endurance training is to increase fitness and thereby increase economy. How do you explain the improved economy? I assume that body composition does not change much. Is their technique changing? Can you see any changes in their distance per stroke, stroke rate, or the velocity of movement? Do you think some characteristic of the muscle is changing to affect energy production?

TROUP: It seems that technique probably has the most important effect on the economy profile. Do you think changes in fiber type recruitment may be affecting economy?

COYLE: Slow twitch (Type I) fibers are much more efficient than fast twitch fibers in cyclists and this plays a very large role in explaining superior performance. I would assume that the same applies in swimming, provided the muscle contraction velocities are slow enough. It may be possible to change the efficiency of ATP hydrolysis at the cross bridges by modifying the type of myosin involved in the contraction.

TROUP: We have not been able to demonstrate a change in efficiency.

MAUGHAN: When I look at fields of top class swimmers, I don't see any blacks. Is that a physiological or social phenomenon?

TROUP: I think it is a socioeconomic phenomenon. Most black children around the world have few opportunities to become involved in swim training programs.

4

Physiology and Nutrition for Wrestling

CRAIG A. HORSWILL, Ph.D.

INTRODUCTION

Wrestling is a sport in which two individuals, matched for body weight, compete for physical control over one another. The ultimate goal of wrestling at the international level and in the USA is to pin the opponent's back (scapulae) to the mat; this is officially known as a fall and immediately ends the match. In the absence of a fall, a scoring system determines the winner; the system is based on points awarded for obtaining degrees of control over the opponent during the match. The scoring system varies for the different levels and styles of competition (Table 4-1), although rule changes in recent years have made international, USA scholastic, and USA collegiate styles almost indistinguishable.

Relatively gross skills, including personal body control and moving or resisting the mass and force of an opponent, are critical for success in this sport. In addition, because competitors are of equal body weight, wrestling demands strength, power, agility, balance, and endurance in proportion to the size of the opposition. The requirement of being equal in weight stresses discipline and planning in nutritional practices for weight reduction and recovery after *making weight* (i.e., attaining a regulation weight, which signifies that opponents are of similar if not identical mass).

In this chapter, we will discuss the physiological characteristics associated with elite wrestling performance (Figure 4-1), the factors associated with fatigue during competition, the methods of training, the practices of nutrition and weight loss, and the potential for problems associated with overtraining. The two recurrent themes in this discussion include 1) the understanding of what is necessary to be successful in this sport, and 2) the identification of where the knowledge of the science of wrestling is limited.

CHARACTERISTICS OF ELITE WRESTLERS

Body Composition and Somatotype

Research supports the stereotype of amateur wrestlers having strong mesomorphic characteristics (low linearity, high muscularity, and low percentage body fat). Table 4-2 presents the percentage body fat of elite wrestlers at various levels of development. Despite the observations that successful high school wrestlers compete closer to their minimum weights (i.e., at lower percentages of body fat) than do less successful wrestlers (Tcheng et al., 1973) and that successful high school wrestlers have lower body fat percentages than do less successful peers (Horswill et al., 1989; Cisar et al., 1987), most studies on collegiate and international caliber wrestlers in the USA show no difference between body fatness of successful and less successful wrestlers (Nagle et al., 1975; Silva et al., 1981; Stine et al., 1979). This similarity in fatness between the two categories of

TABLE 4-1. *Levels and styles of competition of wrestling in which a fall* is the goal*

Level	Age	Styles	Brief Description
Open or Senior	≥17 y	Greco Roman (GR)	Classic style emphasizing wrestling on feet and spectacular throws; defensive or offensive use of legs is illegal; fall time: momentary (<1 s).
		Freestyle (FS)	Like GR (same scoring system and fall time) except legs can be used.
University or Junior World	18–24	FS or GR	Same as Open division.
		Collegiate (C)	Similar to FS but more mat wrestling; fall time: 1 s.
Junior	<20 y	FS or GR	Same as Open division.
		Scholastic	Similar to C but no points for riding time and throws are de-emphasized; fall time: 2 s.
School boy	≤14 y	International	FS or GR rules; shorter match duration.
		Scholastic	Scholastic rules but shorter match duration.

*A fall is the holding of the opponent's scapulae to the mat for a specified time, which varies among the styles.
Adapted from material provided by USA Wrestling, Colorado Springs, CO.

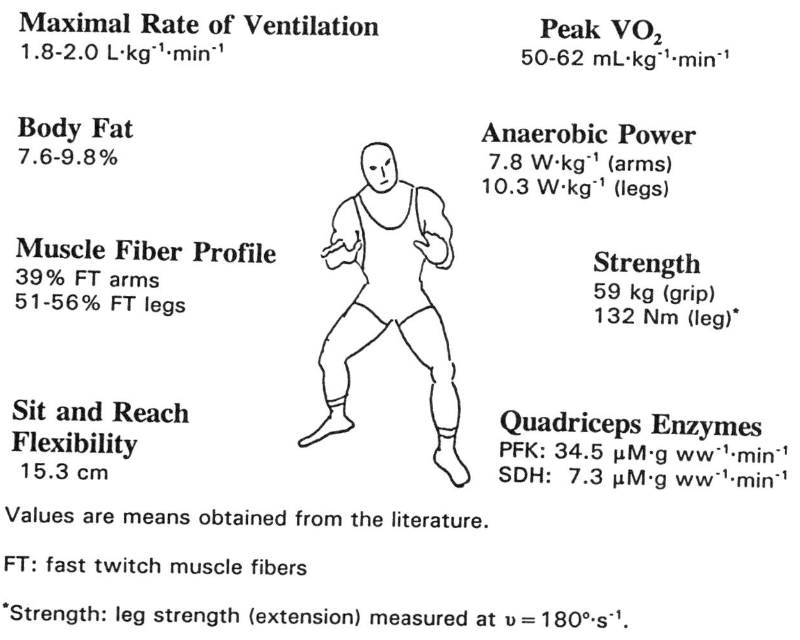

Maximal Rate of Ventilation
1.8-2.0 L·kg⁻¹·min⁻¹

$$\text{1.8-2.0 L}\cdot\text{kg}^{-1}\cdot\text{min}^{-1}$$

Peak VO$_2$
$50\text{-}62 \text{ mL}\cdot\text{kg}^{-1}\cdot\text{min}^{-1}$

Body Fat
7.6-9.8%

Anaerobic Power
$7.8 \text{ W}\cdot\text{kg}^{-1}$ (arms)
$10.3 \text{ W}\cdot\text{kg}^{-1}$ (legs)

Muscle Fiber Profile
39% FT arms
51-56% FT legs

Strength
59 kg (grip)
132 Nm (leg)*

Sit and Reach Flexibility
15.3 cm

Quadriceps Enzymes
PFK: $34.5 \text{ }\mu\text{M}\cdot\text{g ww}^{-1}\cdot\text{min}^{-1}$
SDH: $7.3 \text{ }\mu\text{M}\cdot\text{g ww}^{-1}\cdot\text{min}^{-1}$

Values are means obtained from the literature.

FT: fast twitch muscle fibers

*Strength: leg strength (extension) measured at $v = 180°\cdot\text{s}^{-1}$.

FIGURE 4-1. *Profile of the elite wrestler. Data presented are mean values from the literature.*

TABLE 4-2. *Physical characteristics and body composition of elite wrestlers (mean ± SD)*

	Age (y)	Height (cm)	Weight (kg)	Density (g·mL^{-1})	Fat (%)
Prepubescent[1]	11.3±1.2	141.2±9.2	34.2±5.4	1.070±0.002	12.7±4.0[a]
Adolescent[2]	16.7±0.9	169.9±9.6	64.4±12.4	na	7.2±2.4[b]
Adolescent[3]	16.9±1.2	167.1±7.8	60.2±11.2	1.078±0.014	9.7±5.5[a]
Junior World[4]	18.8±1.1	174.2±10.4	82.1±24.4	na	7.4±0.7[b]
Collegiate[5]	21.3±1.7	179.8±6.6	71.9±11.8	na	3.7±0.5[b]
International[6]	24.3±1.9	175.6±10.8	77.7±16.2	na	8.3±1.0[b]

[a] determined from hydrostatic weighing; [b] estimated from skinfold thickness
[1] Sady et al. (1984) n = 15; [2] Horswill et al. (1988) n = 39; [3] Thorland et al. (1981) n = 18; [4] Silva et al. (1981) n = 8; [5] Stine et al. (1979) n = 6;
[6] Nagle et al. (1975) n = 8

wrestlers may be due to a possible inherent leanness among individuals attracted to the sport, to an inability to attain further leanness, or to the possibility that further leanness offers no additional performance benefits. All wrestlers in the aforementioned studies could be considered successful because they qualified for the corresponding levels of competition, i.e., the Olympics (Nagle et al., 1975), the National Collegiate Athletic Association (NCAA) national tournament (Stine et al., 1979), and the Junior World competition (Silva et al., 1981).

Differences in body fat percentages are more apparent across the weight classes within a group of elite wrestlers than between elite and non-elite wrestlers of similar weight classes. Among successful wrestlers, the lightest are reported to be the leanest (Horswill et al., 1988; de Garay et al., 1974; Song & Garvie, 1980; Tcheng et al., 1973). The direct relationship between fatness and weight class can also be found in non-elite wrestlers (Katch et al., 1971; Tcheng et al., 1973). The relationship between leanness and weight class may be a function of lighter wrestlers attempting to lose more weight than heavier wrestlers (Freischlag, 1984) or inherent differences in athletes of different size. Usually, wrestlers in the heavyweight division have attempted to gain weight, including body fat (Gale et al., 1974), because they thought extra weight offered advantages for success; until recently, heavyweights did not have a maximum weight restriction.

Regarding physique, Olympic wrestlers have high ratings for the mesomorphic characteristics and low endomorphic and ectomorphic characteristics (de Garay et al., 1974; Tanner, 1964). Greco-Roman and freestyle wrestlers together have mean values of 2.3, 6.4, and 1.6 for endomorphy, mesomorphy, and ectomorphy, respectively (de Garay et al., 1974); the ratings were not different between the two styles. Endomorphy and mesomorphy ratings tended to increase and the ectomorphy ratings tended to decrease in progression from the lightest to heaviest Olympic wrestlers (de Garay et al., 1974). Similarly, highly skilled scholastic wrestlers tended to have lower scores for body breadth and linearity-to-fatness, but greater muscularity scores compared to novice wrestlers (Cisar et al., 1987); however, no differences in physique and body composition were found between average wrestlers and the highly skilled wrestlers (Cisar et al., 1987). In contrast, others found that wrestlers were only slightly above average in the mesomorphic rating and did not differ greatly from non-athletic control subjects (Kroll, 1954; Rasch, 1958; Sady et al., 1982). Discrepancies among the study findings (de Garay et al., 1974; Kroll, 1954; Rasch, 1958; Sady et al., 1982; Tanner, 1964) could be in part due to the selection of the subject sample. The top caliber Olympic wrestlers from around the world (de Garay et al., 1974; Tanner, 1964) may differ in physique from wrestlers studied within the USA, who were not necessarily Olympic-level (Kroll, 1954; Rasch, 1958; Sady et al., 1982).

Skeletal Muscle Fiber Type

Description of the histochemical profile of skeletal muscle in elite wrestlers is limited to a few reports (Table 4-3). Overall, the wrestler would not appear to be an exceptionally power-trained or endurance-trained athlete based on peripheral tissue characteristics. The range of published mean values for fast twitch fibers of the lower bodies of wrestlers (gastrocnemius or vastus lateralis) is 51 to 56% (Tesch et al., 1982; Taylor et al., 1979; Sharratt et al., 1986; Bergh et al., 1978). In contrast, fibers from the upper bodies (deltoids) of wrestlers in one study were significantly lower in fast twitch fibers at 39%, compared to 53% in the lower bodies (Tesch et al., 1982). The apparent difference between the upper body and lower body fiber-type distribution in wrestlers may reflect training effects or the natural selection process that attracts an athlete with a genetic disposition for a certain profile of muscle fiber type. In wrestling, the lower body is involved in the explosive and powerful movements of attacking and lifting the opponent. The upper body is used primarily to grasp, hold, and control the opponent in a continuous manner.

Flexibility

The precarious positions that a wrestler experiences in competition suggest that flexibility would be an important attribute in the sport. Also, many wrestlers spend significant amounts of time performing stretching exercises in their warmups before training or competition. Interestingly, research suggests that wrestlers are no more flexible than non-wrestlers. Early studies showed that wrestlers had less flexibility overall than did weightlifters and gymnasts (Leighton, 1957). However, with respect to the specificity of flexibility, wrestlers had greater rotation and abduction/adduction of the shoulders than did non-athletes (Leighton, 1957). Also, flexibility of the neck was great, but wrist flexibility was poor, when wrestlers were compared to non-athletes.

Comparing the successful wrestler to the less successful wrestler,

TABLE 4-3. *Mean percentages of slow twitch fiber type in skeletal muscle of elite wrestlers and other athletes*

	Lower body	Upper body
Swedish wrestlers[1]	44–47	61
Canadian FS wrestlers[2]	48	na
Canadian GR wrestlers[3]	49	na
Cyclists[4]	61	na
Weightlifters[4]	46	na
Kayak paddlers[5]	41	73
Distance runners[5]	67	50

FS: freestyle; GR: Greco Roman
[1]Bergh et al. (1978); Tesch et al. (1982); [2]Sharratt et al. (1986); [3]Taylor et al. (1979); [4]Gollnick et al. (1972); [5]Tesch et al. (1982)

Stine et al., (1979) and Song and Garvie (1980) showed that flexibility might be a discriminating variable. For collegiate wrestlers, the sit-and-reach measurements were slightly greater for the most successful group versus the moderately successful and the least successful wrestlers (Stine et al., 1979). At the international level, the Japanese wrestlers had greater overall flexibility than their Canadian counterparts (Song et al., 1980). Apparently, no relationship exists between flexibility and strength (Song & Garvie, 1980), but the effective combination of the two seems intuitively critical to success in the sport.

Reaction Time and Movement Time

Research indicates that athletes move more quickly in response to a stimulus (i.e., reaction time) than do non-athletes (Keller, 1942). Several reports (Kroll, 1958; Rasch et al., 1961b; Stine et al., 1979) though, do not isolate reaction time or movement time as critical attributes for success in wrestling. No differences in the response time (combined reaction time and movement time) were found in successful and non-successful high school wrestlers for offensive and defensive movements specific to wrestling (Kroll, 1958). Using a standard test to measure both reaction time and movement time, no differences were observed in either for non-wrestlers, collegiate wrestlers, USA national wrestlers, or Japanese team members (Rasch et al., 1961b). A similar lack of differences existed among collegiate wrestlers of various levels of success (placewinners and non-placewinners in the USA national collegiate championship) who performed tests for reaction time and response time for a wrestling-specific movements test (Stine et al., 1979).

In an effort to account for technical skills as well as reaction-movement time, Taylor et al. (1979) developed a battery of tests specifically for wrestling. Because the sample size of eight in this initial study was small and all the wrestlers were of high caliber, it was not possible to correlate technical speed with success on the mat. However, this series of tests could be a promising way to profile champion wrestlers and to monitor technical training in future research.

Muscular Strength

Early studies on wrestlers focused on isometric (static) strength (Nagle et al., 1975; Rasch et al., 1961a). Isometric muscle actions are important in the sport but are associated with holding and controlling the opponent (in many respects, stalling tactics) rather than moving an opponent toward a fall. The development during the 1970s of reliable methods of assessing dynamic strength (i.e., force or torque developed during maximal concentric or eccentric actions) was fortuitous because of concurrent rule changes in the sport that placed an emphasis on continuous aggressiveness and scoring rather than stalling. Nevertheless, definitive studies on the dynamic strength of elite Olympic-caliber wrestlers remain to be done. Strength values of elite and non-elite wrestlers are compared in Table 4-4.

Most research implies that greater strength is advantageous in wrestling. In adolescent wrestlers, a composite of isokinetic strength measurements distinguished the successful wrestler (qualifier for regional or state tournament or winner of a minimum of 67% of bouts) from the least successful (won a maximum of only 33% of matches) (Cisar et al., 1987). A similar although non-significant trend existed for successful collegiate wrestlers (placewinners in the USA collegiate championships) to possess greater isokinetic strength, particularly in the upper body, compared to collegiate wrestlers who were not placewinners (Stine et al., 1979). In contrast, no differences were noted in isometric grip strength between the successful and less successful wrestlers battling for the Junior World games team (Silva et al., 1981) and the 1972 Olympic freestyle team (Nagle et al., 1975). The incongruous findings (Cisar et al., 1987; Nagle et al., 1975; Silva et al., 1981; Stine et al., 1979) could be explained by methodological differences (isokinetic vs. isometric strength testing) and by the style of competitors being studied; USA national style (scholastic and college) performed isokinetic tests, whereas international-style wrestlers performed isometric tests (i.e., Junior World and Olympic).

Of note, the attempt to distinguish differences between successful and less successful wrestlers by using strength scores relative to body

TABLE 4-4. *Mean strength performance of elite wrestlers*

	Grip Strength[A]	Upper Body Strength[B]	Lower Body Strength[C]
Scholastic[1]			
elite	49.2 kg	na[D]	465 kg
non-elite	45.1 kg	na	429 kg
Junior World[2]			
elite	49 kg	na	na
non-elite	51 kg	na	na
Collegiate[3]			
elite	61 kg	592 Nm	783 Nm
non-elite	58 kg	463 Nm	659 Nm
International			
elite	59 kg[4]	62/62.9 Nm[5]	131.5/103 Nm[5]
non-elite	58 kg[4]	na	na

[A]Isometric strength assessed using a grip dynamometer (right hand or unspecified)
[B]The sum of several CYBEX® measurements at $90°\cdot s^{-1}$ (Stine et al., 1979) or peak torque of elbow extension/flexion measured on CYBEX® at $180°\cdot s^{-1}$ (Sharratt et al., 1986)
[C]The isometric leg lift (Kroll, 1958) or the sum of several CYBEX® measurements at $180°\cdot s^{-1}$ (Stine et al., 1979) or peak torque of knee extension/flexion measured on CYBEX® at $180°\cdot s^{-1}$ (Sharratt et al., 1986)
[D]na: not available
[1]Kroll (1958); [2]Silva et al. (1981); [3]Stine et al. (1979); [4]Nagle et al. (1975); [5]Sharratt et al. (1986)

weight does not entirely absolve the influence of body size. Absolute strength is greater in heavier wrestlers compared to lighter wrestlers; however, for relative strength, the lighter the wrestler, the greater the strength (Song & Garvie, 1980). In future studies that attempt to identify factors contributing to success, it might be most accurate to pair successful and less successful wrestlers by weight class, rather than by comparing the relative strengths of the two groups.

Anaerobic Power and Capacity

The ability to produce power may arguably be the most important physiological attribute in wrestling. Successful wrestlers must be able to generate explosive movements for both offensive and defensive purposes. A summary of the anaerobic power in elite wrestlers performing the Wingate test is found in Table 4-5. Using the Margaria stair test, successful adolescent wrestlers generated a mean of 16.5 $W \cdot kg^{-1}$ (Roemmich, 1993), successful collegiate wrestlers (Big 10 Conference and NCAA tournament placewinners) produced a mean of 20.5 ± 1.6 $W \cdot kg^{-1}$ (Horswill, 1979), and selected Olympians generated 17.0 $W \cdot kg^{-1}$ (DiPrampero et al., 1970).

Anaerobic power may be greater in successful wrestlers compared to less successful wrestlers. The anaerobic power and capacities of the upper and lower bodies of elite junior wrestlers measured using the Wingate test were greater by as much as 13% compared to performance tests of non-elite wrestlers of similar weight, age, and wrestling experience (Horswill et al., 1989). This may be due to differences in the relative amount of muscle (Horswill et al., 1989) or to differences in neuromuscular recruitment. Subsequent studies are needed to determine if anaerobic power differences can be found between the successful and less successful wrestlers at the college and international levels.

Because anaerobic power is a local, peripheral characteristic, researchers have begun testing upper body and lower body anaerobic power

TABLE 4-5. *Anaerobic characteristics of elite wrestlers (mean ± SD)*

	Anaerobic Power ($W \cdot kg^{-1}$)*		Anaerobic Capacity ($W \cdot kg^{-1}$)**	
	Arms	Legs	Arms	Legs
Prepubescent[1]	na	7.5#	na	na
Adolescent[2]	7.5	10.6	5.9 ± 0.4	8.6 ± 0.8
International[3]	7.8 ± 1.0	10.3 ± 1.2	6.8 ± 0.9	9.4 ± 0.7

Values shown without ± SD were estimated by dividing the group's mean power by its mean body weight.
*Peak power achieved during a 5-s interval of a 30-s Wingate test.
**Mean power achieved in a 30-s Wingate test.
#Measured during last 5 s of the test.
[1]Sady et al. (1984); [2]Horswill et al. (1988); [3]Horswill et al. (1992c)

separately in elite wrestlers (Horswill et al., 1989; Horswill et al., 1992c). As expected, lower body power is greater by 32–41% than upper body power (Table 4-5). Of note, when anaerobic power is standardized for aerobic power (i.e., anaerobic power/power output at peak $\dot{V}O_2$ measured using similar ergometry), elite senior athletes generate more power in the upper body compared to the lower body (Horswill et al., 1992c). It is not known if this phenomenon is unique to wrestlers because upper body-lower body power comparisons have not yet been made on this basis for athletes engaged in other sports.

The capacity of the muscle to maintain maximum power via anaerobic metabolism (anaerobic capacity) has been assessed in wrestlers primarily with the 30-s Wingate test (Table 4-5). Arguably, a test of such short duration may not quantify the true or total anaerobic capacity (Medbø et al., 1988; Serresse et al., 1988; Simoneau et al., 1983). However, it is likely that anaerobic capacity assessed using the Wingate test would be highly correlated and thus representative of anaerobic capacity determined using longer tests (Bar-Or, 1987). Future research might include measuring power output during longer tests (i.e., longer than 30 s) of high intensity as well as simultaneous assessment of O_2 deficit (Green & Dawson, 1993) in order to define the functional and metabolic anaerobic capacity of wrestlers. Future research also might build on the preliminary studies of ours and others (Hickner et al., 1991; Sharratt et al., 1986) that involved assessing the wrestler's ability to maintain power during repeated, intermittent efforts of high intensity. Because wrestling is usually composed of a series of sporadic, high-power actions, an intermittent protocol may be more relevant to this sport than simply assessing the anaerobic capacity of a single, short-duration, maximum effort.

Cardiopulmonary Fitness and Aerobic Power

A summary of the studies on elite wrestlers (Table 4-6) shows a range of peak $\dot{V}O_2$ values (for running on the treadmill) between 50 and 62 mL·kg^{-1}·min^{-1}. Peak oxygen uptake is likely not a discriminating factor between successful and less successful wrestlers. Within Olympic, collegiate, and scholastic wrestlers, peak oxygen uptake was not statistically different between successful and less successful competitors (Horswill et al., 1989; Nagle et al., 1975; Stine et al., 1979). That a higher peak $\dot{V}O_2$ is not more strongly associated with wrestling success may be a function of the nature of the sport (explosive, powerful, and quick movements) and the duration of competition (only 5–7 min). However, Roemmich (1993) recently reported that successful scholastic wrestlers had higher peak $\dot{V}O_2$ values as estimated from a 15-min run compared to the values estimated for the less successful counterparts. Because peak $\dot{V}O_2$ was estimated and not measured in that study (Roemmich, 1993), the differences could be attributed to other physiological factors, such as differences in anaerobic

TABLE 4-6. *Mean (±SD) peak oxygen uptake (Peak V̇O₂) and maximal minute ventilation (V̇E) of elite wrestlers*

	Peak $\dot{V}O_2$ ($mL \cdot kg^{-1} \cdot min^{-1}$)			
	Arm Cranking	Cycling, Legs	Treadmill Running	max $\dot{V}_E$ ($mL \cdot kg^{-1} \cdot min^{-1}$)*
Prepubescent[1]	na**	na	54.0±4.4	1904
Scholastic[2]	na	na	52.6±8.5	2017
Junior World[3]	na	na	na	1895
Collegiate[4]	40.6	45.4	62.4	na
International[5]	43.7±4.6	50.9±5.1	na	na
International[6]	na	na	60.9±3.6	2015
International[7]	na	na	61.8	1820

*Max $\dot{V}_E$ was calculated using mean values for $\dot{V}_E$ ($L \cdot min^{-1}$) at peak $\dot{V}O_2$ and body weight (kg).
**na: not available

[1]Sady et al. (1984); [2]Horswill et al. (1989); [3]Silva et al. (1981); [4]Seals & Mullin (1982); [5]Horswill et al. (1992c); [6]Nagle et al. (1975); [7]Sharratt et al. (1986)

thresholds, or to psychological factors, such as competitiveness among the wrestlers during the timed run.

Most studies on the peak oxygen uptake of elite wrestlers were conducted before 1980, when matches were longer than present regulations allow. Beginning in 1985, the duration of an international match decreased to a continuous 5-min bout without a rest period, and USA collegiate matches were shortened from 8 to 7 min. With shorter matches, aerobic power and cardiovascular endurance may not be as critical for success as once thought (Sharratt, 1984). Nevertheless, we have recently begun using cycle and arm crank ergometry to assess the peak aerobic capability of wrestlers (Horswill et al., 1990a; Hickner et al., 1991; Horswill et al., 1992c) (Table 4-6). Arm crank and cycle ergometry may be preferred to the running (treadmill) tests used in earlier studies (Gale et al., 1974; Horswill et al., 1988; Nagle et al., 1975; Sady et al., 1984; Sharratt et al., 1986; Stine et al., 1979; Taylor et al., 1979) for several reasons. Ergometry, particularly the arm crank, offers motion that is similar to the movements in wrestling; it isolates the effort to a specific area of the body as wrestling frequently does; and ergometry provides a measure of function (power) at the time peak $\dot{V}O_2$ is estimated to occur (Horswill et al., 1992c).

Mechanical Efficiency—Economy of Movement

The most accomplished wrestlers are often described by fellow competitors as being extremely strong, yet differences in strength between successful and less successful wrestlers are not always measurable (Nagle et al., 1975; Rasch et al., 1961a; Rasch & Kroll, 1964b; Silva et al., 1981). Strength differences may not have been detected because current methods do not include a technical skill component. Superior wrestlers exhibit an economy of movement that allows them to exert a minimum of energy to score control points.

Through technical superiority, the successful wrestler maximizes position and leverage to develop the force, power, or torque necessary to defeat the opponent. Unfortunately, no published research exists on the economy of movement or mechanical efficiency of wrestlers, possibly due to the difficulty of obtaining an accurate estimate of energy expenditure during sporadic, non-steady-state movements of the sport.

Other Factors

While the focus of this book is on the physiological factors that influence sports performance, the psychological factors interwoven with the physiological and biomechanical can not be overlooked. For example, the profile of mood states (POMS) may differ between the elite and non-elite wrestler (Morgan, 1988), and some research indicates that POMS may even have predictive value in determining which wrestlers will be successful (Nagle et al., 1975; Silva et al., 1981). In addition, several studies indicate that wrestlers are more aggressive than other athletes (Husman, 1955; Rasch et al., 1964a), although it is not clear whether this distinction holds up for elite and non-elite wrestlers (Rasch et al., 1964a). Applied research at the international level shows that 80–90% of the time, the first wrestler to score a point in the match ultimately wins the match (Ichiguchi, 1981; Ichiguchi et al., 1978). Similarly, successful scholastic wrestlers get the first takedown 70% of the time and lose the first takedown only 9% of the time (Kroll, 1958). These findings suggest that, besides speed, strength, and technique, aggressiveness contributes to the initial and possibly the overall success of the wrestler.

LIMITATIONS ON A WRESTLER'S PERFORMANCE

Local Energetics and Peripheral Metabolic Factors

The high power output used to complete a single maneuver against an opponent of equal mass, coupled with the repetition of such maneuvers throughout a 5–7 min bout and over several bouts in a day's tournament, place a great demand on all energy-producing systems of a wrestler. Average energy expenditure during intense wrestling is estimated to be 900 to 983 W (AAHPER, 1971; Wilmore et al., 1988). Consequently, the failure to maintain energy output at a sufficiently high rate and the accumulation of metabolites might be the most critical sources of fatigue during performance.

Both aerobic and anaerobic pathways contribute to energy production in wrestling (Rasch & Kroll, 1964b; Sharratt, 1984). During a 6-min, Olympic-style match, muscle glycogen levels of the vastus lateralis were reduced by 21.5%, and the reduction was consistent across muscle fiber types (Houston et al., 1983). It was concluded that wrestling placed similar demands on slow twitch, fast twitch A, and fast twitch B fibers (Houston et al., 1983); however, concluding that recruitment of all fiber types is uniform in wrestling could be erroneous, due to the use of a variety of muscle groups at erratic intensities and to the subjectivity of the methodology employed by the authors (Houston et al., 1983). Comparing the prematch state to almost-immediate postmatch state, venous blood lactate concentrations rose from 1.1 ± 0.4 mmol·L^{-1} to 10.5 ± 1.4 mmol·L^{-1}, and blood pH decreased from 7.31 to 7.06 (Houston et al., 1983). Outside of the confounding effects of weight loss, the accumulation of hydrogen ions (H^+) from lactate production is likely the most significant physiological factor that limits the wrestler during a match. Previous research indicates that the accumulation of H^+ has two effects: 1) it inhibits the cross-linkage between actin and myosin and thereby decreases force production of the muscle fiber (Fabiato & Fabiato, 1978; Hermansen, 1981), and 2) it impairs glycolytic enzyme activity, in particular phosphofructokinase (PFK), and thus decreases ATP production (Dawson et al., 1978; Hermansen, 1981). In addition, under experimental conditions, the buffering of H^+ may minimize fatigue and help maintain performance of high-intensity, intermittent efforts similar to the patterns of activity in wrestling (Gao et al., 1988).

Succinate dehydrogenase (SDH) activity in the vastus lateralis of Olympic-caliber wrestlers has been measured as an index of cellular oxidative capacity (Sharratt et al., 1986). A mean activity of 7.3 μmol·g^{-1} wet weight of muscle·min^{-1} was determined. In comparison, cyclists (endurance-trained) and weightlifters (power-trained) have mean SDH activities of 11.0 μmol·g^{-1} wet weight of muscle·min^{-1} and 3.0 μmol·g^{-1} wet weight of muscle·min^{-1}, respectively (Gollnick et al., 1972). With little more than 50% of the skeletal muscle fibers of wrestlers being fast twitch (Bergh et al., 1978; Sharratt et al., 1986; Taylor et al., 1979), oxidative capacity at the cellular level, at least for the lower bodies of wrestlers, is average compared to that of endurance- and power-trained athletes (Table 4-3).

The limited aerobic capacity of the skeletal muscle of wrestlers, whether due to genetics or training specificity, may place added significance on the capacity for anaerobic metabolism and tolerance to lactate accumulation during a wrestling match. Activity of PFK in wrestlers averaged 34.5 μmol·g^{-1}·min^{-1} (Sharratt et al., 1986), which is reasonably high compared to weightlifters (24.7 μmol·g^{-1}·min^{-1}), cyclists (23.9 μmol·g^{-1}·min^{-1}) (Gollnick et al., 1972), and hockey players (approximately 25.5 μmol·g^{-1}·min^{-1}) (Daub et al., 1982). No research has been done on buffering capacity of wrestlers, but Sharratt (1984) observed that elite Olympic-level wrestlers had maximum minute ventilation values that were low relative to peak $\dot{V}O_2$ values and lactate levels. Sharratt suggested that the Olympic-level wrestlers may hypoventilate during maximal exercise as a result of conditioning over years of restricted breathing during self-generated isometric muscle actions or physical restrictions imposed by opponents, and that successful wrestlers may be more tolerant of lactic acid accumulation compared to less successful wrestlers. Support for this may be inferred from the study of Nagle et al., (1975), in which successful Olympic team contenders had greater dynamic endurance (maximum number of repetitions of bench press performed with a free-weight of 22.7 kg) than did the runners-up for the final team (Nagle et al., 1975). Because blood base excess and lactate concentrations were not measured, superior dynamic endurance in the successful wrestlers may have been due to tolerance of lactate accumulation or the ability to generate energy continuously anaerobically.

Cardiovascular and Pulmonary Factors

Wrestlers spend considerable amounts of time training the aerobic energy system by continuous wrestling, distance running, rope skipping, and stationary cycling (Johnson & Cisar, 1987; Roundtable, 1988a; Roundtable, 1988b). As discussed previously, peak oxygen uptake (peak $\dot{V}O_2$) is not a determinant of success among wrestlers. Furthermore, several studies indicate that peak $\dot{V}O_2$ does not increase with training in wrestlers (Clarke et al., 1984; Herbert et al., 1977; Kelly et al., 1978). The lack of a training effect might be explained by the cardiovascular dynamics in wrestlers. Morganroth et al. (1975) and Cohen and Segal (1985) observed that collegiate wrestlers had left ventricular end-diastolic volumes that were less than those of endurance-trained athletes, but similar to those of non-athletes. The wall and septal thicknesses of the left ventricle were greater in wrestlers compared to non-athletes and endurance athletes. This hypertrophy is likely an adaptation to the increased afterload placed on the heart during isometric muscle actions performed by wrestlers (Huston et al., 1985; Morganroth & Maron, 1977). The volume of the left ventricle is not increased by wrestling training to the extent that it is by lower-intensity aerobic training (Morganroth et al., 1975); thus, maximum cardiac output and stroke volume may not be augmented by wrestling training. Larger septal and posterior walls of the left ventricle have been observed in elite adolescent wrestlers compared to age-matched non-wrestlers (Cohen et al., 1987). Because previous studies were cross-sectional (Cohen & Segal, 1985; Cohen et al., 1987; Morganroth et al., 1975), it is difficult to determine whether the differences are due to training or heredity (Morganroth & Maron, 1977), such that athletes with thicker left ventricle walls have more success and continue in the sport. The lack of an increase in aerobic power despite aerobic training by wrestlers (Clarke et al., 1984; Kelly et al., 1978; Herbert et al., 1977) may be due to genetic limitations or because the stimulus and adaptation from anaerobic training overshadow those of aerobic training.

Regarding pulmonary function, Rasch and Brandt (1957) found mean $\pm SD$ values of 5.2 ± 0.7 L for vital capacity, 4.2 ± 0.4 L for the forced expired volume in 1 sec (FEV$_1$), 6.5 ± 0.8 L for the total lung capacity, and 163.6 ± 0.0 mL for the maximum breathing capacity. Sharratt et al. (1986) found comparable volumes for international competitors on the Canadian national team: wrestlers averaged 4.9 ± 1.0 L for vital capacity and 4.1 ± 0.3 L for FEV$_1$. In comparison, average vital capacity for other athletes was 5.9 L for football (Wilmore & Haskell, 1972), 5.1 L for male marathon runners who had a FEV$_1$ of 84% of $\dot{V}C$ (Mahler et al., 1982), and 5.6 L for male speed skaters (Maksud et al., 1970). In wrestlers (Sharratt et al., 1986), the minute ventilation at peak $\dot{V}O_2$ was 132.5 ± 30 L·min^{-1} (BTPS) and the mean maximum voluntary ventilation measured for 12 s was 181 ± 27 L·min^{-1}; this latter value was similar to the 180 L·min^{-1} recorded for marathon runners (Mahler et al., 1982). The researchers (Rasch & Brandt, 1957; Sharratt et al., 1986) concluded that pulmonary volumes and functions of the wrestlers were greater than those of non-athletes but were average compared to other trained athletes.

At peak $\dot{V}O_2$, the average minute ventilation ranges from 129 ± 23 L·min^{-1} (BTPS) in elite adolescent wrestlers (Horswill et al., 1988) to 156.6 ± 26.5 L·min^{-1} in first-team members of the USA Olympic freestyle team (Nagle et al., 1975). In comparison, for maximum minute ventilation football players average 164 L·min^{-1} (Wilmore & Haskell, 1972), speed-skaters average 128 L·min^{-1} (Maksud et al., 1970), and marathon runners average 155 L·min^{-1} (Mahler et al., 1982). No statistical difference was seen in the maximal minute ventilation of members of the first team (156.6 ± 26.5 L·min^{-1}) and second team (140.3 ± 23.1 L.min-1) vying for an Olympic wrestling team (Nagle et al., 1975). Also, no difference existed between successful (155.7 ± 25.6 L·min^{-1}) and less successful (146.1 ± 22.5 L·min^{-1}) Junior World wrestlers (Silva et al., 1981). In contrast, we did find significant differences in maximal minute ventilation between elite (127 ± 25 L·min^{-1}) and non-elite (111 ± 23 L·min^{-1}) junior wrestlers of similar size (Horswill et al., 1989). Possibly, our subjects were more heterogeneous than the comparatively homogeneous subjects in previous studies (Nagle et al., 1975; Silva et al., 1981).

Hydration and Thermoregulation

Consequent to the rapid weight loss that wrestlers undergo to attain their goal body weights, most methods employed to reduce body weight will affect hydration status, plasma electrolyte concentrations, and possibly the thermoregulatory capacity of the wrestler (Buschschluter, 1977; Short et al., 1983; Woods et al., 1988; Steen & Brownell, 1990; Weissinger et al., 1991). The extent to which these changes affect wrestling performance is unclear. Collegiate and international wrestlers have up to 20 h between the weigh-in and tournament competition; for collegiate dual meet competition, wrestlers have 5 h. In collegiate tournaments, the rapid increases in body weights between the official weigh-ins and the wrestling matchs—an average of 4.8% or 3.2 kg for collegiate wrestlers (Dick et al., 1992; Horswill et al., 1992b)—confirm that wrestlers attempt to rehydrate. The scholastic wrestler, however, usually has only 30–60 min between weigh-in and dual meet competition; therefore, electrolyte losses and dehydration may be causes of fatigue in the younger wrestler. Furthermore, because boys have higher rectal temperatures than do men for the same degree of dehydration (Bar-Or et al., 1980), young wrestlers who dehydrate for competition may be more susceptible to heat illness than older wrestlers.

Mnatzakanian and Vaccaro (1984) found that dehydration in collegiate wrestlers increased serum concentrations of sodium (from 136 to 139 mEq·L^{-1}) and potassium (from 4.4 to 5.3 mEq·L^{-1}), increased hematocrit (from 44 to 47%), and decreased plasma volume (-5.7%). Also, in collegiate wrestlers, a 4% reduction in body weight by acute dehydration led to a decrease in urinary sodium from 132 to 64 mEq·L^{-1} and an increase in the specific gravity of urine from 1.026 to 1.031 g·mL^{-1}. After 5 h of rehydration, during which an average of 1.8 kg were gained (for a net loss of 1.2% of original weight), all hematologic and urinary values returned to normal levels (Mnatzakanian & Vaccaro, 1984).

A minimum duration of 5 h for recovery between the weigh-in and dual meet competition is typical for the collegiate wrestler, compared to only 1 h for scholastic wrestlers. Other studies of collegiate (Vaccaro et al., 1976) and scholastic wrestlers (Zambraski et al., 1975) did not show a reversal of indices of dehydration between the weigh-in and competition (Table 4-7). Despite the physiological evidence, many wrestlers are convinced that they can recover (rehydrate) during the limited time between the weigh-in and the match.

No wrestling-specific research has been conducted on how rapid weight loss affects thermoregulation. In other types of athletes, dehydration decreases blood flow to the skin (Claremont et al., 1976) and muscles

TABLE 4-7. *Weight fluctuations, recovery time, and physiologic perturbations.*

Weight Loss (%)* Initial	Final	Recovery Time	Physiologic Perturbation
4.3	2.6	0.5-1 h†	Exercise heart rate (EHR): ↑ 9%; stroke volume (SV): ↓ 16%; plasma volume (PV): ↓ 4.9%; complete recovery of EHR, SV, PV. (Allen et al., 1977)
9	N.A.	2.5-5 h§	Urinary variables: specific gravity: ↑ 0.4%; K$^+$: ↑ 189%; Na$^+$: ↓ 18%; osmolarity: ↓ 22%; incomplete recovery of all. (Zambraski et al., 1975)
4.7	2.0	5 h**	EHR: ↑ 13%; complete recovery (Ribisl & Herbert, 1970)
6.8	N.A.	5 h	EHR: ↑ 15%; SV: ↓ 21%; (a-v)O$_2$: ↑ 12%; blood pressure: no change; complete recovery of all. (Sproles et al., 1976)
4.0	2.0	5 h	PV: ↓ 17%; incomplete recovery of PV. (Vaccaro et al., 1976)
8.0	4.7	3 h‡	Muscle glycogen: ↓ 46%; incomplete recovery of glycogen. (Houston et al., 1981)

*Initial weight loss was recorded at time of weigh-in; final weight loss after recovery but prior to physiologic testing.
†Period between weigh-in and competition for interscholastic dual meet.
§Approximate period between weigh-in and competition for interscholastic tournament.
**Period between weigh-in and competition for collegiate dual meet.
‡Senior level competitors.
Presently, weigh-ins for college and international tournaments are held one day before competition; no research is available on physiologic recovery for this 20-h period.

(Horstman & Horvath, 1973). Consequently, the sweating threshold is raised, maximal sweat rate is decreased (Sawka et al., 1983), temperature regulation is compromised, and the deep body (core) temperature of the athlete is raised (Claremont et al., 1975). Because wrestlers may not be fully rehydrated by the time they compete (Costill & Sparks, 1973; Vaccaro et al., 1976; Zambraski et al., 1975), the ability to regulate body temperature and dissipate heat might be compromised. Wrestlers who dehydrate to make weight might be at increased risk for heat illnesses (heat exhaustion or heat stroke) during training and competition; however, there are no reports to confirm this risk. Whether impaired thermoregulation limits the wrestler's ability to perform on the mat is not known.

Body Composition and Physical Strength

Strength and power discrepancies that might otherwise occur among wrestling opponents are somewhat limited by the specific body weight requirements. Nevertheless, wrestlers devote significant amounts of time to resistance training to increase relative strength. Isokinetic strength of the shoulders of scholastic wrestlers increases across age (Housh et al., 1989, 1990) and, when corrected for body weight, the shoulder strength measurements exceed those of other athletes and non-athletes (Housh et al., 1990). The strength increases appear to be due to increases in lean tissue mass and possibly to superior ability to recruit muscle fibers (Housh et al., 1989). Neural factors may account for strength increases during the season (Clarke et al., 1984; Freischlag, 1984; Song and Garvie, 1984), whereas increases in muscle mass (measured as an increase in lean body mass) may account for strength increases in the off-season (Kelly et al., 1978; Roemmich et al., 1991). As a wrestler attempts to maintain or reduce body weight during the season, the absence of an increase in anaerobic arm power (Park et al., 1990; Roemmich et al., 1991) and selected measures of strength (Kelly et al., 1978; Rasch et al., 1961a), or a decrease in strength (Kelly et al., 1978; Roemmich et al., 1991) despite rigorous training, may coincide with a stable or declining lean body mass (Kelly et al., 1978; Park et al., 1990; Roemmich et al., 1991; Widerman & Hagen, 1982).

The type of training used by wrestlers during the season may affect strength. Because combinations of training are used (i.e., wrestling, endurance training, and resistance training), it is not possible to determine the training effects of wrestling per se on the development of power and strength. In the past, most wrestlers have been reluctant to undertake resistance training during the season because of time constraints and the weight gain associated with muscle hypertrophy. Concerned that strength may be lost during the season, most coaches now encourage resistance training to continue in-season, but at an attenuated intensity to emphasize muscular endurance (e.g., by lifting light weights for many repetitions). On the other hand, because of perceptions that low-intensity resistance training and wrestling against a partner of equal size violate the progressive overload principle of strength training, some wrestlers have chosen to resistance train at a high intensity throughout the season. Although this may be beneficial to strength and power development, simultaneous muscle hypertrophy may occur and complicate body weight control needed to make weight.

Nutrition and Weight Loss

Faced with having to make a specific weight class, most wrestlers desire to minimize total body weight, which is optimally accomplished by reducing body fat and maintaining muscle mass. Because most wrestlers are fairly lean before the season begins (Tipton & Oppliger, 1984), weight loss ultimately affects some of the non-fat tissues of the body (body water and glycogen stores). The struggle that wrestlers face in having to make weight presents an interesting model for examining the effects of nutritional manipulation on physical performance.

Numerous studies (Ahlman & Karvonen, 1961; Bock et al., 1967; Fogelholm et al., 1993; Horswill et al., 1990a; Houston et al., 1981; Jacobs, 1980; Kelly et al., 1978; Klinzing & Karpowicz, 1986; Serfass et al., 1984; Singer & Weiss, 1968; Tuttle, 1943; Webster et al., 1990; Widerman & Hagen, 1982) have examined the effects of rapid weight loss on physical performance of wrestlers. Contrary to intuition, most studies show no statistically significant effects of dehydration on performance of intense exercise lasting less than 30 s (Fogelholm et al., 1993; Houston et al., 1981; Jacobs, 1980; Serfass et al., 1984; Singer & Weiss, 1968; Tuttle, 1943; Widerman & Hagen, 1982) or on peak $\dot{V}O_2$ (Bock et al., 1967; Kelly et al., 1978; Houston et al., 1981). A plausible reason for the failure of weight loss to adversely affect high-intensity exercise performance is that during such efforts the muscle is relatively independent of blood-borne nutrients such as glucose or oxygen. Consistent with this hypothesis is the finding of normal stores of ATP and phosphocreatine in muscle, even when glycogen has been severely reduced (Houston et al., 1981). Coupled with the ability of myoglobin to provide a limited source of oxygen, these results suggest that a dehydration-induced reduction in oxygen delivery may not be a limitation for brief exertion. Also, it appears that the motor unit in the dehydrated state can still "fire" when recruited, despite imbalances in the electrolyte and water content of the tissues (Costill et al., 1976).

The absence of change in peak $\dot{V}O_2$ after rapid weight loss may be due to the expression of $\dot{V}O_2$ relative to body weight; any reduction in absolute $\dot{V}O_2$ may be masked by the decrease in body weight. As previously recommended (Horswill, 1993), the power output at which peak $\dot{V}O_2$ is achieved should be compared before and after weight loss to determine the impact of weight loss on aerobic performance.

In contrast to brief explosive performance or peak $\dot{V}O_2$, sustained or repeated near-maximal efforts lasting more than 30 s (Horswill et al., 1990a; Klinzing & Karpowicz, 1986; Webster et al., 1990) and prolonged, aerobic efforts (Caldwell et al., 1984; Herbert & Ribisl, 1972; Herbert et al., 1977) seem to be diminished after rapid weight loss in the wrestler. Reduced muscle blood flow in the dehydrated state may slow nutrient exchange, waste removal, and heat dissipation from the muscle during the relaxation period between contractions and thereby impede the muscle's ability to recover. Also, with rapid weight loss of up to 8% of body weight, wrestlers may experience a 46% reduction in muscle glycogen (Houston et al., 1981), which could adversely affect sustained efforts. Finally, the buffering capacity of the muscle and blood may be compromised after rapid weight loss. In previous research (Horswill et al., 1990a), the blood base excess at rest was significantly lower after weight loss. The reduced buffering capacity was dependent upon the type of diet used during weight loss; a high-carbohydrate diet tended to preserve blood base excess. In summary, the weight-reduced wrestler may be unable to recover completely after a flurry of high-power efforts, and subsequent physical performance may be diminished.

Complete rehydration and replenishment of muscle glycogen are thought to occur in 20 h in some athletes (Coyle & Coyle, 1993; Sherman et al., 1983). Therefore, in the international and USA collegiate tournaments, wrestlers may recover adequately. A recent recommendation for maximizing the speed of replenishing muscle glycogen is to consume approximately 50 g of carbohydrate (e.g., the amount in approximately two bananas or in 480 mL [16 oz] of orange juice) every two hours for 20 h (Coyle & Coyle, 1993). The data for this recommendation come from research on athletes in other sports, but the information should presumably also apply to the wrestler, especially since dehydration equivalent to a 5% loss of body weight apparently does not impair glycogen synthesis (Neufer et al., 1991). However, for the USA scholastic or collegiate wrestler who has dehydrated and reduced muscle glycogen to make weight, the 1-5 h duration between the weigh-in and dual meet competition may not be sufficient for complete rehydration and restoration of glycogen stores (Houston et al., 1981; Vaccaro et al., 1976; Zambraski et al., 1976). For these reasons, wrestlers are warned not to lose weight rapidly (American College of Sports Medicine, 1976; Committee on Medical Aspects of Sports, 1967).

Other Factors

Little information exists on how wrestling effectiveness is influenced by biomechanical and psychological factors. Anecdotally, most wrestling coaches would agree that, regardless of the strength, power, or endurance of an athlete, the level of technical skill development is the greatest determinant of success in wrestling competition. Consequently, the vast majority of time in training and supervised practices is spent learning new techniques, drilling, refining familiar skills, and wrestling live (100% effort). How motor learning and skill execution are affected by weight loss or physiological limitations (e.g., diminished strength) is not known.

The psychological factors that limit a wrestler's performance are very complex and should be addressed in conjunction with physiological and nutritional factors. Consistent with this contention is the fact that the profile of mood states (POMS) has been shown to differ between successful and less successful wrestlers at the elite level (Nagle et al., 1975). Also in wrestlers, experimental weight loss of approximately 6.2% of body weight in 4 d increased the POMS ratings of tension, anger, fatigue, depression, and confusion, whereas vigor was reduced (Figure 4-2) (Horswill et al., 1990a). Despite the dramatic shift in moods, the total work performed during sprint intervals of intermittent arm crank ergometry was reduced by only 4% of the capacity before weight loss (Horswill et al., 1990a). As discussed previously (Horswill, 1993), the POMS profile may be affected negatively by weight loss, but other research indicates that weight loss in wrestlers may increase mental concentration (Morgan, 1970), which could enhance the ability to perform. Also, many wrestlers

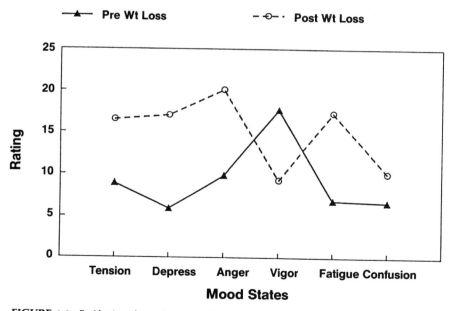

FIGURE 4-2. *Profile of mood states before (Pre Wt Loss) and after (Post Wt Loss) weight reduction in college wrestlers (n=12). Each value represents the mean obtained for two diet treatments (Horswill et al., 1990a). The mood state known as depression is abbreviated Depress.*

subjectively feel that weight loss increases their aggressiveness (Steen & McKinney, 1986). Finally, wrestling produces high levels of pre-competition anxiety (Morgan & Hammer, 1974). The anxiety can have either a positive or negative effect on performance, depending on how the wrestler handles the stress.

BRIEF HISTORY OF TRAINING AND NUTRITIONAL PRACTICES

Training

Over the course of time, the amount of daily training by wrestlers has probably increased, whereas the duration of wrestling matches has been shortened. International matches have ranged from unlimited time in the ancient Olympics to 15-min bouts in the 1950s to 9-min bouts in the 1970s. In 1979, the international governing body of wrestling, Fédération Internationale de Lutte Amateur (FILA), shortened the match duration to 6 min (two 3-min periods separate by a 1-min rest period). FILA justified dropping the third period (last 3 min) because research showed that scoring activity was less frequent during this period; the third period was abolished to make the sport more exciting to spectators. Additional reasons may have played a role; research also showed that the majority of scoring in the third period was achieved by wrestlers from Western countries (e.g., USA and Canada) and, in the matches where such a wrestler defeated a wrestler from an Eastern block country, victory was most likely the result of scores awarded to the Western wrestler during the third period (Sharratt, 1984). Presently, international matches are 5 min long.

Likewise, college matches have been shortened from 10 min in the 1930s to 7 min in the 1990s. Recent restrictions set by the National Collegiate Athletic Association (NCAA—the governing body of collegiate wrestling in the USA) limit supervised practices (i.e., with the head coach or assistant coaches present) to 20 h per week. However, there is no limit on supervised practices for the international wrestler or unsupervised training for the collegiate wrestler.

Regarding the quality of training, a review of research conducted in the 1940s (Rasch & Kroll, 1964b) revealed that scholastic coaches stressed strength training, whereas collegiate coaches emphasized overall conditioning. In general, the college programs compared to the scholastic program included more aerobic conditioning such as running (Rasch & Kroll, 1964b). There are several reasons for this difference. First, in contrast to high schools, most colleges have indoor tracks, which allow athletes in winter sports (e.g., wrestling) to run indoors. Second, college wrestlers appear to practice greater reductions in body weight than do scholastic wrestlers (Steen & Brownell, 1990). Running is used to increase energy expenditure to reduce body fat for long-term weight loss and to increase body heat and sweating for short-term weight loss. Finally, collegiate athletes are likely have more time for supplemental training than do scholastic athletes.

In the early 1970s, the daily amount of training by most USA wrestlers increased due to the exposure and success of the USA Olympic freestyle team and, in particular, 1972 team member Dan Gable. Gable's tireless efforts of wearing down opponents on the mat catapulted continuous, intense wrestling and running as primary methods of conditioning for competition. Presently, while the importance of endurance training is still recognized, the amount of time spent strength training has also increased. Advancements and proliferation of strength-training equipment, the education of coaches as to the importance of muscular strength in performance and injury prevention, the development of strength-training programs by strength-training coaches at the college level, and the shortening of the match duration in collegiate and international wrestling have all probably contributed to an increased emphasis on strength training. Also, because wrestlers often search for additional means of enhancing performance, intense resistance training, particularly during the competitive season, has become a viable option.

Nutrition

The primary nutritional concern of wrestlers is weight reduction for the purpose of being eligible to compete. According to the Committee on Medical Aspects of Sports (1967), the practice of weight loss in wrestlers was first identified in 1930 by H.E. Kenney who noted that the advent of the problem corresponded to the introduction of wrestling as a collegiate sport, around 1903. Methods used to lose weight in wrestlers are categorized in Table 4-8.

The associations governing wrestling at the scholastic and collegiate levels in the USA have attempted legislation to minimize drastic weight reduction by the athletes. Efforts to block drastic weight loss span the late 1960s to the present day (Clark et al., 1993; Tipton et al., 1969) and include the following: 1) weight certification is required for scholastic wrestlers, i.e., a wrestler certifies at one weight class, must wrestle a specific number of times at this weight, and cannot compete at a weight class below the one at which he is certified; 2) the weight classifications were changed (collegiate and scholastic) or supplemented with additional weight classes (scholastic); 3) an allowance for a certain amount of body growth during the season beyond the initial weight class was instituted (scholastic); 4) an early-season allowance was provided for excess body weight while the wrestler slowly lost weight (collegiate); 5) the weigh-in was scheduled the night before tournament competition (collegiate and, in some states, at the scholastic level); 6) standards for minimum wrestling

TABLE 4-8. *Methods of weight loss used by wrestlers*

Method	Example	Compartment of Weight Loss
Negative energy balance		Body cell mass
↑ Energy output	Aerobic training	
↓ Energy intake	Diet, fasting	
Dehydration		Body water
Metabolic	Exercise	
Thermal	Sauna, sweat suit	
Diuresis	High-protein diet, diuretics	
bloodletting		
Purging	Laxatives, vomiting	Gastrointestinal
Other	Haircut	Body cell mass
	Inversion*	Unknown

*Used in the waning moments of a weigh-in, the wrestler stands on his head to redistribute blood and body fluids, which some wrestlers believe affects the scale reading. In reality, the wrestler repositions his body on the scale platform, sometimes at a site that registers a weight slightly lower than that registered prior to inversion.

weight based upon body composition measurement were implemented (scholastic); and 7) educational programs were developed to discourage rapid weight reduction and encourage proper dietary habits. Despite all of these efforts, rapid weight reduction continues among wrestlers.

CONTEMPORARY TRAINING AND NUTRITIONAL PRACTICES

Research-Based Practices

Selection of Athletes. As previously reviewed (Horswill, 1992a), several studies have attempted to develop a comprehensive model for profiling the elite wrestler. Using physiological attributes alone, 45–58% of the variance in success could be accounted for by measures of strength, peak $\dot{V}O_2$ (or maximal minute ventilation), dynamic muscular endurance, and body fat (Nagle et al., 1975; Silva et al., 1981; Stine et al., 1979). Success was defined as those who made the final team for international competition (Nagle et al., 1975; Silva et al., 1981) or those who placed in the USA collegiate national tournament (Stine et al., 1979). A greater portion (79–85%) of the variance in success could be accounted for by combining psychological (profile of mood states) and physiological variables (Nagle et al., 1975; Silva et al., 1981). None of the models has been applied to the actual selection processes perhaps because the investigations were limited in sample size and performance tests (Silva et al., 1981; Stine et al., 1979). The feasibility of such a selection process is also limited by the cost and time associated with the physiological and psychological testing, particularly when the coach realizes that the prediction is not 100% accurate. However, because the top USA wrestlers are now subsidized by USA

Wrestling (USAW), the governing body for international teams from the USA, USAW has considered establishing objective standards of fitness that the salaried athletes must meet. Nevertheless, no physiological or psychological testing has yet been implemented.

Training and Assessment of Progress. No research has been done to systematically evaluate the best method or seasonal plan for training for wrestling. Several studies have evaluated the physiological responses of wrestlers across a season of competition. Testing has included peak $\dot{V}O_2$ (on the treadmill), strength, anaerobic power, and body composition measures (Herbert et al., 1977; Kelly et al., 1978; Park et al., 1990; Roemmich et al., 1991; Shavers, 1974; Song & Garvie, 1984). Positive changes such as increased peak $\dot{V}O_2$, increased strength, and decreased body fat were observed by some researchers (Herbert et al., 1977; Shavers, 1974; Song & Garvie, 1984) (Table 4-9). In contrast, others report no changes in the same variables (Kelly et al., 1978; Park et al., 1990; Roemmich et al., 1991). In those studies in which there is an absence of improvement in the wrestler's fitness following training, the results may be confounded because 1) the wrestlers were already highly trained when tested in the preseason (Kelly et al., 1978) or 2) there were concurrent decreases in body

TABLE 4-9. *Fitness characteristics (means) showing change ($P<0.05$) after training in wrestlers*

Time Interval	Fitness Change	Comment
Pre- to post-season (Clarke et al., 1984)	↑ 17% leg press ↑ 50% arm endurance	No change in weight, skinfolds, or peak $\dot{V}O_2$
Pre- season to next pre-season (Housh et al., 1988)	↑ 21% forearm flexion ↑ 30% forearm extension	↑ weight; ↓ % body fat
Pre- to peak season (Kelly et al., 1978)	↑ 36% muscle endurance ↓ 19% shoulder press (30°/s)	No change in weight, peak $\dot{V}O_2$, or % body fat
Pre- to post-season (Shavers, 1974)	↓ 16% resting heart rate ↓ 3% resting systolic blood pressure ↓ 8% postexercise systolic pressure	No change in diastolic blood pressure; weight and % body fat not reported
Pre- to post-season (Song & Cipriano, 1984)	↑ 11% peak $\dot{V}O_2$ ↑ 4% anaerobic capacity ↑ 3% elbow flexion ↑ 9% trunk extension	↓ body weight and fat-free mass ↑ neck strength
Pre- to peak season (Freischlag, 1984)	↑ 12% grip strength	↓ body weight and % body fat

Endurance was maximal number of repetitions; anaerobic capacity test was 40 s of leg ergometry.

weight, specifically the fat-free weight, that may have offset improvements in fitness variables (Park et al., 1990; Roemmich et al., 1991).

Training varies widely across different weight classes of wrestlers of similar ability. In an unpublished examination of cross-sectional data, we observed a negative correlation ($r = -0.6$, $P<0.05$) between peak $\dot{V}O_2$ (in $mL\cdot kg^{-1}\cdot min^{-1}$) for leg ergometry and body weight of Olympic-level wrestlers (Horswill et al., 1992c). Lightweight wrestlers practice weight reduction to a greater extent than do heavier wrestlers (Freischlag, 1984; Tcheng & Tipton, 1973; Tipton & Tcheng, 1970) and may use more aerobic training as a part of their weight reduction. Whether aerobic training is the most effective use of the lightweight wrestler's training time is open to question; aerobic training may increase endurance and assist in weight loss but restrict simultaneous strength and power development (Dudley & Djmali, 1985, 1987). The most effective training, both in quality and quantity, has yet to be determined for wrestling.

Nutrition and Hydration. Presently, little information is available on the effects of different nutritional practices on the wrestler's recovery of nutrient and fluid balance between the time of the weigh-in and competition. Research has indicated that during a 1-5 h replenishment period, plasma glucose levels can be raised (Fielding et al., 1987; Foster et al., 1979), some muscle glycogen can be restored (Hultman et al., 1971; Ivy et al., 1988), and partial restoration of plasma volume can occur (Allen et al., 1977; Costill & Sparks, 1973), helping to reestablish normal cardiovascular dynamics in wrestlers (Allen et al., 1977). The strategy for nutritional recovery following the weigh-in could have profound implications for performance and on making weight again, especially in a two- or three-day tournament (for NCAA and international tournaments, the weigh-ins occur the afternoon or night before competition for each day that a wrestler advances in the tournament). In fact, the international governing body, FILA, has recently approved a one-time weigh-in for a two-day tournament at the international level. This rule change might encourage further weight reduction for competition in the Olympics and World Games because wrestlers would not need to make weight for the second-day weigh-in of a tournament as they are presently required to do.

Regardless of the approach that wrestlers take to recovering after the weigh-in, they have been encouraged to increase their carbohydrate consumption on a routine basis (Steen & McKinney, 1986). This recommendation is supported by experimental research. Total work performed during maximal-effort arm crank ergometry, which simulated wrestling, was found to be maintained when collegiate wrestlers consumed a high-carbohydrate diet (66% carbohydrate, 23% fat, and 11% protein) (Horswill et al., 1990a). In contrast, the same wrestlers showed a reduction in arm performance when fed a diet lower in carbohydrate (42% carbohydrate, 47% fat, and 11% protein) but equal in calories to the high-carbohydrate treatment. The amount of weight loss was constant for each wrestler during the two treatments (Horswill et al., 1990a).

Other studies support these findings (McMurray et al., 1991; Walberg et al., 1988). Wrestlers who consumed a hypocaloric, high-percentage carbohydrate diet (75% of total calories) for seven days maintained leg anaerobic power determined using a Wingate test after weight loss (3.2%), compared to teammates who had reduced anaerobic power after weight loss of a similar amount using a diet moderate in carbohydrate content (50%) (McMurray et al., 1991). In weightlifters, leg muscular endurance (ability to maintain force during a static contraction) was preserved after subjects consumed a hypocaloric, high-percentage carbohydrate diet (70% of total calories) and lost 4.9% of body weight (Walberg et al., 1988). In contrast, the weightlifters who consumed a diet of 50% carbohydrate demonstrated lowered endurance after reducing weight by a similar amount (4.5%) (Walberg et al., 1988).

The magnitude of weight loss in wrestlers during a brief period suggests that manipulating hydration status is a standard component of making weight. Cohen et al. (1987) reported that of a total weight reduction of 9% of body weight in elite scholastic wrestlers, the majority (6% reduction) is by dehydration just days prior to the weigh-in. Tipton and Tcheng (1970) found that in a period of about 17 d, scholastic wrestlers averaged a 4.9% weight loss and, for those wrestlers in weight classes of 65.8 kg or less, the average loss was at least 5%. In college wrestlers, a 3.6-kg loss in 2.5 d has been reported (Zambraski et al., 1976). Anecdotally, this degree of reduction has occurred in one day for college- and international-caliber wrestlers. In the case study of an international-caliber wrestler, an apparent reduction of 5% of body weight occurred one or two days before the weigh-in (Widerman & Hagen, 1982).

To discourage the practice of dehydration, evaluation of urine specific gravity has been suggested as a method of screening wrestlers (Hursh, 1979). In application, wrestlers would be evaluated at the weigh-in and disqualified if they appeared to have become dehydrated to make weight (Hursh, 1979). However, the wide variability of urine specific gravity, even among well-hydrated subjects (Zambraski et al., 1975), makes this an invalid and unfair test.

Tradition-Based Practices

Selection of Athletes. The selection of athletes for wrestling in the USA usually begins at the grass roots level. In many communities, children of both genders have the opportunity to participate in wrestling clubs. In time, those athletes who have success in competition are most likely to persevere in the sport and continue wrestling at the junior-high and high school level. Infrequently, high school coaches who have trouble finding a wrestler for a particular weight class may recruit a promising candidate because of the student's body build (mesomorphic), exceptional strength, or specific size. Most often, to be successful at the high school level the athlete will have had to enter the sport and assimilate the fundamental skills at an early age.

Selection of wrestlers at higher levels of competition (college and international) depends primarily upon on the individual's prior success. The high school record for state competition and performance on the national level (e.g., annual Junior National tournament) will determine whether a wrestler is invited to walk on or is offered an athletic scholarship to compete on a college team. Even then natural selection, i.e., competitive success and enthusiasm for participation, will play a role in determining those who remain in the sport. Ed Gallagher, the man often regarded as the father of college wrestling, included visual assessments of anthropometry and physiology in his recruitment of wrestlers to Oklahoma State University in the 1920s and 1930s (Dellinger, 1977). Gallagher preferred lean, lanky athletes to stocky, muscle-bound competitors, and he looked for wrestlers with low resting heart rates as a sign of endurance (Dellinger, 1977). Of course, previous wrestling success and the individual's work ethic also played a role in Gallagher's selection.

Wrestlers who have had very successful collegiate careers and were exposed to international style wrestling during their college careers might continue competing after college. Until recently, there was little incentive, aside from personal satisfaction, to do so. In 1989, USA Wrestling, the national governing body of the sport in the United States, began paying salaries to the top three USA wrestlers in each weight class in both styles (freestyle and Greco-Roman) of international wrestling. This change has resulted in more wrestlers continuing to compete after college. For example, in 1992 the USA had its first two two-time Olympic freestyle wrestling champions, and one individual became the USA's first wrestler ever to win three Olympic medals.

The final selection of who steps out on the mat to represent the team at each weight class of competition is almost always determined by a *wrestle-off*. Wrestling is one of the few sports in which coaches can take relief in using such an objective method to select the team. By creating a game-time atmosphere within the practice room, the coach allows wrestlers go head-to-head to determine who is the best competitor at each weight. Depending on the individual coach's philosophy, wrestle-offs may be held weekly throughout the season or only at specific times of the season. To decide the final team members for tournaments and major competitions, many coaches select the winners of two out of three wrestle-off matches.

Training and Assessment of Progress. Most of the training programs developed by coaches are based on years of personal experience and trial-and-error. Because most coaches were wrestlers, practice sessions and the season schedule tend to be structured in the same ways that the coaches participated as athletes. The general approach to training used by scholastic and collegiate wrestlers is found in Table 4-10. Supplemental training outside of wrestling per se includes specific resistance training exercises (Table 4-11), buddy exercises with a teammate of equal mass, running, cycling, and rope skipping.

The scholastic and collegiate seasons typically begin with instruction and learning of technical skills. The strategy most wrestling coaches use for teaching skills is identical to or a variation of that developed by USA Wrestling in the mid 1970s. USA Wrestling's concept is that the seven skills presented in Table 4-12 are the rudimentary techniques that all wrestlers must first learn (Combs, 1980). Once acquired, these fundamentals provide the basis for all specifics maneuvers used in wrestling. Initially, some fitness is required to perform the seven basic skills (Table 4-12); in fact, practicing the basic skills helps develop the necessary fitness. As the wrestler advances to the performance of specific maneuvers and live wrestling with a teammate, fitness requirements change to emphasize speed, strength, and power (Table 4-12). Ultimately, the wrestlers will need the muscular endurance and, to some extent, cardiovascular endurance to execute properly and continuously the maneuvers (and skills) in a dual meet match, in matches during a tournament, and in practices sessions lasting 1–3 h.

TABLE 4-10. *General plan for training scholastic and collegiate wrestlers* (Adapted from Jefferies, 1986).*

Pre-season:		
	3x/wk	resistance training (near-maximum resistance, few reps, several sets) to increase strength, power, and possibly muscle mass
	2–3x/wk	aerobic running or cycling for 20–30 min
Early season		
	5x/wk	technical skill training
	3x/wk	resistance training (as in the pre-season)
	3x/wk	aerobic running, cycling, and mat drills
Mid-season		
	2–3x/wk	technical skill training
	2–3x/wk	begin interval training using wrestling and running: short rest intervals to increase aerobic capacity
	2–3x/wk	continuous wrestling
	2–3x/wk	resistance training to maintain strength (1–2 sets)
Peak season		
	2x/wk	review technical skills
	2–3x/wk	continue interval training using wrestling and running: longer rest intervals to increase anaerobic capacity
	1–2x/wk	resistance training (1 set) to maintain strength
Post-season		
	2x/wk	introduce and develop new technical skills
	2–3x/wk	resistance training (as in the pre-season) to increase strength, power, and possibly muscle mass
	3x/wk	aerobic running, cycling, continuous wrestling, and other novel forms of exercise at a "relaxed" intensity

TABLE 4-11. *Resistance training exercises for developing strength and power in wrestlers*

Lift*	Muscles	Example of Use in Wrestling
Half squat	Quadriceps, gluteus maximus	Double leg lift
Leg extension	Quadriceps	Penetration
Leg flexion	Hamstring group	Leg grapevine (figure four)
Cleans	Quadriceps, deltoids, biceps brachia, trapezius	Almost all lifts
Sit-ups (Curls)	Abdominal group	General trunk support
Deadlifts	Erector spinae, gluteus maximus, quadriceps	Lifting from extending position
Upright rows	Biceps brachia, deltoids, trapezius	Pulling in a single leg
Bent rows	Latissimus dorsi, biceps brachia	Lifting opponent from mat, bear hug
Lat pulldowns	Latissimus dorsi, biceps brachia	Pulling in a single leg
Curls	Biceps brachia	Arm barring
Press	Deltoids, triceps	Pummeling (driving arms)
Neck		Bridging and high arch
Wrist curls	Forearm flexors and extensors	Grasping; locked hands

*Before performing any of these lifts, a wrestler must learn the proper technique to minimize the chances of injury. Also, all resistance training should be performed with a partner (spotter).

Most coaches use some form of interval training to promote the endurance essential for wrestling. One of the most common formats of interval training is to group wrestlers in a triad. While two wrestle, the third rests at the edge of the mat. At the end of the timed interval, wrestling stops, and one wrestler quickly rotates out for a rest while the refreshed wrestler steps on the mat to wrestle against a fatigued wrestler. Each athlete experiences each role (resting, refreshed, and fatigued) over the course of numerous intervals. A modification of this interval approach includes using groups of four for the rotations. In this case, one wrestler remains on the mat while three teammates rotate as sparring partners. For variety or to overcome certain weaknesses, the coach may start each interval with the wrestlers in specific positions or in hypothetical situations (e.g., one wrestler starts on his back, or the fatigued wrestler is behind in points and is given 1 min to score 4 points). To stress the first-team, varsity line-up, the coach may assign only the first-team varsity competitors to the mat for continuous wrestling, whereas the second- and third-string members rotate in the roles of resting and refreshed wrestlers. The rest periods between intervals are systematically modified each week to produce the desired adaptation (e.g., longer rest for anaerobic conditioning as the peak season approaches).

The most popular and practical form of live wrestling is to have athletes wrestle a match with a teammate. The match length may vary from an abbreviation of the official bout duration to a prolonged match that exceeds regulation time, depending on the coach's objective of training

TABLE 4-12. *The basic skills of wrestling and corresponding fitness requirements*

Basic Skills*	Initial Fitness†	Intermediate Fitness	Advanced Fitness
1. Posture or stance	Static (postural) endurance		
2. Motion	Balance, coordination		
3. Changing levels	Strength, flexibility	Speed	Muscular endurance
4. Penetration	Strength	Speed, power	Muscular endurance
5. Lift	Strength, balance	Power	Muscular endurance
6. Back step	Strength, flexibility, coordination	Power	Muscular endurance
7. High Arch	Strength, flexibility, coordination	Power	Muscular endurance

*Adapted from Combs, 1980.
†Initial Fitness characteristics are required to learn basic skills and can be enhanced by performing those skills. Intermediate Fitness characteristics are required, along with initial fitness, during live wrestling in practice. Advanced Fitness characteristics are required, along with initial and intermediate fitness, for competition.

the wrestler for intensity or endurance. A series of matches in the practice room may be employed for interval training.

Coaches have made only limited use of objective methods of assessing physiological progress. Some coaches may test for strength (e.g., 1 repetition maximum for a series of strength-training lifts) or endurance (the time for a standard run). Still, for the most part, subjective assessment is used, such as whether a wrestler appears to tire in the third period of a match. The most objective and detailed assessments taken across a season are the wrestler's win-loss record and individual statistics (e.g., the number of control points scored for takedowns, falls, and near falls). With such data, a coach can determine when the wrestler is scoring points (beginning or end of a match). The individual's statistics must be interpreted with a sense of the caliber of competition that the wrestler has met. Because the competition is fairly uniform for a team, the statistics are best for making comparisons within a team or for an individual across seasons.

Nutrition and Hydration. Despite our current understanding of sports nutrition, wrestling is a sport in which many nutritional myths still exist. For example, a notion has existed among some wrestlers that body fat could be broken down by avoiding water ingestion for one hour after training. Also, a misconception has persisted that wrestlers are fat in the pre-season and can afford large reductions in body weights. Recommendations for increasing carbohydrate consumption during heavy training are seldom practiced. Research indicates that USA collegiate wrestlers consumed about 45% of their total calories as carbohydrate during the season (Steen & McKinney, 1986). Scholastic wrestlers fared only slightly better, by consuming approximately 51% of their total calories as carbohydrate; however, in absolute terms, this amounted to only 3.4 $g \cdot kg^{-1} \cdot d^{-1}$ (Horswill et al., 1990b). Nevertheless, even during weight loss, it is possible for wrestlers to maintain a negative energy balance and still increase carbohydrate intake by decreasing the intake of fat (Fogelholm et al., 1993), which comprises roughly 35% of the daily energy consumed by wrestlers (Horswill et al., 1990b; Short & Short, 1983; Steen & McKinney, 1986).

Regarding other nutrients, USA collegiate and scholastic wrestlers consume an adequate amount of protein on a daily basis, i.e., about 1.0 $g \cdot kg^{-1}$ or 13–15% of the total calories, during the season (Horswill et al., 1990b; Steen & McKinney, 1986). Of the micronutrients, the wrestler's dietary intakes appear to be low for vitamin C, vitamin A, thiamin, niacin, riboflavin, iron, zinc, calcium, and magnesium (Short & Short, 1983; Steen & McKinney, 1986). Recent research (Fogelholm et al., 1993) shows that with relatively slow weight loss (5% of body weight over three weeks), the wrestler may be susceptible to diminished vitamin B_6 and magnesium status. Interestingly, when wrestlers lost the same amount rapidly (5% in

2.4 d), trends for diminished vitamin B_6 and magnesium status did not appear.

On one hand, it may be beneficial for the wrestler to take a multivitamin supplement to ensure meeting the RDA for the limited nutrients. Such practice has been recommended previously (Henson, 1971) to guarantee adequate amounts of the B vitamins and thereby help optimize fat metabolism for weight loss. Furthermore, particularly in light of recent research showing the value that vitamin C and vitamin A serve as antioxidants, vitamin and mineral supplements have a plausible role in preventing overtraining (Panel Discussion, 1993).

On the other hand, a wrestler in the dehydrated state might be at increased risk for side effects if megadoses of vitamins are ingested (e.g., kidney stones formed from calcium oxalate, the oxalate being derived from vitamin C [Baker et al., 1966]). Presently, there are no data to support the encouragement or discouragement of micronutrient supplementation in wrestlers.

Contrary to all recommendations, wrestlers restrict fluid intake as a technique for rapid weight loss. Although dehydration is usually delayed until 1–2 d before the weigh-in, many wrestlers will slowly decrease fluid intake during the week preceding the weigh-in. Dehydration makes for uncomfortable practice sessions and poor training efforts because of the intolerance to the hot temperature (often in excess of 32° C) in the wrestling room and intolerance to fatigue associated with reduced body water and plasma volume. Immediately following the weigh-in, fluids are rapidly replenished; carbohydrate-electrolyte solutions are quite popular for this purpose (Short & Short, 1983). It is common for a USA college wrestler to drink almost a full gallon within 5 h of the weigh-in. Despite warnings that rapid weight loss has ill effects on performance and despite the evidence that some forms of performance show measurable decrements (discussed earlier), we have not been able to detect a relationship, negative or positive, between rapid weight fluctuation and performance on the mat (Horswill et al., 1992b). In fact, a recent preliminary report revealed a positive correlation ($r = 0.7$) between the percentage weight loss and the season record (wins as a percentage of total matches) in 23 collegiate wrestlers (Reimers et al., 1993).

The meal that receives the most attention by wrestlers is the prematch meal. In the 1920s and 1930s Ed Gallagher realized the importance of sugar as a fuel and encouraged his wrestlers to keep carbohydrate in the diet (Dellinger, 1977). However, pre-event meals for wrestlers have usually consisted of foods such as steak, eggs, and salad, and been devoid of foods high in carbohydrate. Even with the explosion of information on sports nutrition in the mid 1970s, wrestlers apparently have not begun eating high-carbohydrate foods between the weigh-in and competition (Steen & McKinney, 1986; Wolf et al., 1979). However, dietary practices may vary for different teams, and with limited data (Horswill et al., 1990b; Short & Short, 1983; Steen & McKinney, 1986), it is obviously impossible to conclude that no wrestlers emphasize carbohydrates in the prematch meal.

The coach's subjective assessment of a wrestler's poor performance in a match, e.g., noticeable fatigue, windedness, and an inability to score or be aggressive in the third period, should lead the coach to investigate the wrestler's dietary practices. More often than not, the coach mistakes this type of performance as being out-of-shape rather than out of fuel and fluid. Some coaches use preseason assessments of body fat percentages to project minimal weights for their wrestlers. In Wisconsin, minimal weight class determinations using body composition assessments independent of the coach's measurements are required of scholastic wrestlers (see Figure 4-3 for flow chart of the program); several other states are experimenting with this approach.

Along with the assessment of minimal weight class, nutritional information for weight loss and match preparation may be provided hopefully, to help minimize drastic weight loss among wrestlers. Programs that offer nutritional education may also help minimize the incidence of eating disorders among wrestlers. Such disorders are uncommon among most male athletes, but wrestlers appear to make up a large portion of those presenting eating abnormalities (Enns et al., 1987; Lakin et al., 1990). Between 2% and 4% of wrestlers may exhibit the classic criteria for bulimia (Enns et al., 1987; Oppliger et al., 1993), and up to 45% present one or more behaviors associated with this disorder (Oppliger et al., 1993). It is unresolved as to whether eating disorders continue to plague the wrestler after the conclusion of a season or career.

As the level of awareness grows among coaches and as incentives are created for continued education of coaches, more coaches will apply sports nutrition and sports medicine knowledge in the preparation of their athletes. Table 4-13 summarizes various programs that offer continuing education in sports medicine for the wrestling coach. It could be argued that those coaches who apply the latest information in sport science are likely to also be successful on a win-loss basis.

OVERTRAINING

No published research is available on overtraining in wrestling. Yet, wrestlers are probably susceptible to overtraining for the following reasons: 1) wrestlers train rigorously, and the season for scholastic and collegiate wrestling is longer than for most other sports (with international competition, wrestlers often train year-round); 2) wrestlers may be misinformed as to how much and what type of training is needed to achieve peak performance; 3) because wrestlers must repeatedly make weight,

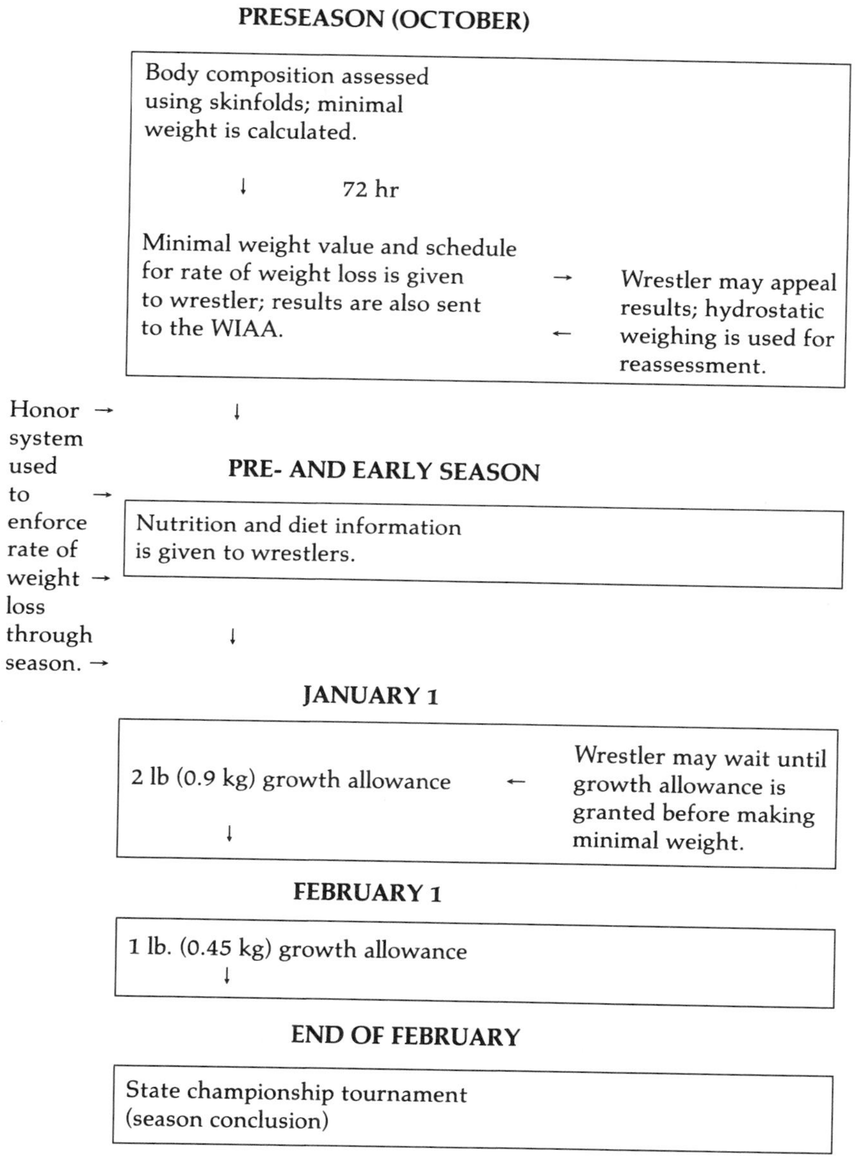

PRESEASON (OCTOBER)

Body composition assessed
using skinfolds; minimal
weight is calculated.

↓   72 hr

Minimal weight value and schedule
for rate of weight loss is given   →   Wrestler may appeal
to wrestler; results are also sent   results; hydrostatic
to the WIAA.   ←   weighing is used for
                                           reassessment.

Honor →   ↓
system
used   **PRE- AND EARLY SEASON**
to   →
enforce   Nutrition and diet information
rate of   is given to wrestlers.
weight →
loss
through   ↓
season. →

JANUARY 1

2 lb (0.9 kg) growth allowance   ←   Wrestler may wait until
                                      growth allowance is
         ↓   granted before making
                                      minimal weight.

FEBRUARY 1

1 lb. (0.45 kg) growth allowance
         ↓

END OF FEBRUARY

State championship tournament
(season conclusion)

FIGURE 4-3. *Flow chart of the minimal weight program required by the Wisconsin Interscholastic Athletic Association (WIAA) for scholastic wrestlers.*

TABLE 4-13. *Programs of continuing education for the wrestling coach**

Program	Description and comments
American Coaching Effectiveness Program (ACEP)	Progressive levels offered; required by USA Wrestling to coach international teams; originally designed for the club or youth coach.
Athletic Health Care System	Designed for the scholastic coach; general program.
BASIC	Designed for club or youth coach; emphasizes injury prevention.
CAPS	Designed for club or youth coach.
Coach Effectiveness Training Program	Designed for club or youth coach.
National Youth Sport Coaches Association	Designed for club or youth coach.
Program for Athletic Coaches' Education (PACE)	Designed for scholastic coach.

*Some states require scholastic coaches to have teaching certificates to coach; however, depending on the state high school association, certification may be waived if one of the programs listed above is completed.

they do not take time off, or taper, during the season; and 4) because of diet restrictions for making weight, wrestlers may suffer from the depletion of carbohydrate or other critical nutrients. Carbohydrate depletion may be both a cause as well as a symptom of overtraining (Costill et al., 1988).

Plausible evidence of overtraining in wrestlers can be drawn from the literature. In wrestlers studied at the end of a competitive season, initial muscle glycogen levels averaged 62 mmol·kg^{-1} wet weight of muscle (Houston et al., 1981). This concentration, which represented baseline levels before the experimental procedures, was extremely low compared to baseline concentrations reported for other athletes (Costill et al., 1988; Kirwan et al., 1988; Sherman et al., 1983), suggesting that wrestlers experience chronic muscle glycogen depletion over the course of the season.

During the season, a loss of fat-free mass (FFM) has been reported in high school wrestlers (Freischlag, 1984; Park et al., 1990; Roemmich et al., 1991), in collegiate wrestlers (Song & Cipriano, 1984; Strauss et al., 1985), and in an international wrestler (Widerman & Hagen, 1982). Loss of FFM might coincide with a fall in the wrestler's serum testosterone or insulin-like-growth-factor-1, which may decrease due to a restricted diet (McMurray et al., 1991; Strauss et al., 1985) or possibly to overtraining.

Further evidence for diminished protein nutritional status that could be related to overtraining includes decreased concentrations of two plasma proteins, thyroxin-binding prealbumin and retinol-binding protein, in scholastic wrestlers (Horswill et al., 1990b) whose dietary habits were fairly consistent with the recommendations of the American College of Sports Medicine (1976).

Wrestlers do not appear to suffer a greater number of illnesses during the season compared to non-wrestling controls (Freischlag, 1984) or compared to athletes competing in sports during the same season of the year (Strauss et al., 1988); however, more research is needed on how overtraining and weight loss might affect the wrestler's immune system.

Coaches must be better educated to avoid overtraining in their wrestlers. When the performance of a wrestler slips, the frustrated coach should not automatically assume that the problem is one of a lack of fitness that can only be cured by making practice sessions harder. Overtraining may occur in the hardest working, most dedicated athlete, not in the one who loafs. Longer and harder practices may simply exacerbate the problem.

To reduce the chances of overtraining, the coach should provide variety in practice, use some type of modified taper, have a definite but limited number of times to peak during the season, and provide information on proper nutrition. The coach who uses a training program that emphasizes periodization and peaking minimizes the chances of overtraining. Periodization helps the athlete focus on different aspects of fitness and performance as each aspect becomes most important during the season (e.g., starting the season by emphasizing training to increase peak oxygen uptake and muscular strength; developing the anaerobic capacity and muscular endurance in the middle of the season; and, finally, developing speed and refining technique while maintaining endurance at the end, or peak, of the season).

To treat the overtrained wrestler, the coach is best advised to reduce the training load. The coach might even change the activities used for training. The athlete could do some novel but mild training (swimming, water polo, cross-country skiing, cycling) during the recovery period. A complete break from all training is also plausible. The coach might also investigate and attempt to reduce the psychological stresses that the wrestler faces. Competitive anxiety and self-imposed pressure can be physically exhausting to the athlete and may contribute to the overtraining syndrome. A final, but less palatable solution, is to have the wrestler move up a weight class. Raising the wrestler's nutrient intake may be the most important step in avoiding and recovering from the overtraining syndrome.

DIRECTIONS FOR FUTURE RESEARCH

Future research on wrestling should include investigations of factors associated with elite performance and fatigue, such as the role of acid-base balance, hydration status, and muscle glycogen level. The interaction of aerobic and anaerobic energy systems during wrestling and during recovery between matches also should be characterized. Basic research should include examining the influence of wrestling, isolated from other types of training, on peripheral adaptations (anaerobic pathways of energy metabolism) and central adaptations (changes in left ventricle dimensions and changes in peak oxygen uptake of the upper and of the lower body).

A second general area for research is that of the influence of weight loss on the performance and health of the wrestler. Recommendations have been made for wrestlers who want to lose weight for competition (Table 4-14). Although the recommendations may minimize unhealthy weight loss in the wrestler, there is no sound evidence that the recommendations are effective in maintaining the wrestlers performance, normal growth rate, fat-free mass, and well-being. Perhaps more can be done to offer the elite Olympic competitor sound nutrition strategies and yet spare the young wrestler from detrimental dietary practices. In evaluating the weight loss-performance relationship, biomechanical and psychological factors should also be considered as a part of the performance measurement.

A final critical area for future research is that of identifying optimal training regimes for the sport. Most training programs have evolved from trial-and-error rather than from a scientific basis. While the methods may be effective, slight modifications or even total alterations in training patterns could improve preparation for competition and increase the likelihood of success. The incidence, cause, and prevention of overtraining, a potential problem faced by all wrestlers, must be examined as well.

SUMMARY

The descriptive data available on the physiology and nutrition of wrestling demonstrate that power, strength, and muscular endurance relative to body weight are important factors in success. Descriptive information is important and must be frequently collected and analyzed to gain an understanding of how these fitness characteristics change in elite wrestlers across eras and with modifications in the bout duration and scoring system. However, the emphasis of future research on wrestling should be on addressing the effectiveness of training protocols and the extent to which weight loss and nutritional practices affect wrestling ability and success. The concern over the nutrition and dietary practices of wrestlers remains prominent, and procedures are being implemented to limit weight loss in scholastic wrestlers; yet no conclusive evidence exists that weight loss impairs wrestling performance in competitive settings. Until the coach and wrestler are convinced of any negative impact on wrestling performance, rapid weight loss to achieve a lower than normal

TABLE 4-14. *Recommendations for wrestlers who desire to lose weight for competition*

1. In the pre-season, estimate minimal weight as follows:
   a. determine % fat using a method developed specifically for wrestlers (e.g., skinfold equation); calculate fat-free mass (FFM).
   b. calculate minimal weight at 7% fat by dividing FFM by 0.93 for scholastic male wrestlers; collegiate and senior wrestlers can use 5% as minimum body fat (i.e., FFM/0.95).
   c. calculate the amount of weight that can be lost (i.e., the difference between present weight and minimal weight).
2. Begin weight loss early, before the competitive season begins, and progress slowly to optimize fat loss and minimize protein and water loss. The rate of weight loss should not exceed 1.0 kg (2 lb) per week.
3. To increase energy expenditure, train aerobically at least twice per week in the pre-season and early part of the competitive season.
4. Decrease daily energy intake by reducing dietary fat, protein, and carbohydrate; do not eliminate any one of these three. Consume:
   a. at least 1500 calories per day to prevent vitamin and mineral deficiencies.
   b. about 1.0 g protein·kg body weight^{-1}.
   c. at least 55% of daily calories as carbohydrate during weight loss in the early season; increase carbohydrate to 60–65% during peak competition.
5. To reduce caloric intake, use the following suggestions:
   a. avoid desserts, butter and margarine, sauces, gravy, and dressings.
   b. consume complex carbohydrates (fruits, vegetables, whole grain cereals and bread).
   c. to reduce fat, grill, bake, broil or boil food; do not fry.
6. To monitor loss of body water loss, record body weight before and after each practice session. Specifically:
   a. do not restrict water during intense training, especially in hot training environments.
   b. consume water, sports drinks, or other fluids to restore at least 80% of the weight lost in a practice session.
   c. drink fluids low in calories (e.g., skim milk rather than whole milk, diet soda rather than regular soda).
   d. avoid dehydrating; however, if dehydration must be used to make weight, attempt no more than 3–5% reduction for short periods (overnight) to minimize adverse effects.

Adapted from Tipton and Opplinger (1984).

body weight will most likely remain a major element of this sport. Finally, while substantial data exist on the physiologic profiles of successful wrestlers, a multi-disciplinary approach to profiling is needed to integrate technical performance and psychological factors with physiological measures and dietary manipulations to gain a more complete understanding of the science of wrestling.

BIBLIOGRAPHY

AAHPER (1971). *Nutrition for athletics: A handbook for coaches.* Washington, DC: American Association for Health, Physical Education, and Recreation, pp. 26.
Ahlman, K., and M.J. Karvonen (1961). Weight reduction by sweating in wrestlers, and its effects on physical fitness. *J. Sports Med.* 1:58–62.
Allen, T.E., D.P. Smith, and D.K. Miller (1977). Hemodynamic response to submaximal exercise after dehydration and rehydration in high school wrestlers. *Med. Sci. Sports* 9:159–163.
American College of Sports Medicine (1976). Position paper on weight loss in wrestlers. *Med. Sci. Sports* 8:xi–xiii.

Baker, E.M., J.C. Saari, and B.M. Talbert (1966). Ascorbic acid metabolism in man. *Am. J. Clin. Nutr.* 19:371–378.

Bar-Or, O. (1987). The Wingate anaerobic test: an update on methodology, reliability and validity. *Sports Med.* 4:381–394.

Bar-Or, O., R. Dotan, O. Inbar, A. Rotshtein, and H. Zonder (1980). Voluntary hypohydration in 10- to 12-year-old boys. *J. Appl. Physiol.* 48:104–108.

Bergh, U., A. Thortensson, B. Sjodin, B. Hulten, K. Piehl, et al. (1978). Maximal oxygen uptake and muscle fiber types in trained and untrained humans. *Med. Sci. Sports* 10:151–154.

Bock, W., E.L. Fox, and R. Bowers (1967). The effects of acute dehydration upon cardio-respiratory endurance. *J. Sports Med. Phys. Fit.* 7:67–72.

Buschschluter, S. (1977). Games blood-letting. *Swim. Tech.* 13:99.

Caldwell, J.E., E. Ahonen, and U. Nousiainen (1984). Differential effects of sauna-, diuretic-, and exercise-induced hypohydration. *J. Appl. Physiol.* 57:1018–1023.

Cisar, C.J., G.O. Johnson, A.C. Fry, T.J. Housh, R.A. Hughes, A.J. Ryan, and W.G. Thorland (1987). Preseason body composition, build, and strength as predictors of high school wrestling success. *J. Appl. Sport Sci. Res.* 1:66–70.

Claremont, A.D., F. Nagle, W.D. Reddan, and G.A. Brooks (1975). Comparison of metabolic, temperature, heart rate and ventilatory responses to exercise at extreme ambient temperatures (0 and 35 C). *Med. Sci. Sports* 7:150–154.

Claremont, A.D., D.L. Costill, W.J. Fink, and P. Van Handel (1976). Heat tolerance following diuretic induced dehydration. *Med. Sci. Sports* 8:239–243.

Clark, R.R., J.M. Kuta, J.C. Sullivan, W.M. Bedford, J.D. Penner, and E.A. Studesville (1993). A comparison of methods to predict minimal weight in high school wrestlers. *Med. Sci. Sports Exerc.* 25:151–158.

Clarke, D.H., P. Vaccaro, and N.M. Andersen (1984). Physiological alterations in 7- to 9-year-old boys following a season of competitive wrestling. *Res. Quart. Exerc. Sport* 55:318–322.

Cohen, C.R., H.D. Allen, J. Spain, G.R. Marx, R.W. Wolfe, and J.S. Harvey (1987). Cardiac structure and function of elite high school wrestlers. *American Journal of Diseases of Children* 141:576–581.

Cohen, J.L., and K.R. Segal (1985). Left ventricular hypertrophy in athletes: an exercise-echocardiographic study. *Med. Sci. Sports Exerc.* 17:695–700.

Combs, S. (1980). *Winning Wrestling.* Chicago: Contemporary Books, pp. 9–32.

Committee on Medical Aspects of Sports (1967). Wrestling and weight control. *J. Am. Med. Assoc.* 201:131–133.

Costill, D.L., and K.E. Sparks (1973). Rapid fluid replacement following thermal dehydration. *J. Appl. Physiol.* 34:299–303.

Costill, D.L., R. Cote, and W. Fink (1976). Muscle water and electrolytes following varied levels of dehydration in man. *J. Appl. Physiol.* 40:6–11.

Costill, D.L., M.G. Flynn, J.P. Kirwan, J.A. Houmard, J.B. Mitchell, R. Thomas, and S.H. Park (1988). Effects of repeated days of intensified training on muscle glycogen and swimming performance. *Med. Sci. Sports Exerc.* 20:249–254.

Coyle, E.F., and E. Coyle (1993). Carbohydrates that speed recovery from training. *Physician Sportsmed.* 21:111–123.

Daub, W.D., H.J. Green, M.E. Houston, J.A. Thomson, I.G. Fraser, and D.A. Ranney (1982). Cross-adaptive responses to different forms of leg training: skeletal muscle biochemistry and histochemistry. *Can. J. Physiol. Pharmacol.* 60:628–633.

Dawson, J.M., D.G. Gadian, and D.R. Wilkie (1978). Muscular fatigue investigated by phosphorus nuclear magnetic resonance. *Nature* 274:861–866.

de Garay, A.L., L. Levine, and J.E.L. Carter (1974). *Genetic and anthropological studies of Olympic athletes.* New York: Academic Press.

Dellinger, D. (1977). *The Story of Wrestling's Dynasty.* Stillwater, OK: Frontier Printers, pp. 18–19.

Dick, R., C.A. Horswill, and J.R. Scott (1992). Acute weight gain in wrestlers at the NCAA championships (Abstract). *Med. Sci. Sports Exerc.* 24:S52.

DiPrampero, P.E., F.P. Limas, and G. Sassi (1970). Maximal muscular power, aerobic and anaerobic, in 116 athletes performing at the XIXth Olympic games in Mexico. *Ergonomics* 13:665–674.

Dudley, G.A., and R. Djmali (1985). Incompatibility of endurance- and strength-training modes of exercise. *J. Appl. Physiol.* 59:1446–1451.

Dudley, G.A., and S.J. Fleck (1987). Strength and endurance training: Are they mutually exclusive? *Sports Med.* 4:79–85.

Enns, M.P., A. Drewnowski, and J.A. Grinker (1987). Body composition, body size estimation and attitudes toward eating in male college athletes. *Psychosom. Med.* 49:56–64.

Fabiato, A., and F. Fabiato (1978). Effects of pH on the myofilaments and the sarcoplasmic reticulum of skinned cells from cardiac and skeletal muscles. *J. Physiol.* 276:233–255.

Fielding, R.A., D.L. Costill, W.J. Fink, D.S. King, J.E. Kovaleski, and J.P. Kirwan (1987). Effects of pre-exercise carbohydrate feedings on muscle glycogen use during exercise in well-trained runners. *Eur. J. Appl. Physiol.* 56:225–229.

Fogelholm, G.M., R. Koskinen, J. Laakso, T. Rankinen, and I. Ruokonen (1993). Gradual and rapid weight loss: effects on nutrition and performance in male athletes. *Med. Sci. Sports Exerc.* 25:371–377.

Foster, C., D.L. Costill, and W.J. Fink (1979). Effects of pre-exercise feedings on endurance performance. *Med. Sci. Sports* 11:1–5.

Freischlag, J. (1984). Weight loss, body composition, and health of high school wrestlers. *Physician Sportsmed.* 12 (1):121–126.

Gale, J.B., and K.W. Flynn (1974). Maximal oxygen consumption and relative body fat of high-ability wrestlers. *Med. Sci. Sports* 6:232–234.

Gao, J., D.L. Costill, C.A. Horswill, and S.H. Park (1988). Sodium bicarbonate ingestion improves performance in interval swimming. *Eur. J. Appl. Physiol.* 58:171–174.

Gollnick, P.D., R.B. Armstrong, C.W. Saubert, K. Piehl, and B. Saltin (1972). Enzyme activity and fiber composition in skeletal muscle of untrained and trained men. *J. Appl. Physiol.* 33:312–319.

Green, S., and B. Dawson (1993). Measurement of anaerobic capacities in humans. Definitions, limitations and unsolved problems. *Sports Med.* 15:312–327.

Henson, S.W. (1971). The problem of losing weight encountered by young wrestlers. *J. Sports Med. Phys. Fit.* 10–11:49–50.

Herbert, W.G., and P.M. Ribisl (1972). Effects of dehydration upon physical working capacity of wrestlers under competitive conditions. *Res. Quart.* 43:416–422.

Herbert, W.G., C. King, A. Teske, and M. Del (1977). Seasonal changes in physical performance of college wrestlers undergoing repetitive weight reduction (abstract). *Med. Sci. Sports Exerc.* 9:56.

Hermansen, L. (1981). Effect of metabolic changes on force production in skeletal muscle during maximal exercise. In: R. Porter and J. Whelan (eds.) *Human muscle fatigue: Physiological measurements.* London: Pitman Medical, pp. 72–88.

Hickner, R.C., C.A. Horswill, J. Welker, J.R. Scott, and D.L. Costill (1991). Test development for study of physical performance in wrestlers following weight loss. *Int. J. Sports Med.* 12:557–562.

Horstman, D.H., and S.M. Horvath (1973). Cardiovascular adjustments to progressive dehydration. *J. Appl. Physiol.* 35:501–504.

Horswill, C.A. (1979). *An investigation of the correlation between success in college wrestlers and the physiological capacities: maximum aerobic power, maximum anaerobic power, and dynamic endurance.* Unpublished Master's thesis, University of Wisconsin-Madison.

Horswill, C.A., J. Scott, P. Galea, and S.H. Park (1988). Physiological profile of elite junior wrestlers. *Res. Quart. Exerc. Sport* 59:257–261.

Horswill, C.A., J.R. Scott, and P. Galea (1989). Comparison of maximum aerobic power, maximum anaerobic power, and skinfold thickness of elite and non-elite junior wrestlers, *Int. J. Sports Med.* 10:165–168.

Horswill, C.A., R.C. Hickner, J.R. Scott, D.L. Costill, and D. Gould (1990a). Weight loss, dietary carbohydrate modifications and high-intensity, physical performance. *Med. Sci. Sports Exerc.* 22:470–476.

Horswill, C.A., S.H. Park, and J.N. Roemmich (1990b). Changes in the protein nutritional status of adolescent wrestlers. *Med. Sci. Sports Exerc.* 22:599–604.

Horswill, C.A. (1992a). Applied physiology of amateur wrestling. *Sports Med.* 14:114–143.

Horswill, C.A., R. Dick, and J.R. Scott (1992b). Relationship of weight gain to success in tournament competition of collegiate wrestlers (Abstract). *Med. Sci. Sports Exerc.* 24:S52.

Horswill, C.A., J.E. Miller, J.R. Scott, C.M. Smith, G. Welk, and P. Van Handel (1992c). Anaerobic and aerobic power in the arms and legs of elite senior wrestlers. *Int. J. Sports Med.* 13:558–561.

Horswill, C.A. (1993). Weight loss and weight cycling in amateur wrestlers: implications for performance and resting metabolic rate. *Int. J Sports Nutr.* 3:245–260.

Housh, T.J., G.O. Johnson, R.J. Hughes, C.J. Cisar, and W.G. Thorland (1988). Yearly changes in the body composition and muscular strength of high school wrestlers. *Res. Quart. Exerc. Sport* 59:240–243.

Housh, T.J., G.O. Johnson, R.A. Hughes, D.J. Housh, R.J. Hughes, A.S. Fry, K.B. Kenney, and C.J. Cisar (1989). Isokinetic strength and body composition of high school wrestlers across age. *Med. Sci. Sports Exerc.* 21:105–109.

Housh, T.J., R.J. Hughes, G.O. Johnson, D.J. Housh, L.L. Wagner, J.P. Weir, and S.A. Evans (1990). Age-related increases in the shoulder strength of high school wrestlers. *Pediatr. Exerc. Sci* 2:65–72.

Houston, M.E., D.A. Marin, H.J. Green, and J.A. Thomson (1981). The effect of rapid weight loss on physiological function in wrestlers. *Physician Sportsmed.* 9:73–78.

Houston, M.E., M.T. Sharratt, and R.W. Bruce (1983). Glycogen depletion and lactate responses in free-style wrestling. *Can. J. Appl. Sports Sci.* 8:79–82.

Hultman, E., J. Bergstrom, and A.E. Roch-Norlund (1971). Glycogen storage in human skeletal muscle. In: B. Saltin and B. Pernow (eds.) *Advances in experimental medicine and biology. Vol. 11.* New York: Plenum Press, pp. 273–288.

Hursh, L.M. (1979). Food and water restriction in the wrestler. *J Am. Med. Assoc.* 241:915–916.

Husman, B.F. (1955). Aggression in boxers and wrestlers as measured by projective techniques. *Res. Quart.* 26:421–425.

Huston, T.P., J.C. Puffer, and W.M. Rodney (1985). The athletic heart syndrome. *N. Engl. J. Med.* 313:24–32.

Ichiguchi, M. (1981). Analysis of techniques in the World Amateur Wrestling games, freestyle in 1979. *Bull. School Phys. Educ. Tokai Univ.* 11:75–83.

Ichiguchi, M., S. Kasai, T. Nishiyama, T. Takenouchi, T. Mitsukuri, and M. Saito (1978). A basic study on recording method and information analysis of wrestling games. *Bull. School Phys. Educ. Tokai Univ.* 8:31–43.

Ivy, J.L., M.C. Lee, J.T. Brozinick, and M.J. Reed (1988). Muscle glycogen storage after different amounts of carbohydrate ingestion. *J. Appl. Physiol.* 65:2018–2023.

Jacobs, I. (1980). The effects of thermal dehydration on performance on the Wingate anaerobic test. *Int. J. Sports Med.* 1:21–24.

Jefferies, S.C. (1986). *Sport Physiology Course: American Coaching Effectiveness Program, Level 2.* Champaign, IL: Human Kinetics.

Johnson, G.O., and C.J. Cisar (1987). Basic conditioning principles for high school wrestlers. *Physician Sportsmed.* 15:153–159.

Katch, F.I., and E.D. Michael (1971). Body composition of high school wrestlers according to age and wrestling weight category. *Med. Sci. Sports* 3:190–194.

Keller, L.F. (1942). The relation of 'quickness of bodily movement' to success in athletics. *Res. Quart.* 13:146–155.

Kelly, J.M., B.A. Gorney, and K.K. Kalm (1978). The effects of a collegiate wrestling season on body composition, cardiovascular fitness and muscular strength and endurance. *Med. Sci. Sports* 10:119–124.

Kirwan, J.P., D.L. Costill, J.B. Mitchell, J.A. Houmard, M.G. Flynn, W.J. Fink, and J.D. Beltz (1988). Carbohydrate balance in competitive runners during successive days of intense training. *J. Appl. Physiol.* 65:2601–2606.

Klinzing, J.E., and W. Karpowicz (1986). The effects of rapid weight loss and rehydration on a wrestling performance test. *J. Sports Med.* 26:149–156.

Kroll, W. (1954). An anthropometrical study of some Big Ten varsity wrestlers. *Res. Quart.* 25:307–312.

Kroll, W. (1958). Selected factors associated with wrestling success. *Res. Quart.* 29:396–406.

Lakin, J.A., S.N. Steen, and R.A. Oppliger (1990). Eating behaviors, weight loss methods and nutritional practices among high school wrestlers. *J. Commun. Health Nurs.* 7:59–67.

Leighton, J.R. (1957). Flexibility characteristics of three specialized skill groups of champion athletes. *Arch. Phys. Med. Rehab.* 38:580–583.

Mahler, D.A., E.D. Moritz, and J. Loke (1982). Ventilatory responses at rest and during exercise in marathon runners. *J. Appl. Physiol.* 52:388–392.

Maksud, M.G., R.L. Wiley, L.H. Hamilton, and B. Lockhart (1970). Maximal $\dot{V}O_2$, ventilation, and heart rate of Olympic speed skating candidates. *J. Appl. Physiol.* 29:186–190.

McMurray, R.G., C.R. Proctor, and W.L. Wilson (1991). Effect of caloric deficit and dietary manipulation on aerobic and anaerobic exercise. *Int. J. Sports Med.* 12:167–172.

Medbø, J.G., A.C. Mohn, I. Tabata, R. Bahr, O. Vaage, and O.M. Sejersted (1988). Anaerobic capacity determined by maximal accumulated O_2 deficit. *J. Appl. Physiol.* 64:50–60.

Mnatzakanian, P.A., and P. Vaccaro (1984). Effects of 4% thermal dehydration and rehydration on hematologic and urinary profile of college wrestlers. *Ann. Sports Med.* 2:41–46.

Morgan, W.P. (1970). Psychological effect of weight reduction in the college wrestler. *Med. Sci. Sports* 2:24–27.

Morgan, W.P. (1988). Test of champions: The iceberg profile. *Psychol. Today* 20:408–414.

Morgan, W.P., and W.M. Hammer (1974). Influence of competitive wrestling upon state anxiety. *Med. Sci. Sports* 6:58–61.

Morganroth, J., B.J. Maron, W.L. Henry, and S.E. Epstein (1975). Comparative left ventricular dimensions in trained athletes. *Ann. Intern. Med.* 82:521–524.

Morganroth, J., and B.J. Maron (1977). The athlete's heart syndrome: a new perspective. *Ann. NY Acad. Sci.* 301:931–941.

Nagle, F.J., W.P. Morgan, R.O. Hellickson, R.C. Serfass, and J.F. Alexander (1975). Spotting success traits in Olympic contenders. *Physician Sportsmed.* 3:31–34.

Neufer, P.D., M.N. Sawka, A.J. Young, M.D. Quigley, W.A. Latza, and L. Levine (1991). Hypohydration does not impair skeletal muscle glycogen resynthesis after exercise. *J. Appl. Physiol.* 70:1490–1494.

Oppliger, R.A., G.L. Landry, S.W. Foster, and A.C. Lambrecht (1993). Bulimic behaviors among interscholastic wrestlers: a statewide survey. *Pediatrics* 91:826–831.

Panel Discussion (1993). *Antioxidants and the elite athlete.* Unpublished proceedings of the American College of Sports Medicine annual meeting, Dallas, TX.

Park, S.H., J.N. Roemmich, and C.A. Horswill (1990). A season of wrestling and weight loss by adolescent wrestlers: effect on anaerobic arm power. *J. Appl. Sport Sci. Res.* 4:1–4.

Rasch, P.J. (1958). Indices of body build of United States freestyle wrestlers. *J. Assoc. Phys. Mental. Rehab.* 12:91–94.

Rasch, P.J., and J.W.A. Brandt (1957). Measurement of pulmonary function in United States freestyle wrestlers. *Res. Quart.* 28:279–287.

Rasch, P.J., W. Pierson, E.R. O'Connell, and M.B. Hunt (1961a). Effect of training for amateur wrestling on total proportional strength scores. *Res. Quart.* 32:201–207.

Rasch, P.J., W. Pierson, E.R. O'Connell, and M.B. Hunt (1961b). Response time of amateur wrestlers. *Res. Quart.* 32:416–419.

Rasch, P.J., A. Adams, W. Boring, R. Gunnar, M.B. Hunt, G. O'Connell, and P.G. Robertson (1964a). Neuroticism and extraversion in United States intercollegiate wrestlers. *J. Assoc. Phys. Mental. Rehab.* 16:153–154.

Rasch, P.J., and W. Kroll (1964b). *What Research Tells the Coach About Wrestling.* Washington, D.C.: American Association for Health, Physical Education, Recreation and Dance.

Reimers, K., A. Grandjean, G. Tetrault, and K. Stanek (1993). The effects of making weight on performance and health parameters of college wrestlers (abstract). *FASEB J.* 7:A293.

Ribisl, P.M., and W.G. Herbert (1970). Effects of rapid weight reduction and subsequent rehydration upon the physical working capacity of wrestlers. *Res. Quart.* 41:536–541.

Roemmich, J.N. (1993). Differences in physiological capacities of successful and less successful high school wrestlers. *Pediatr. Exerc. Sci.* 5:134–144.

Roemmich, J.N., W.E. Sinning, and S.R. Roemmich (1991). Seasonal changes in anaerobic power, strength and body composition of adolescent wrestlers (abstract). *Med. Sci. Sports Exerc.* 23:S29.

Roundtable (1988a). Strength training and conditioning for wrestling. Part I. *Nat. Strength Cond. Assoc. J.* 10:14–19.

Roundtable (1988b). Strength training and conditioning for wrestling. Part II. *Nat. Strength Cond. Assoc. J.* 10:12–23.

Sady, S.P., W.H. Thomson, M. Savage, and M. Petratis (1982). The body composition and physical dimensions of 9- to 12-year-old experienced wrestlers. *Med. Sci. Sports Exerc.* 14:244–248.

Sady, S.P., W.H. Thomson, K. Berg, and M. Savage (1984). Physiological characteristics of high-ability prepubescent wrestlers. *Med. Sci. Sports Exerc.* 16:72–76.

Sawka, M.N., M.M. Toner, R.P. Francesconi, and K.B. Pandolf (1983). Hypohydration and exercise: effects of heat acclimation, gender, and environment. *J. Appl. Physiol.* 55:1147–1153.

Seals, D.R., and J.P. Mullin (1982). VO$_2$max in variable type exercise among well-trained upper body athletes. *Res. Quart. Exerc. Sport* 53:58–63.

Serfass, R.C., G.A. Stull, J.F. Alexander, and J.L. Ewing (1984). The effects of rapid weight loss and attempted rehydration on strength and endurance of the handgripping muscle in college wrestlers. *Res. Quart. Exerc. Sport* 55:46–52.

Serresse, O., G. Lortie, C. Bouchard, and M.R. Bouley (1988). Estimation of the contribution of the various energy systems during maximal work of short duration. *Int. J. Sports Med.* 9:456–460.

Sharratt, M.T. (1984). Wrestling profile. *Clin. Sports Med.* 3:273–289.

Sharratt, M.T., A.W. Taylor, and T.M.K. Song (1986). A physiological profile of elite Canadian freestyle wrestlers. *Can. J. Appl. Sports Sci.* 11:100–105.

Shavers, L.G. (1974). Effects of a season of varsity wrestling on selected physiological parameters. *J. Sports Med.* 14:141–145.

Sherman, W.M., D.L. Costill, W.J. Fink, F.C. Hagerman, L.E. Armstrong, and T.S. Murray (1983). Effect of a 42.2 km footrace and subsequent rest or exercise on muscle glycogen and enzymes. *J. Appl. Physiol.* 55:1219–1224.

Short, S.H., and W.R. Short (1983). Four-year study of university athletes' dietary intake. *J. Am. Diet. Assoc.* 82:632–645.

Silva, J.M., B.B. Schultz, R.W. Haslam, and D. Murray (1981). A psychophysiological assessment of elite wrestlers. *Res. Quart. Exerc. Sport* 52:348–358.

Simoneau, J.A., G. Lortie, M.R. Boulay, and C. Bouchard (1983). Tests of anaerobic alactacid and lactacid capacities: Description and reliabilty. *Can. J. Appl. Sports Sci.* 8:266–270.

Singer, R.N., and S.A. Weiss (1968). Effects of weight reduction on selected anthropometric, physical, and performance measures of wrestlers. *Res. Quart.* 39:361–369.

Song, T.M.K., and G.T. Garvie (1980). Anthropometric, flexibility, strength, and physiological measures of Canadian wrestlers and comparison of Canadian and Japanese Olympic wrestlers. *Can. J. Sports Sci.* 5:1–8.

Song, T.M.K., and N. Cipriano (1984). Effects of seasonal training on physical and physiological function on elite varsity wrestlers. *J. Sports Med.* 24:123–130.

Sproles, C.B., D.P. Smith, R.J. Byrd, and T.E. Allen (1976). Circulatory responses to submaximal exercise after dehydration and rehydration. *J. Sports Med.* 16:98–105.

Steen, S.N., and S. McKinney (1986). Nutrition assessment of college wrestlers. *Physician Sportsmed.* 14:100–116.

Steen, S.N., and K.D. Brownell (1990). Patterns of weight loss and regain in wrestlers: has the tradition changed? *Med. Sci. Sports Exerc.* 22:762–768.

Stine, G., R. Ratliff, G. Shierman, and W.A. Grana (1979). Physical profile of the wrestlers at the 1977 NCAA Championships. *Physician Sportsmed.* 7:98–105.

Strauss, R.H., R.R. Lanese, and W.B. Malarkey (1985). Weight loss in amateur wrestlers and its effect on serum testosterone levels. *J. Am. Med. Assoc.* 254:3337–3338.

Strauss, R.H., R.R. Lanese, and D.J. Leizman (1988). Illness and absence among wrestlers, swimmers, and gymnasts at a large university. *Am. J. Sports Med.* 16:653–655.

Tanner, J.M. (1964). *The physique of the Olympic athlete*. London: George Allen and Unwin, Ltd.

Taylor, A.W., L. Brassard, and R.D. Proteau (1979). A physiological profile of Canadian Greco-Roman wrestlers. *Can. J. Appl. Sports Sci.* 4:131–134.

Tcheng, T.K., and C.M. Tipton (1973). Iowa Wrestling Study: anthropometric measurements and the prediction of a 'minimal' body weight for high school wrestlers. *Med. Sci. Sports* 5:1–10.

Tesch, P., J. Karlsson, and B. Sjodin (1982). Muscle fiber type distribution in trained and untrained muscles of athletes. In: P.V. Komi (ed.) *Exercise and Sport Biology*. Champaign, IL: Human Kinetics, pp. 79–83.

Thorland, W.G., G.O. Johnson, T.G. Fagot, G.D. Tharp, and R.W. Hammer (1981). Body composition and somatotype characteristics of Junior Olympic athletes. *Med. Sci. Sports Exerc.* 13:332–338.

Tipton, C.M., T.K. Tcheng, and W.D. Paul (1969). Evaluation of the Hall method for determining minimum wrestling weights. *J. Iowa Med. Soc.* 59:571–574.

Tipton, C.M., and T.K. Tcheng (1970). Iowa Wrestling Study: Weight loss in high school students. *J. Am. Med. Assoc.* 214:1269–1274.

Tipton, C.M., and R.A. Oppliger (1984). The Iowa wrestling study: lessons for physicians. *Iowa Med.* 74:381–385.

Tuttle, W.W. (1943). The effect of weight loss by dehydration and the withholding of food on the physiologic responses of wrestlers. *Res. Quart.* 14:158–166.

Vaccaro, P., C.W. Zauner, and J.R. Cade (1976). Changes in body weight, hematocrit and plasma protein concentration due to dehydration and rehydration in wrestlers. *J. Sports Med. Phys. Fit.* 16:45–53.

Walberg, J.L., M.K. Leidy, D.J. Sturgill, D.E. Hinkle, S.J. Ritchey, and D.R. Sebolt (1988). Macronutrient content of a hypoenergy diet affects nitrogen retention and muscle function in weight lifters. *Int. J. Sports Med.* 9:261–266.

Webster, S., R. Rutt, and A. Weltman (1990). Physiological effects of a weight loss regimen practiced by college wrestlers. *Med. Sci. Sports Exerc.* 22:229–234.

Weissinger, E., T.J. Housh, G.O. Johnson, and S.A. Evans (1991). Weight loss behavior in high school wrestling: wrestler and parent perceptions. *Pediatr. Exerc. Sci.* 3:64–73.

Widerman, P.M., and R.D. Hagen (1982). Bodyweight loss in a wrestler preparing for competition: a case report. *Med. Sci. Sports Exerc.* 14:413–418.

Wilmore, J.H., and W.L. Haskell (1972). Body composition and endurance capacity of professional football players. *J. Appl. Physiol.* 33:564–567.

Wilmore, J.H., and D.L. Costill (1988). *Training for Sport and Activity*. Dubuque: W.C. Brown.

Wolf, E.M.B., J.C. Wirth, and T.G. Lohman (1979). Nutritional practices of coaches in the Big Ten. *Physician Sportsmed.* 7:1–9.

Woods, E.R., C.D. Wilson, and R.P. Masland (1988). Weight control methods in high school wrestlers. *J. Adolesc. Health Care* 9:394–397.

Zambraski, E.J., C.M. Tipton, T.K. Tcheng, H.R. Jordon, A.C. Vailas, and A.K. Callahan (1975). Iowa wrestling study: Changes in urinary profiles of wrestlers prior to and after competition. *Med. Sci. Sports* 7:217–220.

Zambraski, E.J., D.T. Foster, P.M. Gross, and C.M. Tipton (1976). Iowa wrestling study: weight loss and urinary profiles of collegiate wrestlers. *Med. Sci. Sports* 8:105–108.

DISCUSSION

BAR-OR: Is there any evidence that a child who participates in wrestling and experiences the repeated cycles of body weight loss and gain will be adversely affected as he matures?

HORSWILL: There has been a lot of speculation about the possibility that there could be a retardation of growth or development in younger wrestlers. In a survey by Nitsche et al., published in the *J. Athletic Training*, the authors reported that in former collegiate wrestlers, there were no apparent long-term problems such as arthritis or obesity that could be attributed to previous wrestling experience. In a similar study by Gunderson and MacIntosh, published only as an abstract, wrestlers later in life were found to be overweight and to exhibit tendencies for higher blood pressure and blood cholesterol. The authors concluded that wrestlers may become obese as a result of weight cycling. Unfortunately, data were only obtained from surveys. Without actual body composition data, it is impossible to know whether these wrestlers were actually obese or, as one might anticipate, simply had a greater muscle mass relative to height than did the controls. It is also possible that wrestlers may develop the habitual exercise patterns that cause them to sustain a larger muscle mass later in life. The long-term effects of wrestling on health remain to be fully explored.

GISOLFI: Considering that the season lasts approximately 6 months, a wrestler who has participated in high school and collegiate wrestling has been exposed to chronic dehydration for about 8 years. Tipton and Zambraski several years ago reported that collegiate wrestlers had significant elevations in urine potassium that were indicative of renal ischemia. Is there any evidence of renal dysfunction later in life as a result of this chronic dehydration that wrestlers seem to be exposed to?

HORSWILL: Nitsche et al. found no difference in the incidence of renal problems in former wrestlers compared to controls. Mysnyck, an orthopaedic surgeon in Iowa, found no long-term renal function problems in an unpublished study of former wrestlers, but his studies are unpublished. Research by Paul Vaccaro showed that after wrestlers rehydrate, their urine electrolyte levels return to normal, indicating the adverse changes were temporary. Nevertheless, there are no definitive studies on this important issue.

CLARKSON: Recent epidemiological data suggest that fluctuations in body weight are related to morbidity and mortality.

HORSWILL: Wrestlers may be quite different from the population studied by Steve Blair, the latter being obese persons who repeatedly lost and regained body fat. There is not much fat being lost by most wrestlers. Dehydration and the loss of muscle glycogen account for most of the weight lost. I am not saying that weight cycling by wrestlers should not be a concern, but the outcomes of this cycling may be quite different from those experienced by obese people.

CLARKSON: We have the same weight cycling problem in ballet dancers. Junior high and high school ballet dancers, who repeatedly lose and regain weight to qualify for auditions or performances, progressively have more difficulty in losing weight; most of them eventually forgo dancing. At the elite level, only dancers who can more easily maintain a low body weight remain active dancers. This may occur with the elite wrestlers as well.

HORSWILL: Cross-sectional work by Steen and Brownell suggested that resting metabolic rates were lower in scholastic wrestlers who practiced weight cycling versus wrestlers who did not weight cycle. However, in collegiate wrestlers, Melby et al., showed that resting metabolic rates were decreased only during the wrestling season (to levels similar to those observed in non-wrestlers); after the season, metabolic rates returned to normal. There may be confounding factors such as maturation level and the natural selection process of the sport that account for these differences in metabolic rate.

EICHNER: If weight cycling reduces resting metabolic rate in wrestlers, it is not clear if the weight cycling is the horse or the cart. Maybe those with low metabolic rates to begin with are forced to cycle to make weight. On another issue, is there any evidence that consumption of sports drinks can accelerate rehydration of wrestlers before competition?

HORSWILL: Oddly enough, most studies of strength and power in dehydrated wrestlers do not show any adverse effects of dehydration; consequently, it is difficult to make a case for better rehydration if strength and power are the dependent variables. Perhaps an endurance variable would be more likely to show an effect of different rehydration or feeding regimens. In intercollegiate and international wrestling tournaments, wrestlers are allowed about 20 h to rehydrate between weigh-in and competition, but they must again be weight-certified for the second and third days of the tournaments. On average, intercollegiate wrestlers bounce up and down in body weight by 3.6 kg (8 lb) within 24 h at major tournaments, and some wrestlers may lose and regain as much as 6.8 kg (15 lb) in 24 h. Intuitively, it seems that there must be an optimal regimen of nutrition and rehydration, but so far, no one has verified such a regimen in the scientific literature.

KRAEMER: Given the glycogen depletion that occurs in wrestlers, it seems to me that carbohydrate ingestion after weigh-in and between matches would be important.

HORSWILL: The nutritional strategies should begin much earlier. More emphasis needs to be placed on carbohydrate intake during training and before the weigh-in. Some of the studies we and others have done indicate that wrestlers tend to maintain muscular endurance after weight loss only if they have consumed a high-carbohydrate diet during weight reduction. There is a misconception among wrestlers that, no matter what they do to lose weight, they can repair everything in that period between the weigh-in and competition. A better approach is for the wrestler to view every meal during the season as if it were a pre-match meal. I can not make any specific recommendation about what should be consumed between bouts, but fluids with a high carbohydrate content are important. Such drinks will at least elevate blood glucose levels if not contribute to the replenishment of muscle glycogen stores.

COYLE: I do not think wrestlers need to avoid dietary carbohydrates to help in the dehydration process to lose weight. The general recommendation is that athletes should ingest 50 g of carbohydrate every 2 h to replenish muscle glycogen after strenuous exercise. Wrestlers could eat carbohydrates such as sugars and starches that contain very little fluid.

The 50 g (less than 2 oz) of weight they will gain is certainly worth the glycogen they will be replenishing. They do not have to sacrifice muscle glycogen in order to maintain body weight if they eat concentrated carbohydrates low in water content.

HORSWILL: I agree with you.

MURRAY: Wrestlers obviously drink a lot of fluids shortly before competition in an attempt to rehydrate themselves. Are there any data indicating which body fluid compartments are most affected by this fluid consumption?

HORSWILL: Unfortunately, there is no research addressing that issue in wrestlers.

GISOLFI: Some years ago, Costill analyzed some muscle biopsy material following dehydration. Using the chloride method, which is a questionable technique, Costill found a reasonable rehydration of the extracellular, but not the intracellular, fluid compartment after 5 h of rehydration.

MAUGHAN: We recently studied the effects of electrolytes in rehydration drinks for subjects who lost 2% of their body weights by exercise-induced dehydration. If we rehydrated with beverages containing either sodium or potassium, we observed the same amount of fluid retained (both drinks caused about 800 mL more fluid retention than did plain water), but we did not see an additive effect when we put both sodium and potassium in the beverage. Thus, it does not appear that the sodium is expanding the extracellular space and the potassium the intracellular space.

HORSWILL: Perhaps the optimal solution for rehydrating wrestlers would contain both sodium and glucose; theoretically, such a solution would not only enhance intestinal fluid absorption, but would also contribute some energy for performance.

KRAEMER: It seems like there is a training/nutrition paradox for wrestlers who want to gain power and strength but do not want the increased muscle mass associated with it. Is there any research on strength training for wrestlers?

HORSWILL: There is no systematic research on that topic. We have done some descriptive research on anaerobic power, as have Roemmich et al., and Song and Cipriano, who showed improvements in strength and peak $\dot{V}O_2$ during the wrestling season. A more systematic approach is needed to determine the best method of weight training for wrestlers. Collegiate coaches are emphasizing weight training more during the season than they previously did, especially for those competitors at higher body weight classes. The lightweight wrestlers may perform more aerobic training to reduce body fat and to induce a heat load for sweating to make weight. Maybe wrestlers in the lower weight classes should be doing more power and muscular endurance training than aerobic training.

MAUGHAN: Craig, you report that the average energy expended by wrestlers is 13–14 kcal/min. That works out to a $\dot{V}O_2$ of about 2.5–3.0 L/min, but the $\dot{V}O_2$max values are 3.5–4.0 L/min, perhaps even slightly higher. Accordingly, relative to $\dot{V}O_2$max, the average intensity during wrestling is not all that high. There are obviously periods of very high intensity activity, which are primarily anaerobic, but overall, there seems to be a large aerobic contribution.

HORSWILL: Based on laboratory data, wrestling is often described as using both anaerobic and aerobic sources of energy. It may be quite a different story on the mat. If a wrestler can throw his opponent for a fall in the first 10 s of the match, the match is over; therefore, great anaerobic power can be vital to success. On the other hand, some wrestlers must rely on endurance; they seem to be losing badly at the initiation of the match, but they eventually win when their more powerful opponents become fatigued. In recent years, the rules have changed such that anaerobic power is emphasized. That is primarily why I have concluded that anaerobic power and anaerobic capacity are more critical for success than are the capacities based on aerobic metabolism.

GISOLFI: Is there any evidence to support the contention that buffering capacity is a potential-limiting factor in wrestling?

HORSWILL: Sharp et al., in Costill's lab found that, with sprint training, the muscle-buffering capacity increased. This raises the question of how best to train to increase buffer capacity. Coyle and Lesmes compared the training effects of two approaches—very short, high-intensity repetitions versus more sustained high-intensity repetitions. The former presumably would promote increases in ATP and phosphocreatine stores, whereas the latter was proposed to increase glycolytic capacity. The very brief, high-intensity repetitions program was more effective for improving power. I would speculate that such intense power training, which induces the synthesis of muscle proteins and induces muscle hypertrophy, might also increase muscle buffering capacity. In contrast, training with sustained high-intensity activity that does not cause muscle hypertrophy might not increase buffering capacity. In fact, if the wrestler is losing weight and muscle mass, muscle buffering capacity may actually decrease.

SPRIET: In support of the notion that buffering capacity may limit performances such as wrestling, it has been shown that ingestion of sodium bicarbonate prior to brief, exhaustive exercise allows one to produce more energy from the glycolytic system before the muscles become fatigued. Also, we should not limit our thinking to just the muscle-buffering capacity. We should also consider what happens when metabolites and ions such as lactate are removed from the muscle. If one is better able to remove lactate from the muscle and possibly out of the plasma space, there will be associated changes in hydrogen ion concentration that favor the continuance of muscle contraction and the energy production by the biochemical pathways that support contraction. I believe the muscles undertake a concerted effort to prevent the muscle from becoming so acidic that it has to shut down.

HORSWILL: I agree with you, but I refer you to the observations of Sharratt, who showed that wrestlers on the treadmill seemed to hypoventilate when they were at peak $\dot{V}O_2$. If hydrogen ions are moving out of muscle into the bloodstream, hyperventilation is eventually necessary to buffer hydrogen ions and minimize the pH changes. Sharratt suggested that the wrestler hypoventilates as a result of some training adaptation. It is unclear whether the adaptation is peripheral, i.e., an improved muscle buffering capacity, or whether there is a psychological adjustment allowing the wrestler to tolerate the pain associate with the pH change.

SPRIET: Hydrogen ions may not need to move from one compartment to another. The concentrations of the other ions in the various compartments will determine the hydrogen ion concentration. We need to investigate the entire picture—lactate, potassium, sodium, and all the other ions that will ultimately influence what the muscle hydrogen ion concentration will be in a given compartment.

LAMB: Are there any adverse effects of dehydration on training for wrestling?

HORSWILL: A single match is quite different from a training session in which wrestlers train up to 2.5 h/d. The sport requires a high degree of skill; if the wrestler is chronically restricting nutrient and fluid intake, he does not have the energy to concentrate on the enhancement of wrestling technique during practice sessions. Therefore, the wrestler may, over the span of his career, stunt his skill development so that he never acquires the skills needed to be among the elite. For example, an adolescent wrestler who is chronically attempting to lose weight may have moderate success despite of or as a result of the weight loss, but he reaches a certain moderate level of skill development that does not allow him to advance to the state tournament or to become a collegiate wrestler. In contrast, a wrestler who focuses on technique enhancement and does not lose as much weight may have less competitive success initially, but he may eventually become very successful. This is a consideration that educators should pass on to coaches and wrestlers who may be considering the chronic weight loss approach to wrestling success. The coach and wrestler must look at the whole span of the career and all the factors that need to be developed for wrestling success.

5

Physiology and Nutrition for Skating

ANN C. SNYDER, Ph.D.

CARL FOSTER, Ph.D.

INTRODUCTION

Competitive skating events include speed skating, ice hockey, and figure skating. Each of these individual sports can also be divided into different activities. For example, speed skating includes long track skating, pack style skating, short track skating, in-line skating, and marathon skating; ice hockey players—forwards, defensemen, and goalkeepers—have different responsibilities in competition; and figure skating includes singles, pairs, and dancing events. Speed skating is rhythmical, continuous, and fast. Ice hockey skating is nonrhythmical, with starts, stops, and directional changes occurring rapidly and often, along with frequent body contact. Figure skating is graceful, rhythmical, and slow for the most part, but its various jumps are particularly important in competition. The common feature of all these activities is that they are performed on ice, and the nature of the skating motion involves action of the hip and knee extensors during both the gliding and push-off phases of the stroke. Due to the diverse nature of the three types of skating, they will be discussed independently in this chapter. While much research has been performed on speed skating, little has been published on ice hockey skating or figure skating. However, the current state of knowledge is presented for all three activities in the hopes of stimulating future research efforts.

SPEED SKATING

Skating and skiing can be traced back to the 1200s. In areas where snowfall was frequent, skiing emerged; in areas with more ice, skating evolved when wooden runners were attached to shoes. Both skiing and skating were principally performed as modes of travel. In 1572, the first iron runners were used on skates, and the first speed skating race took place in 1763, over a distance of 24 km on the Fens River in England.

Since 1909, the 11 cities speed skating race/tour (De Elfstedentocht) has been conducted in a northern province of the Netherlands whenever the channels are frozen over the 200 km course. The 14th and latest race/tour was in 1986, with the skating times ranging from 6.75 to 18 h (van Saase et al., 1990). The number of participants in the 11 cities race/tour is currently limited to 20,000 (van Saase et al., 1990).

Long track skating is performed on a 400-m oval ice rink and has been an Olympic sport since 1924 for men and since 1960 for women. The Olympic long track events for men include the 500, 1,000, 1,500, 5,000, and 10,000 m (approximately 0.62 to 14.20 min) and, for women, the 500, 1,000, 1,500, 3,000, and 5,000 m (approximately 0.67 to 7.53 min) (Table 5-1). Long track events are basically time trials in which only two skaters race simultaneously; the fastest performer among all pairs is declared the winner. Generally, long track skaters select themselves into either sprint (500 and 1,000 m) or all-around (500, 1,500, 3,000/5,000, and 5,000/10,000 m) events, with world championships annually contested in both sprint and all-around disciplines.

Short track skating, performed on an 111-m oval ice rink, was initially an Olympic demonstration sport in 1988, then became an Olympic medal sport in 1992. The Olympic events include the 500- and 1,000-m events for men and women, as well as a 3,000-m relay for women and a 5,000-m relay for men, with multiple skaters on the ice during one race. At world championships for men and women, the 1,500- and 3,000-m events are also performed. In long track meets, usually two events are performed in a day, whereas at short track meets, many heats of one race as well as many races are held in a single day.

Marathon skating generally involves a course of 40 km or longer (1 h or more), either on artificial or real ice (Geijsel, 1979). Thus, speed skating events involve performances ordinarily lasting anywhere from 0.6 min to 18 h. The prominent speed skating activities, however, are the Olympic and World Championship long track races. Research on long track skating is much more prominent in the literature than is research on the non-Olympic speed skating events and the athletes who participate in them.

The general speed skating technique involves a three-part stroke: gliding (0.50–0.75 s), push-off (0.15–0.20 s), and recovery (0.05–0.35 s), with 60–80 strokes performed each minute (de Boer & Nilsen, 1989). Because the hip and leg muscles are active all of the time that the skate is on

TABLE 5-1. *Current world records for long track speed skating events (min:s)*

EVENT	FEMALES	MALES
500 m	0:39.10	0:36.02
1,000 m	1:17.65	1:12.58
1,500 m	1:59.30	1:52.06
3,000 m	4:10.89	
5,000 m	7:14.13	6:36.57
10,000 m		13:43.54

the ice (de Boer, 1986), the duty cycle of speed skating (i.e., muscle action time/total cycle time) is approximately 70% of the activity. The propulsion of the stroke occurs due to a push-off in a sideward direction caused by extension of the hip and knee joint muscles (i.e., gluteus maximus, biceps femoris, semitendinous, vastus medialis, rectus femoris, gastrocnemius, vastus lateralis, tibialis anterior, soleus, vastus intermedius, and the erector spinae). To reduce air friction and increase the duration of the push-off, the hip and knee joint angles prior to the push-off (pre-extension) are as small as possible (approximately 50 and 115°, respectively) (van Ingen Schenau & de Groot, 1983). van Ingen Schenau and de Groot (1983) have shown that the greatest technical difference between male and female speed skaters is in the pre-extension angle of the knee; females obtain an angle that is approximately 11° greater.

Characteristics of Elite Speed Skaters

Body Composition and Anthropometry. For the most part, elite male speed skaters are similar in age (21.5 y), height (177 cm), and weight (74.0 kg) (Maksud et al., 1970; Nemoto et al., 1988; Pollock et al., 1982; Quirion et al., 1988; Smith & Roberts, 1990; van Ingen Schenau et al., 1988) compared to the average young man (Pollock et al., 1976). However, speed skaters have less body fat (~ 10% body fat) and more lean body mass (~ 67 kg) than do their more sedentary counterparts (Nemoto et al., 1988; Pollock et al., 1982; Quirion et al., 1988; van Ingen Schenau et al., 1988).

Less information is available concerning the body composition of elite female speed skaters, but the evidence shows that they weigh approximately 63 kg, which includes 21% body fat, and thus, 50 kg of lean body mass (Maksud et al., 1970; Pollock et al., 1986; van Ingen Schenau et al., 1988, 1992). The development of body weight and lean body mass in junior skaters seems to follow that of sedentary control subjects up to age 13 for males and age 16 for females; afterward, lean body mass is greater for skaters than for sedentary controls (Nemoto et al., 1990). Similarly, the female skaters develop less body fat after age 14 than do sedentary controls. However, such a trend was not observed in the male skaters (Nemoto et al., 1990).

Total body heights of male speed skaters are similar to those of average young men (van Ingen Schenau et al., 1983). Elite speed skaters also have similar total leg lengths, but relatively shorter upper legs, than do moderately trained skaters (van Ingen Schenau et al., 1983). A shorter upper leg length could be beneficial to a speed skater, because hip extension would occur with less muscular force. The isometric component of the gliding phase of speed skating undoubtedly influences blood flow and thus metabolism; therefore, reducing the muscular forces necessary should be beneficial to performance. Male Olympic speed skaters have thigh circumferences similar to those of average young men. However, the Olympians have greater ratios of thigh circumference to thigh skinfold thickness, indicating greater fat-free mass (Pollock et al., 1982). The greater lean mass together with the comparatively shorter thigh length contributes to the popular perception of greater mass in the thighs of speed skaters.

Muscle Strength. Due to the small angles of the hip and knee joints prior to the push-off during speed skating, the hip and knee extensor muscles are very important to performance. United States speed skaters exhibit greater strength relative to body weight in these extensor muscles than do sedentary controls; a difference of 20–35% was observed at 180 and 270°/s, with only a 6% difference observed at 90°/s (Foster & Thompson, 1990). The female speed skaters had slightly greater relative strength differences than did the male speed skaters (Foster & Thompson, 1990). Further increases in muscle strength occur subsequent to training (Foster & Thompson, 1990).

Muscle strength seems to be related to skating posture, as increases in strength of the knee and hip extensor muscles were associated with decreases in the pre-extension joint angles (Foster & Thompson, 1990). Herzog et al. (1991) examined moment-length relationships for a group of speed skaters and cyclists (athletes who also require minimal motion at the hip joint) and for a group of runners (athletes whose movements at the hip joint are much greater). The speed skaters/cyclists were relatively stronger at short muscle lengths, an apparent adaptation to the type of training performed.

Recently, Rajala et al. (1994) noted a relatively greater torque (and calculated power) in speed skaters versus controls at the beginning of the range of motion during high-velocity isokinetic knee extension than during mid-action. The results reinforce the concept that training speed skaters selectively increases their strength at points in the range of motion where most individuals are very weak. Given the high velocity of hip/knee extension during skating, the ability to generate torque at the beginning of the push-off is probably critical (Rajala et al., 1994). Finally, muscle activation patterns of selected hip and knee extensor muscles during the act of speed skating do not differ between elite and non-elite speed skaters (de Koning et al., 1991).

Anaerobic Power and Capacity. Anaerobic power and capacity appear to be important components of at least the sprint events (500, 1,000, 1,500 m) in speed skating (de Koning et al., 1992; Foster & Thompson, 1990; Geijsel et al., 1984). Peak anaerobic power is significantly related to 500-m personal best times ($r = -0.61$); however, no such correlation was observed between anaerobic capacity and 500 m performance (de Koning et al., 1992). Peak power output during a 30-s cycling exercise is 1,120–1,348 W in male skaters (Geijsel et al., 1984; van Ingen Schenau et al., 1988) and 927 W in female skaters (van Ingen Schenau et al., 1988). Average power per body weight for male skaters is 14.2 ± 1.0 W/kg and for female skaters is 12.3 ± 0.4 W/kg (a 13.4% difference); power per lean body mass is 19.58 ± 1.98 W/kg for males and 19.13 ± 1.26 W/kg for females (a 2.3% difference) (van Ingen Schenau et al., 1988). Anaerobic capacity determined during a 2.5-min cycling exercise is approximately 2,100 W (Geijsel et al., 1984). Other reports support the concept that speed skaters have great anaerobic capacity—however measured—compared to other athletes (Medbø et al., 1988).

Average anaerobic power generated during speed skating seems to be lower than that generated during cycling. For example, de Groot et al. (1985) had 25 male all-around speed skaters perform 500- and 1,500-m skating time trials and 30-s and 2.5-min cycling tests and observed that the mean power during the skating events (344 ± 60 W and 283 ± 65 W, respectively) was less than that during the cycling tests (875 ± 86 W and 420 ± 52 W, respectively). Mean power during the 30-s cycling test was more related to performance in the 500-m ($r = -0.782$) and in the 1,500-m ($r = -0.850$) skating events than was mean power during the 2.5-min cycling test ($r = -0.595$ and -0.662, respectively) (de Groot et al., 1985).

While anaerobic power appears to be important to performance of at least the sprint events in speed skating, anaerobic power adaptations to training are quite minimal (Foster et al., 1993b; van Ingen Schenau et al., 1992). However, recent studies of anaerobic capacity using the accumulated oxygen deficit technique have demonstrated significant increases with training, at least in non-athletic subjects (Medbø & Burgers, 1990).

Cardiovascular and Pulmonary Capacities and Aerobic Power. For the most part, speed skaters do not have exceptionally large aerobic capacities. Only a study by Ekblom et al. (1967) reported maximal oxygen uptake ($\dot{V}O_2$max) values significantly greater than 70 mL·kg^{-1}·min^{-1} (running) in male speed skaters. Maksud and colleagues (1970, 1971, 1982), also using treadmill running, demonstrated that male speed skaters had a mean $\dot{V}O_2$max of 63 mL·kg^{-1}·min^{-1}. Cycling tests for maximal aerobic power of speed skaters produced slightly lower values than those obtained during the running tests, i.e., 59 mL·kg^{-1}·min^{-1} for men and 52 mL·kg^{-1}·min^{-1} for women (Pollock et al., 1986).

Maximal values of aerobic power are generally higher in athletes when they perform their specific skills rather than generic skills, but this is not the case with speed skaters. During speed skating tests, athletes reach no more than 85–90% of the $\dot{V}O_2$max that they reach during running or cycling (de Groot et al., 1987; Foster & Thompson, 1990), possibly due to a smaller muscle mass utilized in skating or, more likely, to a reduced blood flow caused by the isometric muscle actions of the hip and knee extensors during the gliding phase of the skating stroke. Although blood flow has not been measured during skating, several factors support this theory. First, EMG data have shown that during 70% of the total skating stroke, the hip and leg muscles on each leg are active (de Boer, 1986). Second, muscle force is relatively high, at least in excess of body weight (de Koning, 1991). Third, blood lactate concentration and heart rate are both higher at a given oxygen uptake during speed skating than during cycling (Snyder et al., 1993). Fourth, during speed skating, blood lactate concentration is elevated (5–7 mM), even at very slow speeds (Foster & Thompson, 1990). Fifth, the rate of muscle glycogen utilization during skating is very high (Green et al., 1978a). Finally, glycogen utilization is greater during exercise when blood flow is reduced (Sundberg et al., 1993). Taken together, these findings are consistent with the hypothesis that relatively low leg blood flow may be a limiting factor in skating performance.

Maximal oxygen uptake is related to skating performance at both 500 m ($r = -0.806$) and 1,500 m ($r = -0.864$). Thus, aerobic ability seems to be an important component of even the sprint events in speed skating (Foster & Thompson, 1990; van Ingen Schenau et al., 1983). On the other hand, only minimal changes were observed in $\dot{V}O_2$max and related variables over the course of a training season during which performance improved (Foster et al., 1993b; van Ingen Schenau et al., 1992).

Heart rates during all skating events (from 500 m to 10,000 m) have been recorded at or near maximal levels (Foster & Thompson, 1990). Maximal heart rates of male skaters are 186–194 beats/min and are independent of the mode of exercise (Kandou et al., 1987; Maksud et al., 1982; Nemoto et al., 1988; Quirion et al., 1988). Maximal ventilation volume of male skaters during exercise is approximately 150 L/min (Maksud et al., 1982; Nemoto et al., 1988; Quirion et al., 1988) but is lower during skating than during cycling (Kandou et al., 1987). The reduced ventilation is proportional to the reduced $\dot{V}O_2$max during skating (Foster & Thompson, 1990).

The so-called aerobic and anaerobic thresholds have been measured in skaters during incremental cycling tests. Although the significance of these measures is controversial, they are discussed here for the sake of completeness. In a group of male skaters, the ventilatory aerobic threshold occurred at approximately 61.1 ± 7.2% of $\dot{V}O_2$max, which corresponded to a heart rate of 142 ± 13 beats/min and a rating of perceived exertion (RPE) of 14.8 ± 1.2 on a 6–20 scale (Nemoto et al., 1988). The anaerobic threshold was similarly determined and occurred at 73.4 ± 5.9% of $\dot{V}O_2$max, a heart rate of 160 ± 11 beats/min, and an RPE of 16.4 ± 1.1 (Nemoto et al., 1988). The anaerobic threshold determined using the 4 mM lactate technique (OBLA) occurred at 73.5 ± 11.9% of $\dot{V}O_2$max and at a heart rate of 140.0 ± 21.0 beats/min (Quirion et al., 1988). The anaerobic threshold occurred at a higher exercise intensity in a group of all-around speed skaters than in sprinters (Nemoto et al., 1988) and was not affected by performance in a cold environment (Quirion et al., 1988).

Hematologic Values. Maksud et al. (1982) reported that a sample of male skaters had a hematocrit of 44.5 ± 0.5% and a serum hemoglobin concentration of 15.2 ± 0.9 g/dL following a dry land training season. Roberts and Smith (1990) followed six male and six female skaters for 2 y; the skaters had normal values for hematocrit, hemoglobin, iron concentration, and total iron binding capacity, and these values were unchanged during the course of the study. Serum ferritin in the females also did not change significantly during 2 y (year 1 = 57 ± 14 μg/L; year 2 = 51 ± 7 μg/L); however, in the males, ferritin decreased from 94 ± 27 μg/L to 72 ± 19 μg/L. It might be speculated that the decreased serum ferritin in the men was associated with the consumption of a modified vegetarian diet, which can reduce serum ferritin levels (Snyder et al., 1989a). Unfortunately, nutrient intakes were not reported by Roberts and Smith (1990).

Potential Limiting Factors

Skating Technique. Long and short track speed skating are high-intensity activities in which three of the five competitive events are completed in less than 2 min; the longer races last less than 8 min for women and less than 15 min for men. The relative contribution of anaerobic energy to the total energy demand for the different speed skating races ranges from 82%–11% (Table 5-2) (van Ingen Schenau et al., 1990). Thus, one would expect high levels of blood lactate at the conclusion of the races. Indeed, blood lactate concentration is greatest after the 1,000- and 1,500-m events (1.25–2 min), with values averaging around 16 mM (Figure 5-1) (Foster & Thompson, 1990; Smith & Roberts, 1990; von Kindermann & Keul, 1980). Slightly lower blood lactate concentrations (13-15 mM) have been reported for the other speed skating events (500, 3,000, 5,000, and 10,000 m) (Foster & Thompson, 1990; Smith & Roberts, 1990; von Kindermann & Keul, 1980). We have recorded postcompetition blood lactate concentrations as high as 24.0 mM following 1,000-m races (Snyder & Foster, unpublished data).

Blood lactate concentrations following the three shortest events were similar for male and female skaters (von Kindermann & Keul, 1980). In the same study, blood lactate concentrations following skating events lasting less than 5 min (500, 1,000, 1,500, 3,000 m) were lower than those recorded after running for similar durations; whereas lactates measured after skating 5,000 and 10,000 m were similar to those following running for comparable durations (von Kindermann & Keul, 1980). The blood lactate concentrations following all of the speed skating events in this investigation were similar to those for comparable swimming events. Furthermore, changes in pH, pCO_2, base excess, and plasma bicarbonate concentrations were all less following the speed skating events than they were after comparably timed running events. The greatest changes were observed following the 1,000-m skating event (males: pH = 7.095 ± 0.029, pCO_2 =

TABLE 5-2. *Anaerobic and aerobic energy contributions to long track speed skating events (van Ingen Schenau et al., 1990)*

EVENT	ANAEROBIC	AEROBIC
500 m	82%	18%
1,000 m	67%	33%
1,500 m	54%	46%
5,000 m	32%	68%
10,000 m	11%	89%

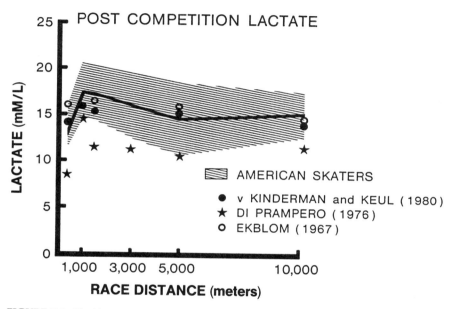

FIGURE 5-1. *Blood lactate concentrations following long track speed skating events.* The shaded area represents ± 1 S.D. of the means for U.S. skaters as recorded by the authors. The data from other investigators are included for comparison purposes (Foster & Thompson, 1990, reprinted with permission).

25.8 ± 1.9 mm Hg, base excess = −21.5 ± 2.2 mEq/L, standard-bicarbonate = 10.0 ± 1.1 mEq/L); similar changes were observed with the females (von Kindermann & Keul, 1980).

Although one might speculate that the lesser magnitude of the above markers of anaerobic activity following skating versus running show that speed skating events are less anaerobic than are comparable running events, we do not believe this to be the case. As described previously, the skating position involves a tightly crouched stance with small pre-extension angles of the knee and hip. To maintain this position, known to skaters as *sitting*, isometric actions of the knee and hip extensor muscles must occur. We hypothesize that the previously described poor local blood flow that is associated with the skating posture slows both the removal of lactate from the muscles and the distribution of that lactate throughout the blood and other extracellular compartments. Thus, the relatively low blood lactate concentrations found after speed skating versus running may actually reflect more profound regional anaerobic metabolism in the muscles of the skaters.

Thermoregulation. Although speed skating is generally performed outdoors (there are only five indoor long track ice ovals in the world) in air temperatures below 5°C (with wind chills even lower), no reports of hypothermia were found for skaters. However, speed skaters who do not dress appropriately during long practice sessions can experience frostbite of the hands and feet; this problem is discussed later in the chapter.

The low incidence of hypothermia during actual competition is probably a function of the warm-up and cool-down practices of the skaters. Before a race, a skater will typically: a) warm-up by jogging or cycling for approximately 30 min, b) stretch for approximately 20–30 min, c) warm-up by skating on the ice for 5-10 min, d) stretch again for approximately 20 min, and e) finally go back on the ice for no more than 5 min before the race. Postevent procedures are almost the reverse of the prerace activities. Almost all of the pre- and postcompetition activities can be performed indoors if the outdoor environment is exceedingly cold. Although the speed skaters compete in skin-tight lycra body suits that offer little protection against the cold, before and after the race itself they can wear more protective clothing. To summarize, speed skaters apparently have no major difficulties with thermoregulation that might limit skating performance.

Gender Limitations. Males and females compete in four of the same events (i.e., 500, 1,000, 1,500, and 5,000 m), with the mean advantages in performance for men during the past two Olympiads being 9.5%, 7.5%, 8.3%, and 7.4%, respectively. Both male (van Ingen Schenau & de Groot, 1983) and female (van Ingen Schenau et al., 1985) skaters seem to change their speeds over the different distances by altering stroke frequency, rather than changing the distance covered per stroke. However, traversing the same (or slightly greater) distance per stroke with a smaller time per stroke dictates that the push-off be proportionately more forceful in the shorter events. As mentioned earlier, two differences between male and female speed skaters are the pre-extension knee and hip joint angles and the percentage of body fat. Because aerobic power and anaerobic power expressed per unit of fat-free mass are similar between males and females (van Ingen Schenau et al., 1988), these characteristics do not appear to explain the gender-associated differences in skating performance.

Rather, van Ingen Schenau et al. (1988, 1990) have attributed about 50% of the apparent gender effect to the fact that women generally have a smaller muscle mass and a greater body fat mass than do men; they hypothesized that skating technique, particularly the strength-dependent pre-extension knee angle, accounts for the remaining 50% of the gender difference in skating performance.

Limitations on Performance Imposed by Air and Ice Resistance. At similar speeds, the energy expended per unit body surface area against air resistance is similar for speed skating, running, and cycling. However, when expressed per unit body mass, energy expenditure is greater for skating and cycling than for running (di Prampero et al., 1976). Due to the high velocities associated with speed skating and cycling, the total resistance attributable to air friction is quite large compared to that for the slower running pace.

Skaters generally accelerate rapidly during the 500- and 1,000-m events; the same rate of acceleration lasts for a shorter time in the longer events (van Ingen Schenau et al., 1990). During the sprint events, the use of a running-like technique to produce a high power output at the start of the race increases the energy lost to air friction, but this is compensated for by slower speeds at the end of the race (van Ingen Schenau et al., 1990). During the longer races, skaters exhibit a more uniform velocity. However, there is still a decrement in velocity as the race progresses, especially in the 1,500-m event (Foster et al., 1993a; van Ingen Schenau et al., 1990).

As altitude is increased, air pressure and resistance are reduced. Four long track ice ovals are at moderately high altitudes, i.e., Alma Ata, Kazakstan (1,700 m); Butte, Montana, USA (5,000 m); Calgary, Alberta, Canada (1,000 m); and Davos, Switzerland (5,000 m). Eight of the ten world record performances were achieved at two of these ovals. The only world records not established at these two ovals are the two longest events for the males (5,000- and 10,000-m).

The condition of the ice can also affect skating performance. Ekblom et al. (1967) reported $\dot{V}O_2$ increases of up to 20% during skating on "bad ice." de Koning (1991) noted that ice temperatures either less than or greater than the optimal $-4°C$, mechanical disruption of the ice surface, and foreign substances on the ice (e.g., snow, ice crystals, and dirt) all increased the coefficient of friction of the ice and thus reduced skating performance.

Brief History of Training Practices

Speed skaters, like most winter sports athletes, face unique training problems due to a lack of year-round venue availability. Even though there are now five indoor 400-m ice ovals in the world, none of the venues has ice throughout the year. In fact, the venues are generally open only from September through March. Thus, multiple dry-land training techniques are needed if training is to continue during the warmer months. In general with speed skaters, a training year is broken down into three phases: a) transition, b) preparation, and c) competition (Crowe, 1990; van Ingen Schenau et al., 1992). The transition phase is that period after the competitive season (generally about mid-March) to the beginning of the preparation phase (May/June). During the transition phase, participation in activities other than skating is encouraged. During the preparation phase (May/June to late October), training progresses from general conditioning to more specific skating techniques. Finally, during the competition phase (November to March), the general conditioning aspects are maintained while skating technique (now with on-ice drills) is emphasized. As would be expected, significantly greater ratings of perceived exertion (RPE) have been reported at the end of the preparation phase than at the beginning, indicating an increase in perceived training intensity; no gender-related differences in RPE were observed (Gutmann et al., 1986).

Gutmann et al. (1986) reported that the moods of skaters improved during the preparation phase, while vigor and fatigue remained constant. There were no differences in the psychological profiles between males and females, but younger athletes had higher scores for anger, fatigue, and total mood disturbances and lower scores for vigor (Gutmann et al., 1986).

Training and Nutrition Practices

Testing Protocols for Speed Skating. The authors believe that an exercise test can benefit an athlete and coach only if it meets three criteria: a) there must be a high correlation between the test measure and subsequent competitive performance; b) the test must be able to detect changes in the competitive fitness of the athlete; and c) the test must allow the athletes to set goals (Foster et al., 1993b).

In an attempt to find such an exercise test, we and others have tested and followed athletes using a number of protocols. Initially, we measured $\dot{V}O_2$max, first by running and then by cycling; $\dot{V}O_2$max was related to skating performance in the 1,500-m event ($r = -0.75$), but it did not change from the beginning to the end of the preparation phase of training (Foster et al., 1993b). In these initial observations and those that followed, we chose to relate the test performance with that of skating a 1,500-m event. Our rationale for this choice was that most skaters, whether they skate the all-around or sprint program, will perform the 1,500-m event. Also, the event is more of an endurance event than the 500-m event (included in both the all-around and sprint programs).

Next, we examined whether power output at the onset of blood lactate accumulation (OBLA) during a cycle ergometer test was related to skating performance and if improvements occurred during the skating season. Significant improvements in power output at OBLA occurred during the preparatory phase (3.55 ± 0.24 to 3.80 ± 0.22 W/kg), and the power output was related to 1,500-m performance ($r = -0.77$) (Foster et al., 1993b). While the test met two of the criteria we had established, the athlete was able neither to set any goals during the test nor see any actual improvement, other than what the scientist divulged.

Because most speed skating events utilize anaerobic energy production quite extensively, we next tested speed skaters using the 30-s Wingate test. Again, a good correlation was obtained between power output and 1,500-m skating performance ($r = -0.79$), but no change in Wingate test results occurred when athletes were followed from June to November (Foster et al., 1993b). Similarly, van Ingen Schenau et al. (1992) tested athletes at four time points throughout a season using a Wingate-type 30-s sprint test and a 2.5-min supramaximal test and observed no seasonal changes in elite junior male and female skaters.

Geijsel (1979) developed a cycle ergometer endurance test with male marathon skaters. The athlete was required to ride the cycle ergometer at an exercise intensity of 5 W/kg body weight to exhaustion. Since marathon speed skaters generally skate at around 75–90 strokes/min, the athletes were required to cycle at this cadence. Endurance times of the skaters increased during the preparation phase and could be used by the athletes as indicators of increased competitive fitness. Geijsel (1980) then had some of the best and worst marathon speed skaters perform the test. Significant differences were recorded between the best and worst skaters, with the best skaters performing 14.0 min of exercise and the worst skaters only 5.8 min. Thus, within a group of well-trained athletes, the 5 W/kg test not only indicated increases in competitive fitness, but also discriminated between best and worst performers.

We have since adopted the Geijsel test for use with long track speed skaters by requiring them to cycle at 60 RPM to more closely simulate their 60 strokes/min skating cadence. Using this procedure, we have observed performance increases in males from 6.5 ± 4.0 min to 12.0 ± 5.8 min during the preparation phase of training, as well as a relationship with performances in a 1,500-m event ($r = -0.79$) (Foster et al., 1993b). We initially also had the female skaters perform the 5 W/kg endurance test, but we were observing short endurance times and small improvements. The aerobic requirement of the 5 W/kg is approximately 65 mL· $kg^{-1} \cdot min^{-1}$ (approximately 100% and 116% of mean $\dot{V}O_2$ max for male and female speed skaters, respectively). Adjusting for gender specific differences in $\dot{V}O_2$ max, we now have the female skaters perform a 4.3 W/kg endurance cycle ergometer test. The results of this test with the females proved to be quite comparable to those demonstrated by the males, with performances improving from 5.0 ± 1.6 min to 12.5 ± 4.5 min and the relationship to 1,500-m performances being r = −0.80 (Foster et al., 1993b).

Even though the cycling endurance test proved to be a successful exercise test for us and others because it tracked competitive fitness and was related to skating performance, the test had its drawbacks. First, while some goal setting is produced by the test (i.e., the skater can try to last longer than during a previous test or longer than a teammate), such goals are unlike competitive goals (i.e., how fast an event can be completed). Second, the equipment necessary to perform the test (an electrically braked cycle ergometer) is heavy and expensive and not easily transported to training camps where the athletes are to be tested. Finally, when endurance greater than about 15 min is achieved, the test loses its predictive ability (Foster et al., 1993b) and becomes boring for the athlete (Geijsel, 1980).

We next developed a 10-km cycling time-trial test (Foster et al., 1993b). The 10-km test was performed with a skater's personal bicycle attached to a portable windload simulator and set at the highest gear possible (Figure 5-2). The reproducibility of the exercise testing set-up had been established previously by Dengel et al. (1990). The 10-km test proved to be: a) related to 1,500-m performance (r = −0.81); b) an indicator of competitive fitness (times improved from 16.1 ± 2.5 min to 15.1 ± 2.4 min during the course of the preparation phase); 3) goal oriented; and 4) perceived by the skaters as requiring exertion quite similar to that in skating competitions.

Training Practices. During the preparation phase, approximately 14 exercise sessions are performed per week. These sessions include a total training time of about 30–35 h/wk, counting stretching and warm-up activities (Pollock et al., 1982; van Ingen Schaneu et al., 1992). The training is conducted almost entirely away from the ice and can be categorized into: a) primarily aerobic activities (40%), including distance running and cycling; b) primarily anaerobic activities (20%), including high-intensity interval running and cycling; c) weight training (15%), both for strength and local muscular endurance; and d) training specific to skating movements (25%), including low walking (i.e., walking while in the skating position), slide board exercising, roller skating, and dry skating, which involves sideward push-offs with alternating legs, allowing little or no change in the center of gravity (Pollock et al., 1982) (Figures 5-3, 5-4, 5-5).

During this preparation phase, the skaters follow a 4-wk macro cycle, i.e., 3 wk of intensive training are followed by 1 wk of easier training (Knapp et al., 1986; van Ingen Schenau et al., 1992). The aerobic activities are quite similar to those performed by runners and/or cyclists and are intended to prepare the athlete for higher intensity conditioning. The anaerobic and strength activities consist primarily of tempo and high-

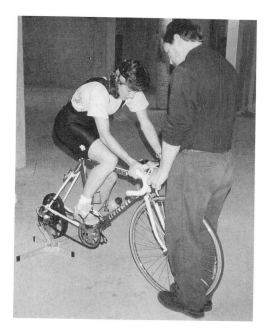

FIGURE 5-2. *Cycling time trial (10 km) with skater's bicycle attached to a portable wind load simulator.*

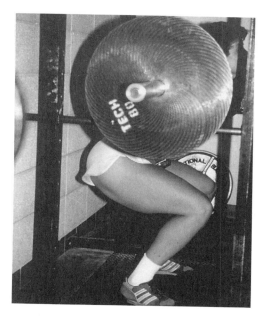

FIGURE 5-3. *Heavy resistance training performed by a long-track speed skater (from Foster & Thompson, 1990, reprinted with permission).*

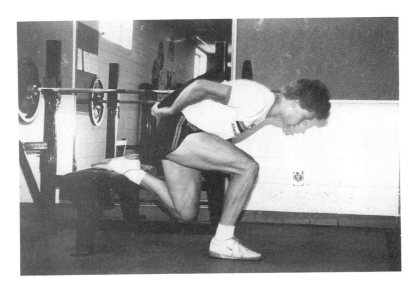

FIGURE 5-4. *Light resistance training performed by a long-track speed skater.*

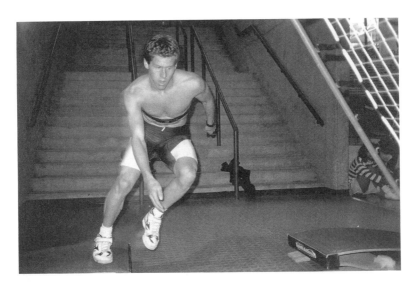

FIGURE 5-5. *Plyometric jumps from boards performed by a long-track speed skater.*

intensity (or heavy resistance), low-repetition exercises, stressing mainly the hip and knee extensor muscles. Three different types of anaerobic and strength activities are typically performed by the speed skaters; these are shown in Table 5-3.

TABLE 5-3. *Resistance training activities performed by longtrack speed skaters*

HEAVY RESISTANCE
Activities: Leg Curls and Squats
Volume: 5 sets of 5 repetitions
Resistance: Men—2.5 × body weight
Women—2.0 × body weight

LIGHT RESISTANCE
Activity: One Legged Squats
Volume: 3 sets of 50 – 100 repetitions
Resistance: 10 – 20 kg weight on back

PLYOMETRICS
Activities: Jumps with counter movements
Jumps without counter movements
Jumps from boards

As previously mentioned, long track speed skaters face lack of ice availability. During the preparation phase, some ice is available in short track venues (hockey or figure skating rinks). However, short track skate blades are 30 cm long, 15 cm shorter than long track skate blades. Short track skaters compete on smaller ovals and use shorter blades to accomplish higher turns than those performed on 400-m tracks. Many long track skaters refuse to skate on short course tracks because they are convinced that using the shorter blades changes their "feel" for the ice. Thus, other non-ice activities must be used to simulate the speed skating motion.

Much debate and concern has arisen over whether the dry-land activities are specific enough to benefit the speed skater. Many different activities have been tried with different degrees of efficacy. Dry skating and low walking need no special equipment. However, the speed skater usually performs low walking while traversing up a hill (Figure 5-6). Low walking produces $\dot{V}O_2$max levels that are similar to those produced while skating, but maximal heart rates, respiratory exchange ratios, and ventilation volumes that are higher (De Boer et al., 1987b). In the same study, dry skating produced lower $\dot{V}O_2$max levels and ventilation volumes, but comparable maximal respiratory exchange ratios and heart rates when compared to speed skating. Biomechanically, stroke frequency was greater during low walking and lower during dry skating than during speed skating (de Boer et al., 1987b). Also, the joint angles and the movement patterns at the knee and hip joints were different in dry skating and low walking compared with actual speed skating on the ice (de Boer et al., 1987b). Thus, while many skaters use dry skating and low walking as specific dry-land skating activities, de Boer and colleagues (1987b) and de Groot et al. (1987) suggested that they not be included in a training program, but that more specific activities such as board skating or roller skating be used.

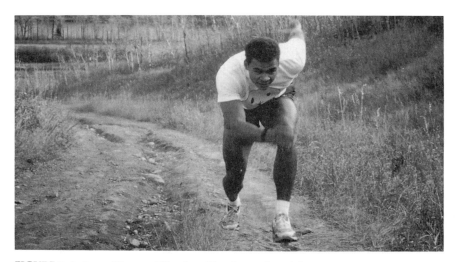

FIGURE 5-6. *Low walking up a hill performed by a long track speed skater.*

A slide board is a 0.5 X 2.0 X 2.5-m board covered with formica that has been polished to promote sliding. The skaters generally wear socks over their shoes, to maximize sliding ability (Figure 5-7). Kandou et al. (1987) observed extensive similarities between speed skating and slide board exercise in the biomechanics of the movements of the hip and knee joints, as well as in $\dot{V}O_2$max, heart rate, and respiratory exchange ratio (Kandou et al., 1987). Similar biomechanical results were observed by de Boer et al. (1987a). Furthermore, we recorded similar blood lactate concentrations following 15 min of either slideboard exercise or continuous speed skating when both were completed at similar intensities (slideboard = 4.8 ± 1.2 mM, speed skating = 5.1 ± 1.0 mM) (Snyder et al., 1989b).

Roller skating with in-line skates (skates with a single row of four or five wheels) is also performed by speed skaters as a specific training protocol. The $\dot{V}O_2$max levels, ventilation volumes, and heart rates were comparable in both roller skating and speed skating, whereas the maximal respiratory exchange ratios were greater during roller skating (de Boer et al., 1987c). The two types of skating produce similar values for work per stroke and stroke frequency, except that the pre-extension knee angle is smaller during speed skating (de Boer et al., 1987a, 1987c). During roller skating, the total power to overcome the air and surface resistance was comparable to that for speed skating; however, the surface resistance was greater and the air resistance less during roller skating (de Boer et al., 1987c). Maximal speeds in the two activities were different; therefore, de Boer et al. (1987c) suggested using heart rate rather than speed as an indicator of exercise intensity. Hoffman et al. (1992) and Snyder et al. (1993)

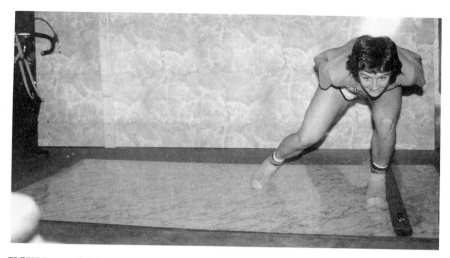

FIGURE 5-7. *Slide board exercise performed by a long track speed skater (from Foster & Thompson, 1990, reprinted with permission).*

cautioned about the high speeds that might be necessary for trained individuals to obtain cardiovascular benefits from the use of roller skating. One technique that might be used to reduce the speed of the activity would be to roller skate up hills.

Once the skater begins training on the ice, technique and skating endurance should be important goals. Training efficacy for improving endurance can be monitored by following changes in the lactate profile of the skater, i.e, changes in the concentration of blood lactate observed during progressive increases in skating velocity. The general protocol for establishing the lactate profile begins by asking the skater to skate 1,200–2,000 m at a set speed; heart rate, RPE, and blood lactate concentration are recorded immediately following the skating task. The exercise is then repeated 4–5 times at incrementally higher velocities. The lactate profiles show that: a) as expected, blood lactate concentration increases in a curvilinear fashion as the skating velocity increases, and b) once the skater assumes the correct skating posture, i.e., with low pre-extension angles of the knee and hip, blood lactate concentrations of at least 5–7 mM can be expected, no matter how slow the skating velocity (Foster & Thompson, 1990). The lactate profile shifts rightward both when the athlete becomes better trained and when the glycogen concentration in the skater's muscles is low at the start of the exercise (Foster et al., 1988). Finally, blood lactate concentrations progressively and linearly increase during simulated roller skating at distances comparable to 3,000 and 5,000 m on the ice (Crowe et al., 1986).

Nutrition Practices. Because skaters perform intense, prolonged training on a daily basis, it is possible that their muscles may become relatively depleted of glycogen stores, as shown by Costill et al. (1971) in runners. When we first measured the food intake of skaters in 1983, we observed that the skaters consumed primarily a high-fat (50%), low-carbohydrate (30%) diet. By 1989, after extensive nutritional education and the provision of carbohydrate supplements, many of the same skaters were consuming a diet containing 57% (women) or 49% (men) carbohydrates, even without the use of supplements (Snyder et al., 1989c). If carbohydrate supplements were added to the dietary record, the carbohydrate percentages were 63% for the females and 56% for the males. Thus, with the use of carbohydrate supplements, the speed skaters were consuming the minimal amount typically recommended (Costill & Miller, 1980).

Because of the erratic availability of skating venues and high quality coaching, skaters typically spend a maximum of 4–8 wk at any given location; this reduces the athletes' familiarity with local sources of healthful foods. Furthermore, to maximize training time when they gain access to a skating venue, the skaters often spend little time on food preparation. Coaches and trainers should make special efforts to ensure that the skaters' diets contain adequate nutrients, including at least 60% of energy intake as complex carbohydrates. The recommended daily dietary protein intake is roughly 1.6 g/kg body weight, but most athletes routinely consume at least this much protein because their total energy intakes are so great (Walberg et al., 1988). A meal containing about 300–400 g of carbohydrate consumed approximately 4 h prior to competition may improve performance (Sherman et al., 1989), and, if time permits between events, a light carbohydrate snack might be useful to help replenish glycogen stores in liver and muscle. Also, studies with cycling exercise suggest that muscle glycogen replenishment can be maximized by consuming 100 g of carbohydrates (liquid or solid form) within 2 h after the completion of an exercise bout and a total of about 8–10 g of carbohydrate per kilogram of body weight during the 24 h following exhaustive training or competition (Ivy et al., 1988a, 1988b).

Fluid should be made available at all exercise and competition sites and should be consumed as needed. Monitoring of body weight before and after practice sessions can be used to detect weight loss due to dehydration.

Medical Considerations

As speed skating by necessity requires a great deal of cross-training, injuries common to running and cycling can also occur in speed skaters, but will not be discussed here (see chapters 7 and 8). Long track speed skating itself has historically involved few injuries, probably due to the minimal stress placed on the joints and muscles during the skating motion and to the fact that only two skaters compete at a time (Woods, 1990). The most common injuries to speed skaters involve back pain (caused by the skating position), laceration and stab wounds (primarily during the start of the race), strain of the leg adductor muscles (again at the start of the race), and foot injuries caused by the boot (Woods, 1990). Prevention of the back and adductor muscle injuries is probably best achieved by exercise training, flexibility training, and warm-up activities.

Many injuries occur during short track skating because many skaters compete simultaneously on a small ice oval. Short track speed skaters wear helmets and elbow and knee pads during competition; some skaters concerned about lacerations also wear protection around the neck. Injuries during short track speed skating can include lacerations, bruised body parts, concussions, and fractures.

The fact that ice skating is performed in a cold environment leads to two other potential medical problems—frostbite and postcompetition exercise-induced bronchospasm. (As mentioned previously, hypothermia is generally not a major problem with speed skating because the skaters wear warm clothing both before and after races.) In speed skaters, frostbite commonly occurs on the toes and on uncovered hands and noses (Woods, 1990). Speed skaters usually do not wear socks and wear boots that are 1–2 sizes smaller than the shoes they wear so that the skating blade becomes an extension of the foot. Accordingly, skaters are prone to calluses, tendinitis, and frostbite of the foot. Finally, following races lasting 1–4 min, many athletes experience a persistent cough for about 2 d (Woods, 1990). This exercise-induced bronchospasm has been associated with abnormalities observed in pulmonary function tests after competition that are consistent with mild obstructive airway disease (Wiley et al., 1992). Probably the low temperature and low relative humidity in the environment contribute to the development of this illness.

As with any athlete, the speed skater can become overtrained. Our experience indicates that the skaters are most vulnerable from the beginning to the middle part of the preparation phase, especially during Olympic years. We also believe that athletes who are at critical points in their careers (e.g., club skaters attempting to qualify for national teams or national team skaters attempting to qualify for an Olympic team) and who thus have incentives for more serious training are particularly subject to the overtraining syndrome. During these circumstances, training intensity and competitiveness appear to be maximized. While the exact cause of the overtraining syndrome is not yet known, the outcome is generally a decrement in performance. A sufficient number of recovery days during a training program appears to be an important consideration in the prevention of overtraining.

ICE HOCKEY

Ice hockey originated in Canada in the early 1800s and has been an Olympic sport since 1920. Ice hockey is played on an ice oval that measures approximately 61 m X 30.5 m and is generally played indoors. The ice hockey game takes place in three 20-min periods, with 12-min intermissions between periods. Ice hockey teams generally have about 15 players and two goalkeepers, with three forwards, two defensemen, and one goalkeeper on the ice at one time. A team generally has 3–4 lines (or shifts) of forwards and two or three lines of defensemen.

Time-motion analysis showed that a shift for the average player usually involved 39.7 s of uninterrupted play followed by 27.1 s of play stoppage, repeated 2.3 times (Green et al., 1976). As the recovery time between shifts was 3.8 min, the total playing time was 24.5 min (Green et al., 1976). Because there are fewer of them, defensemen generally play for more minutes than do forwards, but also tend to skate at a slower velocity (62% of the velocity of forwards).

The ice hockey skate is very different from the speed skate, having a shorter blade and a stiffer/taller boot. The ice hockey skating stroke, like that of the speed skater, involves three components: a) a glide with single leg support, b) propulsion with single leg support, and c) propulsion with double leg support (Marino & Weese, 1979). The propulsion occurs from about half-way through the single leg support through the end of the double leg support.

Characteristics of Elite Ice Hockey Players

Because there is apparently no published information on women ice hockey players, the following discussion relies solely on reports on men.

Body Composition and Anthropometry. Defensemen tend to be taller ($\sim$ 180 cm) and heavier ($\sim$ 85 kg) than forwards ($\sim$ 176 cm, 77 kg) and goalkeepers ($\sim$ 176 cm, 74 kg) (Agre et al., 1988; Green & Houston, 1975; Houston & Green, 1976; Orvanova, 1987). In general, elite hockey players are endomorphic mesomorphs (Orvanova, 1987) with approximately 10% body fat (Agre et al., 1988; Green & Houston, 1975; Green et al., 1979; Houston & Green, 1976; Montgomery, 1988; Montgomery & Dallaire, 1986; Orvanova, 1987). Thus, the average lean body mass of hockey players is approximately 70 kg.

Muscle Fiber Type Profile. Green et al. (1979) examined the muscle fiber type profiles in elite ice hockey players from university, junior, and professional divisions. Tissue samples were taken from the vastus lateralis muscle. No significant differences were observed among the muscle samples from the athletes playing in the different leagues. The fiber type distribution was typical of that of an untrained individual; i.e., 49.6 $\pm$

2.7% slow twitch (Type I); 38.0 ± 2.3% fast twitch, oxidative-glycolytic (Type IIA); and 12.2 ± 2.5% fast twitch, glycolytic (Type IIB). Relative muscle fiber area followed the distribution of muscle fiber type and was 47.1 ± 3.2% Type I, 40.4 ± 2.5% Type IIA, and 12.5 ± 2.8% Type IIB. Finally, the activities of the enzymes phosphorylase, phosphofructokinase, and lactate dehydrogenase were all similar to those observed in control subjects (Green et al., 1979). However, activities of 3-hydroxyacyl CoA dehydrogenase and succinate dehydrogenase were significantly greater in the hockey players than in the control subjects.

Flexibility and Muscle Strength. The flexibility of forwards is similar to that of defensemen, but goalkeepers had greater ranges of motion for trunk flexion, shoulder extension, and hip abduction than did either forwards or defensemen (Agre et al., 1988; Montgomery & Dallaire, 1986).

When expressed on an absolute basis, grip strength and maximal bench press were greater in defensemen (69.4 kg and 101 kg, respectively) than in forwards (65.3 kg and 89.6 kg, respectively) (Montgomery & Dallaire, 1986; Orvanova, 1987). However, when strength was expressed per unit of body mass, strength differences were not significant.

Anaerobic Power and Capacity. Due to the high intensity and short duration of hockey skating, high anaerobic power and a large anaerobic capacity would seem to be important. For the most part, three different tests—the Wingate test, an intermittent cycle ergometer test, and a 2 × 60-s cycle test—have been used to measure anaerobic power and capacity. In the intermittent cycle test, six 15-s repetitions are performed with a 15-s recovery following each exercise bout (Gamble & Montgomery, 1986). During the 2 × 60-s cycle test, a 60-s all-out effort is followed by a 3-min recovery period, which is then followed by a second 60-s all-out effort (Montgomery, 1988). Independent of the test used, forwards and defensemen had similar anaerobic abilities when expressed per unit of body mass (Montgomery, 1988; Montgomery & Dallaire, 1986). Because defensemen weigh more than forwards, defensemen had greater absolute anaerobic abilities than forwards (Montgomery, 1988; Montgomery & Dallaire, 1986). Montgomery (1988) reported peak power for ice hockey players in the Wingate test to be 11.0 ± 0.8 W/kg, whereas mean power was 8.8 ± 0.6 W/kg.

Cardiovascular and Pulmonary Capacities and Aerobic Power. Even more so than speed skaters, ice hockey players tend to have relatively ordinary aerobic abilities. Values for $\dot{V}O_2$max ranging from 4.3–4.7 L/min (53–57 mL·kg^{-1}·min^{-1}) have been reported for ice hockey players who completed treadmill running tests (Agre et al., 1988; Green & Houston, 1975; Houston & Green, 1976; Montgomery & Dallaire, 1986; Rosentswieg et al., 1979). Montgomery (1988) reported that a group of ice hockey players had mean values for $\dot{V}O_2$max of 57.2 mL·kg^{-1}·min^{-1} during running tests, 53.4 mL·kg^1·min^{-1} during cycling tests, and 55.5 mL·kg^{-1}·min^{-1} during skating tests. As expected, the running test produced slightly greater ($\sim$ 7%) $\dot{V}O_2$max levels than did the cycling test, with the skating test values falling between running and cycling. Defensemen have lower $\dot{V}O_2$max values than do forwards, with goalkeepers generally having the lowest $\dot{V}O_2$max values (Agre et al., 1988; Green & Houston, 1975; Houston & Green, 1976; Minkoff, 1982).

Maximal heart rates during running tests ranged between 185 and 197 beats/min, with goalkeepers having slightly higher maximal heart rates than forwards and defensemen (Agre et al., 1988; Green & Houston, 1975; Houston & Green, 1976). Maximal ventilation volume averaged 130 L/min STPD and was not different among the three different playing positions (Green & Houston, 1975; Houston & Green, 1976). No investigations have examined the anaerobic threshold of ice hockey players.

Visual Ability. Ice hockey is not only a high-intensity activity, but one that also requires a great deal of accuracy. Minkoff (1982) performed visual testing on ice hockey players during preseason examinations and showed that total eye score rating (a composite of the scores of the tests performed) was strongly related to shot accuracy. Furthermore, vision span was related to shot accuracy and success during face-offs, whereas vision speed was not related to shot accuracy. Goalkeepers and all-star performers achieved better scores on the vision tests than did forwards, defensemen, and non all-stars.

Potential Limiting Factors

Limitations Imposed by Energy Metabolism. In an ice hockey game, the length of a shift can vary from several seconds to greater than 2 min (Green, 1979); during this time, high-intensity exercise with few breaks is performed. Blood lactate concentrations of $\sim$12 mM have been observed after one period of play (Watson & Hanley, 1986). The high intensity and intermittent nature of the activity can produce two metabolic problems: a) depletion of muscle glycogen, and b) slow recovery from metabolic acidosis.

Green (1978) had ice hockey players skate either continuously for 60 min ($\sim$55% of $\dot{V}O_2$max) or perform intermittent exercise (ten 1-min bouts with 5-min recovery between each, $\sim$ 75% of $\dot{V}O_2$max). Biopsies from the vastus lateralis muscle and blood samples were obtained following 30- and 60-min of activity. During the intermittent activity, blood glucose, lactate, glycerol, pyruvate, plasma free fatty acids, and hematocrit were all increased significantly at both the 30 and 60 min measurement periods. During the continuous skating, only blood glucose (30 and 60 min) and lactate (30 min) showed small, but significant, increases. Within the muscle, decreases in adenosine triphosphate (18%) and phosphocreatine (37%)

occurred during the intermittent exercise, whereas muscle lactate concentration was 10-fold higher following the intermittent exercise than following the continuous exercise. Muscle glycogen was reduced 29% by the continuous exercise; with the intermittent exercise, glycogen was reduced by 45% after 30 min and by 70% after 60 min. Following the intermittent exercise, the greatest depletion of muscle glycogen occurred in the Type I muscle fibers, but some depletion also occurred in the Type II fibers. Thus, at least during a simulated hockey competition, carbohydrate metabolism was used extensively, and depletion of muscle glycogen did occur (Green, 1978; Montpetit et al., 1979).

Green (1978) measured blood lactate levels of 10.9 ± 1.2 mM following 30 min and 13.3 ± 0.6 mM following 60 min of intermittent exercise. Similar blood lactate values were observed by Watson and Hanley (1986), who collected samples during two periods of simulated ice hockey play. One of the problems associated with lactate accumulation in ice hockey players is that the lactate is metabolized only slowly when the skaters sit on the bench between shifts on the ice. Watson and Hanley (1986) examined blood lactate concentrations following participation in a variety of activities during the 15-min intermission periods to see if blood lactate concentration could be reduced. The subjects spent the first 3 min sitting, the next 10 min in either active or passive recovery, and the last 2 min sitting. The active recovery consisted of either a) bench stepping (with skates removed) at a cadence required to produce a heart rate of 120 beats/min, or b) continuous skating at a heart rate of 120 beats/min. Post-recovery blood lactate levels were slightly lower following bench stepping (6.1 ± 2.2 mM) than following continuous skating (6.7 ± 1.4 mM) and significantly lower than following passive rest (8.1 ± 1.6 mM). Perhaps gliding was the main activity during the low-intensity skating so that relatively little lactate was metabolized (Watson & Hanley, 1986). Still, it appears that ice hockey players might be well advised to perform low-intensity physical activities rather than sit during the intermission periods if they wish to reduce blood lactate concentrations before the next shift on the ice.

Disturbance in Temperature Regulation. Even though ice hockey is played on ice and in a cool environment, the players can lose 2–3 kg of body weight over the course of a game despite *ad libitum* fluid intake (Green et al., 1978b; MacDougall, 1979). Associated with this loss of body fluid is at least a 2% increase in hematocrit following a single period of play (Green et al., 1976; 1978b). The reason hockey players lose so much weight during play is that heat dissipation is limited by their protective clothing so that core temperature rises and stimulates excessive sweating. To reduce this effect of clothing on fluid loss, MacDougall (1979) suggested the following: a) removal of helmet and gloves between shifts, b) encouragement of greater intake of liquids, c) wearing of underwear made from polypropylene or other fabrics that "wick" sweat away from the skin, and d) use of open neck porous jerseys.

Training and Nutrition Practices

Testing Protocols. Testing of ice hockey players has included measures of anthropometry, anaerobic power and capacity, cardiovascular fitness, and musculoskeletal strength and flexibility, but many of the testing protocols have not been specific to ice hockey. Anthropometric measures generally obtained on ice hockey players include height, weight, percent body fat, lean body mass, and body surface area. Cardiovascular fitness has usually been tested on a treadmill or cycle ergometer, with very few actual skating tests having been performed. Flexibility has been tested at the shoulder, hip, and knee joints, and strength measures have included grip strength, maximal bench press, or isokinetic determination of knee and shoulder strength.

Most tests specific to ice hockey have measured variables related to anaerobic metabolism. Among the tests used have been the Sargeant Anaerobic Skate test (SAS_{40}), which consists of players skating back and forth along pylons placed a distance of 55 m on the ice for a total of 40 s; the Reed Repeat Sprint Skate test (RSS), which requires players to skate 55 m six times every 30 s; the Wingate test lengthened to 40 s (WAT_{40}); and a cycle ergometer test of six 15-s exercise:rest periods (RCE) (Gamble & Montgomery, 1986; Watson & Sargeant, 1986). Mean anaerobic capacity scores for the four tests were: SAS_{40} = 9.7 ± 0.8 W/kg; RSS = 9.3 ± 0.8 W/kg; WAT_{40} = 7.7 ± 0.2 W/kg; and RCE = 8.2 W/kg (Koziris & Montgomery, 1991; Watson & Sargeant, 1986). Blood lactate concentrations following the performances of these anaerobic tests ranged from 10.7 to 13.7 mM (Koziris & Montgomery, 1991; Watson & Sargeant, 1986). As might be expected, Watson and Sargeant (1986) observed that the results for the RSS and SAS_{40} were more related to each other than either of these variables was to WAT_{40}.

Other skill-specific tests have been developed to monitor the progress of ice hockey players. Such tests as the skating agility test, Hansen puck control test, and the backward skating agility test are described by Macnab (1979) and Montgomery (1988). The results of the study by Macnab (1979) showed that performances on the fitness tests as well as the skating agility tests improved as young players aged, and that the tests may be used to track changes in a skater's ability.

Training Practices. The duration of a typical ice hockey season is 5–8 months and includes at least 100 games. However, very little scientific literature exists concerning proper preparation for the season. During a season, 2–3 games are generally played per week; practices are held on non-game days. Because games are so frequent during a season, practice sessions are typically designed to develop skill and to prepare for the next game.

A typical practice lasts about 1.5–2 h and consists of a short warm-up period, repeat bouts of high-intensity skating, instruction, special plays, and controlled scrimmages (Daub et al., 1982). The majority of the appropriate studies show that aerobic power, anaerobic capacity, and muscular strength are either unchanged or reduced during the ice hockey season (Cotton et al., 1979; Daub et al., 1983; Green & Houston, 1975; Green et al., 1979; Johansson et al., 1989; Posch et al., 1989; Quinney et al., 1982). In examining the characteristics of the muscle fibers before and after a season of ice hockey, Green et al. (1979) observed an increase in the percentage of Type IIA fibers and decreases in both the percentage of Type IIB fibers and the percentage of the total fiber area devoted to Type IIB fibers. Two muscle enzymes—phosphofructokinase and phosphorylase—were significantly reduced, while 3-hydroxyacyl CoA dehydrogenase was significantly greater following the hockey season (Green et al., 1979). The activities of succinate dehydrogenase and lactate dehydrogenase were unchanged (Green et al., 1979). In a similar study, Daub et al. (1982) observed minimal muscle adaptations following a season of hockey playing.

A few studies have attempted to increase the aerobic power and/or anaerobic capacity of hockey players through additional on-ice or non-ice training (Greer et al., 1992; Hollering & Simpson, 1977; Hutchinson et al., 1979). While the duration of the added training program was brief in all cases (6–7 wk), improvements in aerobic power (Hutchinson et al., 1979) and skating speed and acceleration (Greer et al., 1992) were achieved. On the other hand, Daub et al. (1983), found no change (relative to control subjects) in the maximal or submaximal skating abilities of players who incorporated low-intensity ($\sim$74% $\dot{V}O_2$max) cycling exercise into a hockey training program.

Nutrition Practices. Little information exists in the scientific literature pertaining to the food intake of ice hockey players. Houston (1979) had seven players complete a 7 d diet survey and reported that on a daily basis they consumed 2.8 servings of meat or equivalent, 2.3 servings of milk or equivalent, 1.6 servings of vegetables, 1.2 servings of fruit, 4.6 servings of grain, 2.1 servings of pop and candy, and 3.0 servings of alcohol. The intake of grain was mainly as breads, crackers and pasta, whereas about half of the vegetable servings were in the form of french fries. Houston (1979) also reported that informal discussions with the ice hockey players suggested that the reported alcohol consumption was probably only about 60% of the actual consumption. The players averaged 2.4 meals/d, with 45% of the meals eaten away from home. Finally, 67% of the time the players skipped breakfast.

Rehunen and Liitsola (1978) had a group of ice hockey players consume 360 g of carbohydrate as a supplement for 3 d prior to a championship series and reported muscle glycogen levels twice as high as those of players who did not consume the supplement. Similar to the suggestions for speed skaters, regular consumption of high-carbohydrate supplements may be necessary to insure normal glycogen levels for competition.

As with speed skaters, ice hockey players probably need to consume sufficient carbohydrate (~60% of dietary energy intake) and protein (~1.6 g/kg body weight) to ensure strength maintenance and development and the replenishment of glycogen stores. Fluid intake, especially during and immediately after a game, should also be encouraged to replace body fluid lost during practice or competition.

Medical Considerations

Ice hockey is a sport in which aggressive behavior can affect performance positively, e.g., it can cause more goals to be scored and more shots on goal to be attempted (McCarthy & Kelly, 1978). Injuries are quite common in all levels of ice hockey, especially as the intensity of the game increases. Moore reported in 1980 that injured players missed 11% of their teams' games. According to Moore (1980), 21.9% of the injuries occurred when a skater was being checked, 17.8% while carrying or passing the puck, 15.2% while gaining possession of the puck, and 14.8% during checking. Posch et al. (1989) observed no association between the injury rate and the decrease in muscle strength that occurred during an ice hockey season. Of the 68 injuries noted by Posch et al. (1989) the head, neck, face, shoulder, upper arm, thorax, abdomen, back, forearm, hand, thigh, knee, lower leg, and foot were affected. Because the injuries usually involve contact with another player, a stick, the ice, and/or the boards, the exact types of injuries and treatments to be performed are too numerous to discuss here.

No long-term studies have examined health problems of ice hockey players who have completed their playing careers. However, to the extent that participants in ice hockey and American style professional football are exposed to common physical, psychological, and social stressors, results of a recent symposium concerning former professional football players in the United States may be instructive (Cantu, 1993). Apparently, these athletes had reduced longevity, continued chronic injuries from their playing days, and increased substance abuse when compared to society in general (Cantu, 1993). Similar health problems might be expected to occur in post-career ice hockey players.

In the one study that examined respiratory infections in young (12 y) ice hockey players, other athletes, and sedentary controls, no intergroup differences were detected (Osterback & Qvarnberg, 1987). The common cold accounted for 91% of the infections in all groups.

FIGURE SKATING

Figure skating includes four events: women's singles (an Olympic sport since 1920), men's singles (an Olympic sport since 1908), pairs (an Olympic sport since 1920), and ice dancing (an Olympic sport since 1976). Figure skating is performed on a rink (usually indoors) that has maximal dimensions of 60 X 30 m. The figure skate blade is narrow (~3 mm wide), and the leather boot extends above the ankle joint. Figure skaters perform two programs: a short program (maximum time 2.5 min) and a long program (maximum time 4.0 min).

Characteristics of Elite Figure Skaters

The average ranges in height and weight for elite men and women figure skaters are 167–173 cm/60–66 kg and 158–161 cm/49–51 kg, respectively; body fat percentages range between 5–9% for men and 9–12% for women (Brock & Striowski, 1986; Niinimaa, 1982). For the most part, the elite figure skater is lighter and leaner than the average sedentary person.

Like the speed skaters and ice hockey players, figure skaters were initially described as having fairly unremarkable maximal values for aerobic power (i.e., 58.5 ± 2.4 mL·kg^{-1}·min^{-1} for men and 48.9 ± 4.5 mL·kg^{-1}·min^{-1} for women) (Niinimaa, 1982). More recently, men and women Danish figure skaters have achieved $\dot{V}O_2$max values of 66.7 ± 1.3 mL·kg^{-1}·min^{-1} and 56.8 ± 1.0 mL·kg^{-1}·min^{-1}, respectively (Kjaer & Larsson, 1992). Maximal heart rates for both male and female Danish skaters were about 200 beats/min; maximal ventilation rates for the men and women were 138 ± 8 and 88 ± 5 L/min, respectively (Kjaer & Larsson, 1992).

Training and Nutrition Practices

Training practices. Typically, a figure skater spends between 30–33 h/wk training, most of which is spent skating (Brock & Striowski, 1986; Niimimaa, 1982; Smith & Ludington, 1989). Of this time, approximately 5.6 h/wk are spent completing strength and aerobic activities, 0.2 h/wk doing pre-skating warm-up, and 27 h/wk performing on-ice activities (Brock & Striowski, 1986). Similarly, Smith and Micheli (1982) reported that a group of elite figure skaters spent less than 5 min in off-ice and on-ice warm-up activities before each training session.

Figure skaters' heart rates increased at rest when the skaters moved from the off-ice area to the ice (Woch et al., 1979). During figure skating performances, heart rates are approximately 92% of the maximal values (Kjaer & Larsson, 1992), with greater heart rates observed as skills become more difficult (Woch et al., 1979). Oxygen uptakes during figure skating programs are approximately 80% of $\dot{V}O_2$max for men and 75% for women (Niinimaa, 1982).

Much of figure skating performance involves jumps, and a higher jump may produce greater scores for technical merit (Podolsky et al., 1990). Therefore, muscular strength and power are important to the figure skater. Podolsky et al. (1990) found a significant linear relationship between maximal knee extension force and jump height for the single and double axel. In fact, knee extension force accounted for 77–79% of the variance in the jumps. Shoulder abduction strength accounted for the next greatest percentage (5.5–7.8%) of the variance in the jumps. However, figure skaters traditionally have performed very little strength training off the ice. Rather, most of their strength training is performed on the ice through repetitions of the jumps (Podolsky, et al., 1990).

McMaster et al. (1979) added a 3-month on-ice and off-ice conditioning program to the traditional skating program of figure skating to enhance aerobic capacity, muscular strength, and flexibility. Values for $\dot{V}O_2$ max of the figure skaters increased 9% following the additional training program, while the subjects also reported that they were less fatigued at the end of their skating programs (McMaster et al., 1979).

Nutrition Practices. Rucinski (1989) examined the nutrition practices of 17 male and 23 female figure skaters using a diet record for 3 d and the Eating Attitude Test (EAT). The daily caloric intake was 4.9 ± 1.9 MJ for the females and 12.1 ± 4.5 MJ for the males. The females consumed less than 60% of the U.S. Recommended Dietary Allowance (RDA) for iron (47%), vitamin D (18%), vitamin B-6 (46%), folacin (26%), vitamin B-12 (56%), pantothenic acid (43%), and calcium (55%), whereas the males consumed less than 60% of the U.S. RDA for only folacin (56%). Finally, based on the EAT scores, 48% of the females were within the anorexic range.

Similar to the speed skaters and ice hockey players, figure skaters perform demanding exercise sessions throughout a very long season. Unlike other skaters, however, figure skaters, especially female figure skaters, have to be conscious of their body weights and physiques. Still, the best dietary advice for figure skaters is the same as that previously described for other skaters.

Medical Considerations

Figure skaters sustain many types of injuries (Brock & Striowski, 1986; Kjaer & Larsson, 1992; Pecina et al., 1990; Smith & Ludington, 1989; Smith & Micheli, 1982; Smith et al., 1991), including overuse injuries such as low back pain (Smith & Micheli, 1982) and stress fractures (Pecina et al., 1990), and more acute injuries such as fractures and sprains (Brock & Striowski, 1986). Poor ice conditions and problems with skates may be related to the incidence of injuries, but there seems to be no association between injury occurrence and the time during practice when the injury happens (Brock & Striowski, 1986).

Even though no studies were found that addressed the incidence of amenorrhea in women figure skaters, low body weights, leanness and a relatively high incidence of anorexia suggest that the incidence of amenorrhea is also quite high. Because athletes who are amenorrheic may not produce sufficient bone mass to protect them from osteoporosis in later years, an amenorrheic figure skater could be risking future bone health. Amenorrheic and/or anorexic athletes should receive medical attention as soon as possible.

DIRECTIONS FOR FUTURE RESEARCH IN SKATING

One of the main areas of concern in skating is the reduced leg blood flow caused by the skating techniques. Future research should examine the degree to which blood flow is reduced and the effects of reduced blood flow on cardiac output, peripheral resistance, and blood pressure. Strategies for minimizing the consequence of the poor muscle blood flow need to be examined. Certainly, experimental studies of several basic variations in training patterns need to be evaluated. Would skaters benefit by doing more strength training, allowing speed skaters a greater distance per stroke with a longer recovery phase for blood flow? Alternatively, are they better advised to try strategies designed to promote better local blood flow? Other research ideas include the following:

- More strength training of ice hockey players might minimize the reductions in muscle strength seen as the season progresses.
- More information on the optimal warm-up would be beneficial.
- Are there dietary strategies that might improve buffering characteristics of the blood and/or muscle without resorting to bicarbonate ingestion?
- Would the use of a face mask during training reduce the incidence of exercise-induced bronchospasm?
- Is it cost-effective for hockey players and figure skaters to invest time and energy to undertake more of the fitness training characteristically used by speed skaters?
- More nutritional information is necessary in all three types of skating. Energy expenditure and intake should be characterized for ice hockey players and figure skaters. Also, much work is needed to assess the value of fluid replacement for ice hockey players to counteract the dehydration caused by excessive sweating.

SUMMARY

Skating performance encompasses a variety of activities, many of which require large expenditures of energy produced anaerobically. Skaters often must turn to dry-land activities for a large portion of their training, and that training should be designed to be as specific to skating movements as possible and should overload both anaerobic and aerobic energy systems. Diets high in carbohydrate and adequate fluid intake are important for good skating performances. Finally, proper strength development, flexibility exercises, and warm-up and cool-down activities are valuable in the overall program of a skater.

ACKNOWLEDGEMENTS

Most of our work with speed skaters has been funded by the United States Olympic Committee and the United States International Skating Association. We also acknowledge the assistance and cooperation of the coaches (Mike Crowe, Susan Sandvig, Dianne Holum, and Stan Klotkowski) and athletes who not only allowed us to test them over the past years, but also allowed us to learn from them. Finally, we thank Nancy Thompson, Matt Schrager, and Ralph Welsh, who assisted us in the testing of the athletes.

BIBLIOGRAPHY

Agre, J.C., D.C. Casal, A.S. Leon, C. McNally, T.L. Baxter, and R.C. Serfass (1988). Professional ice hockey players: Physiologic, anthropometric, and musculoskeletal characteristics. *Arch. Phys. Med. Rehabil.* 69:188–192.

Brock, R.M., and C.C. Striowski (1986). Injuries in elite figure skaters. *Phys. Sportsmed.* 14:111–115.

Cantu, R.C. (1993). Football: Life on the edge. *Med. Sci. Sports Exerc.* 25:XXII.

Costill, D.L., R. Bower, G. Branham, and K. Sparks (1971). Muscle glycogen utilization during prolonged exercise on successive days. *J. Appl. Physiol.* 31:834–838.

Costill, D.L., and J.M. Miller (1980). Nutrition for endurance sport: Carbohydrate and fluid balance. *Int. J. Sports Med.* 1:2–14.

Cotton, C.E., A. Reed, H. Hansen, and R. Gauthier (1979). Pre and post seasonal muscular strength tests of professional hockey players. *Can. J. Appl. Sport Sci.* 4:245.

Crowe, M. (1990). Year-round preparation of the winter sports athlete. In: M.J. Casey, C. Foster, and E.G. Hixson (eds.) *Winter Sports Medicine.* Philadelphia, F. A. Davis Co., pp. 7–13.

Crowe, M., C. Foster, N.N. Thompson, J. Phul, C. Baldwin, and A. Katz (1986). Blood lactate and perceptual responses during simulated competition (abstract). *Med. Sci. Sports Exerc.* 18:59.

Daub, W.B., H.J. Green, M.E. Houston, J.A. Thompson, I.G. Fraser, and D.A. Ranney (1982). Cross-adaptive responses to different forms of leg training—skeletal muscle biochemistry and histochemistry. *Can. J. Physiol. Pharmacol.* 60:628–633.

Daub, W.B., H.J. Green, M.E. Houston, J.A. Thompson, I.G. Fraser, and D.A. Ranney (1983). Specificity of physiological adaptations resulting from ice-hockey training. *Med. Sci. Sports Exerc.* 15:290–294.

de Boer, R.W. (1986). *Training and technique in speed skating.* Amsterdam: Free University Press.

de Boer, R.W., G. de Groot, and G.J. van Ingen Schenau (1987a). Specificity of training in speed skating. In: B. Jonsson (ed.) *Biomechanics X-B.* Champaign, IL; Human Kinetics Publishers, pp. 685–689.

de Boer, R.W., G.J.C. Ettema, B.G.M. Faessen, H. Krekels, A. P. Hollander, G. de Groot, and G. J. van Ingen Schenau (1987b). Specific characteristics of speed skating: implications for summer training. *Med. Sci. Sports Exerc.* 19:504–510.

de Boer, R.W., E. Vos, W. Hutter, G. de Groot, and G.J. van Ingen Schenau (1987c). Physiological and biomechanical comparison of roller skating and speed skating on ice. *Eur. J. Appl. Physiol.* 56:562–569.

de Boer, R.W., and K.L. Nilsen (1989). The gliding and push-off technique of male and female Olympic speed skaters. *Int. J. Sport Biomech.* 5:119–134.

de Groot, G., R.W. de Boer, and G.J. van Ingen Schenau (1985). Power output during cycling and speed skating. In: D.A. Winters, R.W. Norman, R.P. Wells, K.C. Hayes, and A.E. Patla (eds.) *Biomechanics IX.* Champaign, IL: Human Kinetics Publishers, pp. 555–559.

de Groot, G., A.P. Hollander, A.J. Sargeant, G.J. van Ingen Schenau, and R.W. de Boer (1987). Applied physiology of speed skating. *J. Sport Sci.* 5:249–259.

de Koning, J.J. (1991). *Biomechanical aspects of speed skating.* Amsterdam: Free University Press.

de Koning, J.J., G. de Groot, and G.J. van Ingen Schenau (1991). Coordination of leg muscles during speed skating. *J. Biomech.* 24:137–146.

de Koning, J.J., G. de Groot, and G.J. van Ingen Schenau (1992). A power equation for the sprint in speed skating. *J. Biomech.* 25:573–580.

Dengel, D.R., R.E. Graham, M.E. Jones, K.I. Norton, and K.J. Cureton (1990). Prediction of oxygen uptake on a bicycle wind-load simulator. *Int. J. Sports Med.* 11:279–283.

di Prampero, P.E., G. Cortili, P. Mognoni, and F. Saibene (1976). Energy cost of speed skating and efficiency of work against air resistance. *J. Appl. Physiol.* 40:584–591.

Ekblom, B., L. Hermansen, and B. Saltin (1967). *Hastighetsakinng pa skridsko: Idrottsfysiologi rapport nr 5.* Stockholm: Trygg-Hansa.

Foster, C., J. Hare, and L. Meyer (1984). Practical demonstrations of nutritional support in elite athletes (abstract). *American Alliance for Health, Physical Education, Recreation, and Dance Abstracts.* Washington, D.C.: AAHPERD.

Foster, C., A.C. Snyder, N.N. Thompson, M.A. Green, M. Foley, and M. Schrager (1993a). Effect of pacing strategy on cycle time trial performance. *Med. Sci. Sports Exerc.* 25:383–388.

Foster, C., A.C. Snyder, N.N. Thompson, and K. Kuettel (1988). Normalization of the blood lactate profile in athletes. *Int. J. Sports Med.* 9:198–200.

Foster, C., and N. Thompson (1990). The physiology of speed skating. In: M.J. Casey, C. Foster, and E.G. Hixson (eds.) *Winter Sports Medicine.* Philadelphia: F.A. Davis Co., pp. 221–240.

Foster, C., N.N. Thompson, and A.C. Snyder (1993b). Ergometric studies with speed skaters: Evolution of laboratory methods. *J. Strength Cond. Res.* 7:193–200.

Gamble F., and D.L. Montgomery (1986). A cycling test of anaerobic endurance for ice hockey players (abstract). *Can. J. Appl. Sport Sci.* 11:14P.

Geijsel, J.S.M. (1979). Training and testing in marathon speed skating. *J. Sports Med.* 19:277–284.

Geijsel, J.S.M. (1980). The endurance time on a bicycle ergometer as a test for marathon speed skating. *J. Sports Med.* 20:333–340.

Geijsel, J., G. Bomhoff, J. van Velzen, G. de Groot, and G.J. van Ingen Schenau (1984). Bicycle ergometry and speed skating performance. *Int. J. Sports Med.* 5:241–245.

Green, H.J. (1978). Glycogen depletion patterns during continuous and intermittent ice skating. *Med. Sci. Sports.* 10:183–187.

Green, H.J. (1979). Metabolic aspects of intermittent work with specific regard to ice hockey. *Can. J. Appl. Sport Sci.* 4:29–34.

Green, H.J., P. Bishop, M. Houston, R. McKillop, R. Norman, and P. Stothart (1976). Time-motion and physiological assessments of ice hockey performance. *J. Appl. Physiol.* 40:159–163.

Green, H.J., B.D. Daub, D.C. Painter, and J.A. Thompson (1978a). Glycogen depletion patterns during ice hockey performance. *Med. Sci. Sports.* 10:289–293.

Green, H.J., and M.E. Houston (1975). Effect of a season of ice hockey on energy capacities and associated functions. *Med. Sci. Sports.* 7:299–303.

Green, H.J., M.E. Houston, and J.A. Thompson (1978b). Inter- and intragame alterations in selected blood parameters during ice hockey performance. In: F. Landry and W.A.R. Orban (eds.) *Ice Hockey.* Miami, FL: Symposia Specialists Inc., pp. 37–46.

Green, H.J., J.A. Thompson, W.D. Daub, M.E. Houston, and D.A. Ranney (1979). Fiber composition, fiber size and enzyme activities in vastus lateralis of elite athletes involved in high intensity exercise. *Eur. J. Appl. Physiol.* 41:109–117.

Greer, N., R. Serfass, W. Picconatto, and J. Blatherwick (1992). The effects of a hockey-specific training program on performance of bantam players. *Can. J. Sport Sci.* 17:65–69.

Gutmann, M.C., D.N. Knapp, C. Foster, M.L. Pollock, and B.L. Rogowski (1986). Age, experience, and gender as predictors of psychological response to training in Olympic speedskaters. In: D. Landers (ed.) *Sport and the Elite Performer.* Champaign, IL: Human Kinetics Publishers, pp. 97–102.

Herzog, W., A.C. Guimaraes, M.G. Anton, and K.A. Carter-Erdman (1991). Moment-length relations of rectus femoris muscles of speed skaters/cyclists and runners. *Med. Sci. Sports Exerc.* 23:1289–1296.

Hoffman, M.D., G.M. Jones, B. Bota, M. Mandli, and P.S. Clifford (1992). In-line skating: Physiological responses and comparison with roller skiing. *Int. J. Sports Med.* 13:137–144.

Hollering, B.L., and D. Simpson (1977). The effects of three types of training programs upon skating speed of college ice hockey players. *J. Sports Med.* 17:335–340.

Houston, M.E. (1979). Nutrition and ice hockey performance. *Can. J. Appl. Sport. Sci.* 4:98–99.

Houston, M.E., and H.J. Green (1976). Physiological and anthropometric characteristics of elite Canadian ice hockey players. *J. Sports Med. Phys. Fit.* 16:123–128.

Hutchinson, W.W., G.M. Maas, and A.J. Murdoch (1979). Effect of dry land training on aerobic capacity of college hockey players. *J. Sports Med.* 19:271–276.

Ivy, J.J., A.L. Katz, C.L. Cutler, W.M. Sherman, and E.F. Coyle (1988a). Muscle glycogen synthesis after exercise: Effect of time on carbohydrate ingestion. *J. Appl. Physiol.* 64:1480–1485.

Ivy, J.J., M.C. Lee, J.T. Brozinick, and M.J. Reed (1988b). Muscle glycogen storage after different amounts of carbohydrate ingestion. *J. Appl. Physiol.* 65:2018–2023.

Johansson, C., R. Lorentzon, and A.R. Fugl-Meyer (1989). Isokinetic muscular performance of the quadriceps in elite ice hockey players. *Am. J. Sports Med.* 17:30–34.

Kandou, T.W.A., I.L.D. Houtman, E.V.D. Bol, R.W. de Boer, G. de Groot, and G.J. van Ingen Schenau (1987). Comparison of physiology and biomechanics of speed skating with cycling and with skateboard exercise. *Can. J. Sport Sci.* 12:31–36.

Kindermann, M., C. Foster, and J. Keul (1993). Overtraining in endurance athletes: a brief review. *Med. Sci. Sports Exerc.* 25:854–862.

Kjaer, M., and B. Larsson (1992). Physiological profile and incidence of injuries among elite figure skaters. *J. Sports Sci.* 10:29–36.

Knapp, D.N., M.C. Gutmann, B.L. Rogowski, C. Foster and M.L. Pollock (1986). Perceived vulnerability to illness and injury among Olympic speedskating candidates: Effects on emotional response to training. In: D. Landers (ed.) *Sport and the Elite Performer.* Champaign, IL: Human Kinetics Publishers, pp. 103–112.

Koziris, L.P., and D.L. Montgomery (1991). Blood lactate concentration following intermittent and continuous cycling tests of anaerobic capacity. *Eur. J. Appl. Physiol.* 63:273–277.

MacDougall, J.D. (1979). Thermoregulatory problems encountered in ice hockey. *Can. J. Appl. Sport Sci.* 4:35–38.

Macnab, R.B.J. (1979). A longitudinal study of ice hockey in boys aged 8-12. *Can. J. Appl. Sport Sci.* 4:11–17.

Maksud, M.G., P. Farrell, C. Foster, M. Pollock, M. Hare, J. Anholm, and D. Schmidt (1982). Maximal oxygen uptake, ventilation and heart rate of Olympic speed skating candidates. *J. Sports Med.* 22:217–223.

Maksud, M.G., L.H. Hamilton, and B. Balke (1971). Physiological responses of a male Olympic speed skater—Terry McDermott. *Med. Sci. Sports.* 3:107–109.

Maksud, M.G., R.L. Wiley, L.H. Hamilton, and B. Lockhart (1970). Maximal oxygen uptake, ventilation and heart rate of Olympic speed skating candidates. *J. Appl. Physiol.* 29:186–190.

Marino, G.W., and R.G. Weese (1979). A kinematic analysis of the ice skating stride. In: J. Terauds and H.J. Gros (eds.) *Science in Skiing, Skating and Hockey.* Del Mar, CA: Academic Publishers, pp. 65–74.

McCarthy, J.F., and B.R. Kelly (1978). Aggression, performance variables, and anger self-report in ice hockey players. *J. Psych.* 99:97–101.

McMaster, W.C., S. Liddle, and J. Walsh (1979). Conditioning program for competitive figure skating. *Am. J. Sports Med.* 7:43–47.

Medbø, J.I., and S. Burgers (1990). Effect of training on anaerobic capacity. *Med. Sci. Sports Exerc.* 22:501–507.

Medbø, J.I., A.C. Mohn, I. Tabata, R. Bahr, O. Vaage, and O.M. Sejersted (1988). Anaerobic capacity determined by maximal accumulated O_2 deficit. *J. Appl. Physiol.* 64:50–60.

Minkoff, J. (1982). Evaluating parameters of a professional hockey team. *Am. J. Sports Med.* 10:285–292.

Montgomery, D.L. (1988). Physiology of ice hockey. *Sports Med.* 5:99–126.

Montgomery, D.L., and J.A. Dallaire (1986). Physiological characteristics of elite ice hockey players over two consecutive years. In: J. Broekhoff et al. (eds.) *Sport and elite performers.* Champaign, IL: Human Kinetics Publishers, pp. 133–143.

Montpetit, R.R., P. Binette, and A.W. Taylor (1979). Glycogen depletion in a game-simulated hockey task. *Can. J. Appl. Sport Sci.* 4:43–45.

Moore, M. (1980). Fighting NHL brawling with suspensions. *Phys. Sportsmed.* 8:19.

Nemoto, I., K. Iwaoka, K. Funato, N. Yoshioka, and M. Miyashita (1988). Aerobic threshold, anaerobic threshold, and maximal oxygen uptake of Japanese speed-skaters. *Int. J. Sports Med.* 9:433–437.

Nemoto, I., H. Kanehisa, and M. Miyashita (1990). The effect of sports training on the age-related changes of body composition and isokinetic peak torque in knee extensors of junior speed skaters. *J. Sports Med. Phys. Fit.* 30:83–88.

Niinimaa, V. (1982). Figure skating: What do we know about it? *Phys. Sportsmed.* 10:51–56.

Niinimaa, V., Z.T. Woch, and R.J. Shephard (1979). Intensity of physical effort during a free figure skating program. In: J. Terauds and H.J. Gros (eds.) *Science in Skiing, Skating and Hockey.* Del Mar, CA: Academic Publishers, pp. 75–81.

Orvanova, E. (1987). Physical structure of winter sports athletes. *J. Sports Sci.* 5:197–248.

Osterback, L., and Y. Qvarnberg (1987). A prospective study of respiratory infections in 12-year-old children actively engaged in sports. *Acta Pediatr. Scand.* 76:944–949.

Pecina, B., I. Bojanic, and S. Dubravcic (1990). Stress fractures in figure skaters. *Am. J. Sports Med.* 18:277–279.

Podolsky, A., K.R. Kaufman, T.D. Cahalan, S.Y. Aleshinskky, and E.Y.S. Chao (1990). The relationship of strength and jump height in figure skaters. *Am. J. Sports Med.* 18:400–405.

Pollock, M.L., C. Foster, J. Anholm, J. Hare, P. Farrell, M. Maksud, and A. Jackson (1982). Body composition of Olympic speed skating candidates. *Res. Quart.* 53:150–155.

Pollock, M.L., C. Foster, D. Pels, and D. Holum (1986). Comparison of male and female speed skating candidates. In: D. Landers (ed) *Sports and the Elite Performer.* Champaign, IL: Human Kinetics Publishers, pp. 143–152.

Pollock, M.L., T. Hickman, Z. Kendrick, A. Jackson, A.C. Linnerud, and G. Dawson (1976). Prediction of body density in young and middle-aged men. *J. Appl. Physiol.* 40:300–304.

Posch, E., Y. Haglund, and E. Eriksson (1989). Prospective study of concentric and eccentric leg muscle torques, flexibility, physical conditioning, and variation of injury rates during one season of amateur ice hockey. *Int. J. Sports Med.* 2:113–117.

Quinney, H.A., A. Belcastro, and R.D. Steadward (1982). Seasonal fitness variations and pre-playoff blood analysis in NHL players (abstract). *Can. J. Appl. Sport Sci.* 7:237.

Quirion, A., A. Therminarias, E. Pellerei, D. Methot, L. Laurencelle, M. Tanche, and P. Vogelaere (1988). Aerobic capacity, anaerobic threshold and cold exposure with speed skaters. *J. Sport Med.* 28:27–34.

Rajala, G.M., D.A. Neumann, C. Foster, and R.H. Jensen (1994). Quadriceps muscle performance in male speed skaters. *J. Strength Cond. Res.* 8:48–52.

Rehunen, S., and S. Liitsola (1978). Modification of the muscle-glycogen level of ice-hockey players through a drink with high carbohydrate content. *Z. Sportsmed.2* 26:15–25.

Roberts, D., and D. Smith (1990). Serum ferritin values in elite speed and synchronized swimmers and speed skaters. *J. Lab. Clin. Med.* 116:661–665.

Rosentswieg, J., D. Williams, C. Sandburg, K. Kolten, L. Engler, and G. Norman (1979). Perceived exertion of professional hockey players. *Percep. Motor Skills* 48:992–994.

Rucinski, A. (1989). Relationship of body image and dietary intake of competitive ice skaters. *J. Am. Diet. Assoc.* 89:98–100.

Sherman, W.M., G. Brodowicz, D.A. Wright, W.K. Allen, J. Simonsen, and A. Dernbach (1989). Effects of 4 h preexercise carbohydrate feedings on cycling performance. *Med. Sci. Sports Exerc.* 21:598–604.

Smith, A.D., and R. Ludington (1989). Injuries in elite pair skaters and ice dancers. *Am. J. Sports Med.* 17:482–488.

Smith, A.D., and L.J. Micheli (1982). Injuries in competitive skaters. *Phys. Sportsmed.* 82:36–47.

Smith, A.D., L. Stroud, and C. McQueen (1991). Flexibility and anterior knee pain in adolescent elite figure skaters. *J. Pedatric Orthopaed.* 11:77–82.

Smith, D.J., and D. Roberts (1990). Heart rate and blood lactate concentration during on-ice training in speed skating. *Can. J. Sport Sci.* 15:23–27.

Snyder, A.C., L.L. Dvorak, and J.B. Roepke (1989a). Influence of dietary iron source on measures of iron status among female runners. *Med. Sci. Sports Exerc.* 21:7–10.

Snyder, A.C., C. Foster, N.N. Thompson, and P.J. Van Handel (1989b). Blood lactate accumulation during ice speed skating, roller skating and slideboard exercise. *Proc. First IOC Congress Sports Sci.*

Snyder, A.C., K.P. O'Hagan, P.S. Clifford, M.D. Hoffman, and C. Foster (1993). Exercise responses to in-line skating: comparisons to running and cycling. *Int. J. Sports Med.* 14:38–42.

Snyder, A.C., L.O. Schulz, and C. Foster (1989c). Voluntary consumption of a carbohydrate supplement by elite speed skaters. *J. Am. Diet. Assoc.* 89:1125–1127.

Sundberg, C.J., M. Viru, M. Esbjornsson, E. Jansson, and L. Kaijser (1993). The influence of reduced blood flow on glycogen breakdown during exercise in man (abstract). *Med. Sci. Sports Exerc.* 25:S2.

van Ingen Schenau, G.J., F.C. Bakker, G. de Groot, and J.J. de Koning (1992). Supramaximal cycle tests do not detect seasonal progression in performance in groups of elite speed skaters. *Eur. J. Appl. Physiol.* 64:292–297.

van Ingen Schenau, G.J., R.W. de Boer, J.S.M. Geysel, and G. de Groot (1988). Supramaximal test results of male and female speed skaters with particular reference to methodological problems. *Eur. J. Appl. Physiol.* 57:6–9.

van Ingen Schenau, G.J., and G. de Groot (1983). On the origin of differences in performance level between elite male and female speed skaters. *Hum. Movement Sci.* 2:151–159.

van Ingen Schenau, G.J., G. de Groot, and R.W. de Boer (1985). The control of speed in elite female speed skaters. *J. Biomech.* 18:91–96.

van Ingen Schenau, G.J., G. de Groot, and A.P. Hollander (1983). Some technical, physiological and anthropometrical aspects of speed skating. *Eur. J. Appl. Physiol.* 50:343–354.

van Ingen Schenau, G.J., J.J. de Koning, and G. de Groot (1990). A simulation of speed skating performances based on a power equation. *Med. Sci. Sports Exerc.* 22:718–728.

van Saase, J.L.C.M., W.M.P. Noteboom, and J.P. Vandenbroucke (1990). Longevity of men capable of prolonged vigorous physical exercise: a 32 year follow up of 2259 participants in the Dutch eleven cities ice skating tour. *Br. Med. J.* 301:1409–1411.

von Kindermann, W., and J. Keul (1980). Anaerobic supply of energy in high-speed skating. *Deutsche Z. Sportmedizin.* 5:142–147.

Walberg, J.L., M.K. Leidy, D.J. Sturgill, D.E. Hinkle, S.J. Ritchey, and D.R. Sebolt (1988). Macronutrient content of a hypoenergy diet affects nitrogen retention and muscle function in weight lifters. *Int. J. Sports Med.* 9:261–266.

Watson, R.C., and R.D. Hanley (1986). Application of active recovery techniques for a simulated ice hockey task. *Can. J. Appl. Sport Sci.* 11:82–87.

Watson, R.C., and T.L.C. Sargeant (1986). Laboratory and on-ice test comparisons of anaerobic power of ice hockey players. *Can. J. Appl. Sport Sci.* 11:218–224.

Wiley, J.P., W.H. Meeuwisse, M.D. Montgomery, and I. Paul (1992). Athlete's hack may be associated with transient bronchospasm. *Med. Sci. Sports Exerc.* 24:S143.

Woch, Z.T., V. Niinimaa, and R.J. Shephard (1979). Heart rate responses during free figure skating manoeuvres. *Can. J. Sport Sci.* 4:274–276.

Woods, M.P. (1990). Medical aspects of speed skating. In: M.J. Casey, C. Foster, and E.G. Hixson (eds.) *Winter Sports Medicine.* Philadelphia: F. A. Davis Co., pp. 248–253.

DISCUSSION

SPRIET: Can you explain how Eric Heiden could win all the speed skating gold medals from the sprint (~35 sec) to the 14-min race? That kind of dominance over such a wide range of durations does not seem to happen in any other sport. Is technique so important in this sport that a world class skater can excel in both aerobic and anaerobic events?

SNYDER: Technique is certainly critical, but Heiden seemed to be uniquely blessed physiologically to be a great competitor at almost any sport he chose.

KNUTTGEN: Without detracting from Eric Heiden's performances, it should be pointed out that the pool of speed skaters, both internationally and in the USA, is extremely small. When compared to running, for example, it is much easier for a good athlete to be successful in skating events of different distances.

HAGERMAN: In the late 1970s Ed Burke and I studied both Eric Heiden and Greg Lemond at the US Olympic Training Center at Squaw Valley. They performed so well on all of our tests, both aerobic and anaerobic, that we were convinced they could be outstanding in nearly any sport they chose. They both performed at the top of the pack in tests not related to either cycling or skating.

BURKE: A lot of people do not realize that Eric's sister, Beth Heiden, who was outstanding in Olympic speed skating at racing distances of 3000 m or less, gave up skating and won the women's cycling road race in France in 1980. Then she got tired of cycling and went on to win the NCAA cross-country skiing championships. Eric, who we all think of as the typical explosive athlete, rode in the Tour de France and also won the Four States Road Race, which is approximately 150 miles long. This shows the importance of good genes and being raised in a family that encouraged participation in sports.

GISOLFI: Over 40 y ago, Sid Robinson addressed the issue of pacing in middle-distance runners. He performed an experiment where he had subjects a) start quickly and finish slowly, b) start slowly and finish quickly, or c) run at a constant speed. The data were rather convincing that if you started fast and finished slowly, you had the greatest oxygen requirement and blood lactates. The implication was that if you started slowly and finished rapidly or if you ran at a constant speed, you would be able to run faster.

COYLE: Sports like speed skating and bicycling with the events lasting 1–2 min are very different than running because the skaters and cyclists are going much faster than the runners and are therefore encountering much higher wind resistance, which is the greatest force that they have to overcome. When sprint cycling and speed skating for 1 min, it may be advantageous for the athletes to go out very hard and to sprint from the very onset. They don't want to have a lot of kinetic energy left at the finish. They produce great kinetic energy initially to accelerate themselves, and they seem to be decelerating at the finish. If they had very high velocities at the finish, there would be a lot of stored kinetic energy that would not be applied to the event. Therefore, I think the strategy of going out very hard from the onset for these high velocity skating and cycling events may be reasonable.

GISOLFI: Is there any evidence to support that notion?

SNYDER: We did one study on skaters and found that sprinting from the onset resulted in the best performance.

COYLE: van Ingen Schenau (*Int. J. Sports Med.* 13:447–451, 1992) developed a mathematical model of anaerobic energy distribution, claiming it is best to sprint maximally from the beginning of a 1,000-m track cycling event requiring 64 s.

HORSWILL: Is there any evidence regarding the use of bicarbonate loading by skaters?

SNYDER: To my knowledge, the skaters do not bicarbonate load at all.

EKBLOM: It is fairly obvious that blood flow to the muscles of speed skaters is impaired because there are very high blood lactate concentrations at any given oxygen uptake during speed skating. If you have high blood pressure and high lactates at a given oxygen uptake, it is a good indication of a reduction in blood flow. Also, the rather low values you have given for $\dot{V}O_2$max in speed skaters is an artifact of the expression of $\dot{V}O_2$max per kg body mass. In the case of large, muscular athletes, this method of expression is not reflective of their true cardiovascular fitness. Expressing $\dot{V}O_2$max per $kg^{2/3}$ of body mass (preferably lean body mass) gives a more realistic value for $\dot{V}O_2$max for this and many sports.

SNYDER: I agree.

COYLE: Which muscle groups generate most of the power in speed skating? Are these the muscles that use the most glycogen?

SNYDER: The muscles of the thighs, hips, and the low back are most critical. The arms are also heavily involved, depending on the event.

EKBLOM: We took vastus lateralis biopsies immediately following 2,000-m races and recorded almost the highest muscle lactates that we ever measured. The knee extensors are obviously very important muscles in speed skating.

BURKE: The large body masses of speed skaters are probably important to performance for the same reason they are in flat course cycling. Body volume increases to a greater extent than does body surface area; therefore, a larger speed skater compensates for increased wind resistance caused by a greater surface area by gaining relatively more power from a larger volume of muscle, from a larger heart, etc.

MAUGHAN: In ice hockey, you showed that active recovery between shifts would use the blood lactate faster, and you implied that active recovery would be a good idea between shifts. But I wonder if your logic is sound. Active recovery decreases the blood lactate quickly because lactate is such a good substrate for the muscle. But is there any evidence that lactate or the acidosis per se is a limitation in hockey? I do not think so. It seems to me that by performing active recovery, the hockey player is eliminating lactate that could be used for energy to conserve glycogen during subsequent play. If glycogen depletion is a limiting factor to hockey performance, active recovery could hasten eventual fatigue.

SPRIET: I am not sure I agree with Ron on this point. The amount of glycogen spared by metabolizing lactate that might have been used during a recovery period is not enough to make much of a difference for future exercise. On the other hand, if acidosis in the muscle is great at the end of a shift, removing lactate from the extracellular space during active recovery will enhance its removal from muscle and leave the muscle in a more favorable acid-base status prior to skating again. However, there are some sports where acidosis will not be a problem and there will be no need to reduce the lactate.

MAUGHAN: Which category does hockey fall in?

SPRIET: It depends on how much the player is skating, e.g., whether he has been on the bench for the last 2–3 min of the period. I agree that studies are needed to determine whether lactate removal is an issue during ice hockey.

MAUGHAN: So we should not automatically assume that removing lactate by performing active recovery is necessarily a good thing?

SPRIET: That is true.

BAR-OR: Has anyone compared different warm-up routines and their effects on performance in skating? The warm-up routine Ann describes seems very long.

MAUGHAN: Some sprinters and hurdlers warm up for 2 h for an event that lasts 10–14 s. It seems that the shorter the event, the longer the warm-up. There probably is not any scientific underpinning to this prolonged warm-up, but it does not particularly surprise me that skaters do it.

GREGG: Given that many of the competitive events for swimming and skating are of similar duration, it is of interest to me that both skaters and swimmers spend similar amounts of time training, but the type of training is much different. Swimmers spend a lot of time training in the water, and maybe that is important for technique development. However, skaters do not seem to spend as much time on the ice because of lack of venue availability. Swimmers seem to swim and train more aerobically at lower intensities; skaters spend more time on relatively high intensity power training. I wonder which group is using the right type of training. Also, can someone tell me what anaerobic training is?

SPRIET: Anaerobic training involves activity for which anaerobic energy sources must be called upon to provide a substantial portion of the energy requirement. Thus, anaerobic training activities require a greater power output than can be provided aerobically. Anaerobic training may be invoked continuously in short-duration, high-power efforts, or may be involved intermittently, e.g., at the beginning or end of longer duration activities.

GREGG: What are the adaptations to anaerobic training?

SPRIET: The anaerobic training studies suggest that the only system that can increase its capacity is the glycolytic system, and that is on the order of 10–20%. This improvement often does not reach statistical significance, but I suppose it can be significant for performance. Athletes already engaging in so-called anaerobic activities do not increase their anaerobic ability with further anaerobic training. They usually start out with an anaerobic capacity that is 20–30% higher than that in people who are not engaged in these events. There must be a genetic component to their ability, but there does appear to be a small improvement that can be gained from this type of training in the "anaerobically naive."

6

Physiology and Nutrition for Rowing

FREDRICK C. HAGERMAN, Ph.D.

NUTRITIONAL CONSIDERATIONS

INTRODUCTION

The first written documentation of the sport of rowing appeared early in the 18th century when professional boatmen in England raced on the river Thames, and there is some evidence that ancient mariners may have competed on a friendly basis when they were not engaging in trade or war (Gardner, 1965). The oldest continuous rowing competition dates from 1829 with the inaugural Oxford-Cambridge boat race (Dodd, 1983); the most famous rowing regatta has been held at Henley, England, since 1839 (Cleaver, 1957). The Yale-Harvard race was introduced in 1852 (Mendenhall, 1980), and the first intercollegiate athletic association in the U.S.—the Intercollegiate Rowing Association—was organized at about this time; this association still exists independently of the National Collegiate Athletic Association.

Many technical improvements were made on racing boats and oars during the 19th century. Important changes included the oarlock-mounted outrigger, the rotating oarlock, boats without keels, and especially the development of the sliding seat. The 20th century saw the design and production of more hydrodynamically efficient boats of light synthetic materials; experimentation with and development of fiberglass oars; the use of various blade designs, including the recent introduction of the more efficient "hatchet" or "big blade;" the design and use of rowing ergometers; and standardization of the 2000-m racing course.

Rowing was introduced as an Olympic sport at the revival of the Olympic Games in 1896 and has grown into a prominent international sport with annual World Championships and a quadrennial Olympic regatta; at the 1992 Olympic Regatta in Banyoles, Spain, 48 countries and more than 700 rowers competed. (Women's rowing became a permanent Olympic sport in 1976.) In Olympic sports, the total number of rowing competitors ranks second only to the number of competitors in track and field (athletics).

The sport of rowing is divided into two distinct categories: sweep rowing and sculling. Both sweep and sculling boats are sleek, streamlined, and hydrodynamically designed. Although some are still constructed from a light wood, most boats are now made of lightweight synthetic polymers. Single sculls weigh between 10 and 15 kg; larger eight-oared boats range from 88 to 98 kg. Sweep boat competition may involve as few as two rowers or as many as eight, excluding the coxswain, who steers the boat. Sculling events include single, double, and quadruple sculls, all without coxswains. Sweep rowing requires each competitor to row with a single long oar on one side of the boat, whereas scullers use two shorter oars and pull on them simultaneously. The standard competitive distance for international and most national rowing regattas is a 2000-m course with no water current.

The differences in biomechanics, gender, and number of competitors in the various boats competing at international regattas (eight events for men—five sweep and three sculling; six for women—three sweep and three sculling) obviously affect the specific physiological demands of each event. With the exception of the Olympic Games Regatta, international competition for both men and women is conducted in two divisions: an open division with no weight classifications and a restricted weight class category for lightweights. In January 1993, the international governing body of rowing, Fédération Internationale des Sociétés d'Aviron or International Rowing Federation (FISA), voted to include lightweight rowing in the 1996 Olympic Regatta. The mandatory weight limit for lightweight men is 72.5 kg; for lightweight women it is 59 kg. Both lightweight men and women compete in two sculling and two sweep events. Junior World Championships are conducted annually for rowers under 19 years of age in sculling and sweep events that are similar to those in the open division for seniors.

International races for men in the open division last between 5.5 min and 7.2 min, whereas those for women last between 5.7 min and 7.4 min. These time variations are affected by the number of competitors in a specific boat and by environmental conditions, including wind, temperature, humidity, and water depth. Despite the year-to-year differences in environmental conditions, competitive results for many years improved by about 0.7 s/y (Schwanitz, 1991; Secher, 1973). However, more recent performance times have improved at a more rapid rate (Table 6-1). The average improvement in the five men's events from 1968 to 1992 was 7.7% per Olympic year; single scullers showed the most marked improvement. Percent improvement from 1968–1992 ranged from 9–15%; double sculls improved the least and pair-oared without coxswain the most.

Although women have now been competing in the 2000-m for over 12 y (primarily in World Championships), Olympic competition for this distance has been conducted only twice (Table 6-1), and the four-oared-without-coxswain event was not introduced until 1992. Average improvement for the women in four events from 1988 to 1992 was almost 17 s; single sculls and pair-oared without coxswain showed the greatest improvements.

Because there are very few comparative Olympic data for men and

TABLE 6-1. *A comparison of Olympic Games performance times over 2000 m for five common rowing events for men and women (1968–1992).*

			EVENT		
Year	Single Scull	Double Sculls	Pair-Oared Without Coxswain	Four-Oared Without Coxswain	Eight-Oared With Coxswain
MEN					
1968	7:48	6:52	7:26	6:39	6:07
1972	7:10	7:02	6:53	6:24	6:09
1976	7:29	7:13	7:23	6:37	5:58
1980	7:10	6:24	6:48	6:08	5:49
1984	7:00	6:36	6:45	6:03	5:41
1988	6:50	6:21	6:37	6:03	5:46
1992	6:51	6:17	6:28	5:55	5:29
WOMEN*					
1988	7:47	7:01	7:28	6:56[a]	6:15
1992	7:26	6:49	7:06	6:31	6:03

*Women rowed 1000 m prior to 1988.
[a]Olympic competition not held until 1992.

women, it is difficult to explain the apparent gender-related differences. However, it is clear from Table 6-1 that women improved substantially from 1988 to 1992. For the events analyzed in Table 6-1, the men were 11.4% faster than the women in 1988, but this had decreased to 9.3% faster in 1992; the one exception was the eight-oared event, in which the men demonstrated more improvement between 1988 and 1992 than did their female counterparts. Performance improvements for both men and women over the years have been a result of better equipment, more experienced athletes, and improved training programs. However, it appears that women are now improving at a faster rate than men; this can probably be accounted for primarily by the fact that better athletes are being attracted to the women's sport than was previously the case. Also, women have had less experience rowing 2000 m than men; as they continue to train for this distance, the women's performance times should continue to improve.

For the reader who is not familiar with the sport of rowing, it may seem to be primarily an upper body activity. However, because all competitive rowing boats are equipped with sliding seats, the major rowing muscles are those of the quadriceps femoris that forcibly extend the knee. During the rowing stroke, the explosive extension of the legs is accompanied by a vigorous extension of the back, with a smaller power contribution coming from the arms at the end of the stroke. Rowing is also different from most aerobic activities in that it is performed in a sitting position with the athlete's back facing the direction of movement. Unlike running and cycling but similar to swimming, almost every major muscle group is used during rowing. It has been estimated that the most successful elite rowers produce about 75% of their rowing power with their legs and 25% with their arms. The legs provide a greater proportion of the power (80%) for rowing the faster boats, such as those powered by an eight-oared crew, whereas the legs contribute as little as 65% of the power produced by a single sculler or a paired-oared crew with coxswain.

Biomechanically, competitive rowing is an exercise of contrasts. During the initial "catch" phase of the rowing stroke, when the blade is placed in the water, the muscles of the arms and back perform a *static* exercise, whereas the remainder of the stroke is dynamic. The quadriceps muscles (Figure 6-1) are stretched during leg flexion as the body coils with a slightly curved upper body and, as the rower's arm muscles pull on the oars, the legs and back are forcibly extended (Figure 6-2) so that when the stroke is finished (Figure 6-3), the legs are extended and the back is extended beyond vertical. The body is then prepared to roll forward on the sliding seat to assume another catch (Figure 6-4).

Rowing differs from other types of human locomotion because, unlike the alternate force application of the limbs during running, cycling, and some swimming strokes, the limbs are used simultaneously during rowing. Rowing is also unique because it is the only predominantly aerobic sport in which, for all events except the single scull, there are multiple participants. Thus, a specific boat and its crew are only as strong as the weakest link.

The physiology of rowing was previously reviewed by Törner (1959) and more recently by Hagerman (1984), Körner and Schwanitz (1985), Secher (1983, 1990, 1993), Steinacker (1987), and Zsidegh (1981). It is the purpose of this chapter to review and summarize physiological data relating to men's and women's rowing. Pertinent anthropometric, muscular,

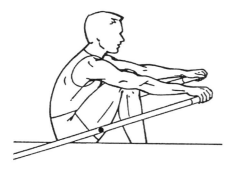 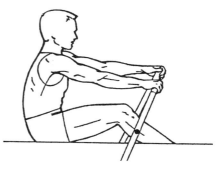

FIGURE 6-1. *The initial "catch" phase of the rowing stroke.* Reproduced with permission from R. Chen et al., *Instructor Manual, Level I, USRowing Coaching Education Program*, Indianapolis: United States Rowing Association, 1994.

FIGURE 6-2. *The early power "mid-drive" phase of the rowing stroke.* Reproduced with permission from R. Chen et al. *Instructor Manual, Level I, USRowing Coaching Education Program*, Indianapolis: United States Rowing Association, 1994.

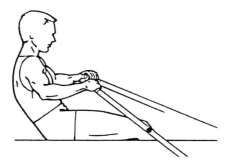

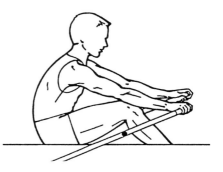

FIGURE 6-3. *End of the late power "drive" phase of the rowing stroke.* Reproduced with permission from R. Chen et al. *Instructor Manual, Level I, USRowing Coaching Education Program,* Indianapolis: United States Rowing Association, 1994.

FIGURE 6-4. *The "mid-recovery" phase of the rowing stroke serves as preparation for the next stroke.* Reproduced with permission from R. Chen et al. *Instructor Manual, Level I, USRowing Coaching Education Program,* Indianapolis: United States Rowing Association, 1994.

respiratory, cardiovascular, and metabolic data will be discussed along with applied information concerning power output, energy expenditure, caloric input, mechanical efficiency, training, testing procedures, environmental factors, overtraining, injuries, and nutrition.

CHARACTERISTICS OF ELITE ROWERS

Body Composition and Anthropometry

There is a wide range of ages, 18–38 y (excluding coxswains), for international caliber oarsmen and oarswomen competing in the open division. Rowers tend to be tall, muscular, and lean (deGaray et al., 1974; DeRose et al., 1989; Hebbelinck et al., 1980; Khosla, 1983). Data from more than 3000 rowers studied in our laboratory since 1964 have shown that open division or heavyweight oarsmen average 192 cm in height and 88 kg in body weight, whereas their female counterparts average 180 cm in height and 77 kg in weight. Percent body fat has steadily decreased for men and women since earlier investigations so that men now average about 8–10% fat, and women about 15–17% body fat. Lightweight men and women are leaner, with averages of 6–8% fat for men and 12–14% for women. Physical characteristics of the 1992 Olympic team are summarized in Table 6-2.

Muscle Qualities

Recent muscle biopsy data revealed that highly trained oarsmen have a significant representation of slow twitch or Type I muscle fibers in the major power muscles for rowing. Muscle samples obtained from the vastus lateralis and deltoideus have shown a dominance of oxidative fibers

	N	Age (y)	Ht (cm)	Wt (kg)	Body Fat (%)
Women	25	24 (1.13)	178.6 (1.43)	73.6 (2.41)	15.4 (0.36)
Men	35	26 (1.86)	194.1 (1.19)	88.1 (2.36)	8.7 (0.29)

(Bonde-Peterson et al., 1975; Hagerman & Staron, 1983; Larsson & Forsberg, 1980; Mickelson & Hagerman, 1982; Roth et al., 1983; Secher et al., 1981). The results of these studies indicate that the relative proportions of fiber types in oarsmen are similar to those found in other elite endurance athletes (Costill et al., 1976; Saltin et al., 1977).

Mean percentages of 70–75% for slow twitch or Type I fibers have been consistently observed in the vastus lateralis of oarsmen as opposed to controls, who have about 40% slow twitch fibers (Figure 6-5). Fast twitch IIA fibers have accounted for 20–25% of the fibers in the vastus lateralis of oarsmen, whereas fast twitch IIB fibers are usually represented by less than 3% of the total fiber population. However, these average values are somewhat misleading; a summary of representative individual fiber proportions (Table 6-3) indicates that most elite oarsmen have few, if any IIB fibers in the vastus lateralis and that the mean values for IIB fibers are strongly influenced by a few subjects having 5–10% Type IIB fibers.

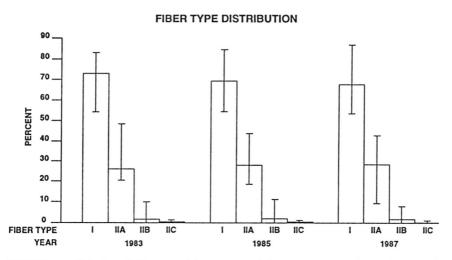

FIBER TYPE DISTRIBUTION

FIGURE 6-5. *Skeletal muscle fiber types of elite oarsmen studied in 1983, 1985, and 1987 (n = 30/y).* These are previously unpublished data from the author's laboratory.

Subject	Percent Fiber Type			
	I	IIA	IIB	IIC
01	67.5	32.5	0.0	0.0
02	70.1	29.2	0.0	0.7
03	55.0	43.4	1.0	0.6
04	55.9	44.1	0.0	0.0
05	80.7	19.2	0.0	0.1
06	74.6	25.4	0.0	0.0
07	73.1	26.0	0.0	0.9
08	69.8	26.6	2.1	1.5
09	81.3	17.5	0.8	0.4
10	61.1	34.0	4.9	0.0
11	64.1	35.9	0.0	0.0
12	67.9	31.6	0.5	0.0
13	55.2	32.8	10.0	2.0
14	75.1	24.1	0.0	0.8
15	74.5	24.5	0.0	1.0
$\bar{X}$ =	68.4	29.8	1.4	0.4
SD =	8.36	7.45	2.80	0.60

Larsson and Forsberg (1980) and Roth et al. (1983) have observed similar proportions of fast vs. slow twitch fibers in oarsmen's leg muscles. These groups have also reported percentages of slow twitch fibers ranging from 73% to 76% in the deltoid muscles of elite oarsmen. It is noteworthy that results of serial biopsy analyses of 15 oarsmen over an 8 y period and four oarsmen over a 12 y period have shown consistent fiber proportion responses. Most of these subjects were initially sampled at age 20 or younger and, with no exception, displayed the same fiber proportions year after year (Table 6-3). Despite changes in training and the possible cumulative effects of training over these periods, fiber type proportions remained stable.

Only limited biopsy sampling has been conducted with women rowers. Clarkson et al. (1984) found the ratio of slow to fast twitch fibers in the vastus lateralis to be about 60:40; the 55:45 ratio in the biceps brachii was only slightly different, again favoring slow twitch fibers. An earlier study reported slightly higher slow to fast ratios in these same muscles, i.e., 68:30 for the vastus lateralis and 60:40 for the biceps brachii (Pohlentz, 1980).

In a more recent study, Type I fibers were 62% of all fibers in the vastus lateralis of male elite rowers, Type IIA fibers were 30%, and IIB fibers were only 2.5%; transitional subtypes IC, IIC, and IIAB collectively represented about 5% of all fibers, with IIAB being the dominant type of this grouping (Hagerman et al., 1993, unpublished data). In this same study, the elite women showed the following representation of fiber types in the vastus lateralis: 55% Type I, 30% Type IIA, 10% Type IIB, and 5%

for the remaining transitional fibers, which were again dominated by the IIAB fibers. These relative fiber populations are similar to those reported by Clarkson et al. (1984) and Pohlentz (1980).

The presence of greater numbers of IIB fibers in highly trained women rowers may account for both diminished absolute power outputs and lower aerobic capacities in comparison to their male counterparts. As shown in recent studies (Staron et al., 1989, 1991) the Type IIB fiber, if found in large proportions, usually indicates that the athletes are less well-trained. The IIB population is only reduced by increasing the intensity and duration of exercise to induce the conversion of IIB to IIA fibers (Staron et al., 1989, 1991).

We have also observed a significantly greater mitochondrial size and density and increased activities of oxidative enzymes in muscles of rowers when compared with untrained muscles and muscles of elite power lifters (Hagerman & Staron, 1983). These findings help explain the extreme aerobic capacities of elite rowers that may allow them to more rapidly and efficiently oxidize large quantities of lactic acid during and following exercise and help raise the rowers' anaerobic thresholds (Mickelson & Hagerman, 1982). Roth et al. (1983) found increased activities of aerobic enzymes in rowers' muscles but activities of anaerobic enzymes were the same as for control subjects. It is clear from the results of these studies that the muscles primarily responsible for generating power in rowing are dominated by oxidative Type I and Type IIA muscle fibers.

Both fast twitch and slow twitch fiber types in rowers show abnormally large cross-sectional areas when compared with the same fiber types in other endurance athletes (Hagerman & Staron, 1983; Larsson & Forsberg, 1980). Slow twitch (Type I) fibers are appreciably larger in diameter than are those reported for other athletes and controls (Prince et al., 1976). We have measured fiber areas in excess of 8000 μm^2 for slow twitch fibers and 11000 μm^2 for fast twitch (IIA) fibers in elite oarsmen. Elite oarswomen's fibers are somewhat smaller, with some Type I and IIA fibers measured in excess of 7000 μm^2. Type IIB fibers in rowers are the smallest in both men and women, i.e., 5000–8000 μm^2. A summary of cross-sectional fiber areas observed in our laboratory is presented in Table 6-4. In the deltoid muscle of oarsmen, Roth et al. (1983) measured fiber diameters of 9000 μm^2, whereas Larsson and Forsberg (1980) observed smaller fibers of 3580 μm^2.

These cross-sectional areas seem unique for the endurance athlete. However, when one carefully examines the biomechanical and physiological demands of rowing, it becomes clear why a rower's vastus lateralis exhibits extreme oxidative properties and, at the same time, displays large fiber diameters. The extremes of aerobic capacity and muscular power necessary to insure success in rowing are probably influenced by both inherited muscle quality and a high intensity of training and competition. Al-

TABLE 6-4. *Mean cross-sectional areas of muscle fiber types in elite rowers. Data were compiled in the author's laboratory from 1978–1992. Maximal values are shown in parentheses.*

Gender	Cross Sectional Area (μm^2)		
	Type I	Type IIA	Type IIB
Male	6,000–8,000	7,000–10,000	5,000–8,000
(n = 300)	(8,000[+])	(11,000[+])	(8,000[+])
Female	5,000–6,000	5,000–7,000	5,000–7,000
(n = 80)	(7,000[+])	(8,000[+])	(7,000[+])

though fiber type proportions did not appear to change in the oarsmen we studied repeatedly over several years, the cross-sectional areas and both mitochondrial and aerobic enzyme profiles of oxidative fibers did improve.

Bergh et al. (1975) have shown a positive relationship between high aerobic capacity and an abundance of slow twitch fibers in muscles of elite endurance athletes. Secher (1983) suggested that the absence of fast twitch fibers in oarsmen may be due to the specificity of the exercise. He suggested that the generation of a typical rowing stroke cycle during racing permits adequate time for the slow twitch fibers to generate maximum force, thus delegating major contractile responsibility to the IIA fibers and to some degree the IIB fibers only during the initial phase of each stroke.

Increased oxidative capacity in the muscles of oarsmen was also substantiated by Larsson and Forsberg (1980), who reported capillary densities in trained rowers' muscles that were nearly double those observed for the same muscles of untrained subjects (Anderson, 1975; Ingjer, 1979). This great capillary density could obviously facilitate greater delivery of oxygen to highly aerobic muscle fibers.

A simple muscle tissue spectrophotometer has been adapted to measure recovery time (T_R) for hemoglobin/myoglobin (Hb/Mb) desaturation in the capillary bed of exercising muscle (Chance et al., 1988). This technique was applied to the study of the quadriceps femoris in elite male and female rowers (N = 22) for two separate all-out 2000-m rowing ergometer efforts (Chance et al., 1992). Because T_R reflects the balance of localized 0_2 delivery and 0_2 demand in the muscles, T_R can be interpreted as a measure of the time for mitochondrial repayment of 0_2 and energy deficits accumulated during intense exercise. An analysis of T_R after submaximal and high-intensity exercise in conjunction with plasma lactate, power output, and oxygen uptake, may lead to suggestions for improving performance.

Magnetic resonance imaging techniques applied to muscles of highly trained rowers have reflected this trained state by displaying smaller exercise-induced decreases in pH and smaller increases in ratios of free phosphate (P_i) to creatine phosphate (PCr) than are characteristic of untrained subjects (Fountain & McCully, 1988; McCully et al., 1989). Elite rowers also normalized their P_i/PCr ratios more rapidly following exercise than did the controls.

Muscle Strength and Power

Although peak forces during competitive rowing are not very high when compared to those in other sports, average force must be maintained at a high level for about 200 strokes to compete successfully over 2000 m. Isometric strength (Yamakawa & Ishiko, 1966) and isokinetic strength (Pyke et al., 1979) have been correlated with performance on a rowing ergometer, but others have found only poor correlations between strength and rowing performance (Bloomfield & Roberts, 1972; Kramer et al., 1991; Secher, 1975). High-velocity resistance training in one study did increase peak torque at high-velocity resistances, and low-velocity training increased peak torque at low-velocity testing; however, the resistance training did not improve anaerobic rowing power (Bell et al., 1989).

Because strength or power measured in non-rowing circumstances often seems to have little value when applied to rowing, it has been suggested that only strength training involving the rowing motion be recommended for rowers (Bompa & Roaf, 1977). Since the leg drive during the pulling phase of the stroke is the major source of power, developing force and increasing the velocity of contraction in the quadriceps muscle group become primary goals. However, rowers, unlike other elite endurance athletes, develop force using both legs; thus, force and power correspond to the sum of their combined efforts (Secher, 1975; Secher et al., 1988).

Isokinetic strength of high performance rowers is comparable to that of other elite athletes (Clarkson et al., 1984; Hagerman & Staron, 1983; Larsson & Forsberg, 1980). Peak isokinetic strength for the knee extensors of oarsmen was recorded at 0.5 rad/s and averaged 319 Nm (Hagerman & Staron, 1983). Clarkson et al. (1984) tested female rowers at 0 rad/s (isometric actions) and observed a peak strength of 220 N for the knee extensors.

Muscle strength-velocity curves representing some endurance-trained elite athletes are displayed in Figure 6-6. With the exception of the two greatest velocities of contraction, oarsmen exhibited the highest absolute strength. At the two greatest velocities, male swimmers and canoeists exceeded oarsmen at 4.2 and 5.3 rad/s and also showed lesser strength decrements. This finding may be accounted for, at least in part, by the differences in muscle fiber type proportions found in the quadriceps of these athletes. The predominance of slow twitch fibers in rowers may be responsible for the reduced muscular performances at faster contraction velocities. The higher absolute strength values for oarsmen also probably reflect their larger muscle masses. With the exception of some swimmers, the data shown in Figure 6-6 were recorded for athletes who were considerably shorter in stature and had much less lean body mass than elite rowers.

Absolute strength for oarswomen is lower at all test velocities than that of their male counterparts (Figure 6-6) (Hagerman, 1984). However, leg strength per kg of lean body mass, i.e., relative strength, for the oarswomen whose absolute strength data are shown in Figure 6-6 is equal to or greater than that for their male counterparts. This finding is consistent with relative leg strength data reported previously for untrained men and women by Wilmore (1974) and for elite Alpine and cross-country skiers by Haymes and Dickinson (1980).

Muscular power (W) was measured isokinetically for the knee extensors and flexors of oarsmen for 1 min at 3.2 rad/s (Hagerman & Staron, 1983). This velocity was used because the velocity of leg extension during the pulling or drive phase of the rowing stroke was estimated at or slightly above 3.2 rad/s (Mickelson & Hagerman, 1982). Oarsmen achieved an average power of 660 W, whereas other elite male athletes we studied averaged 550 W. Relative values for power favored elite cyclists (7.59 W/kg), with oarsmen slightly lower at 7.30 W/kg. The relative power values for canoeists and swimmers were 7.25 and 7.11 W/kg, respectively.

Ishiko (1968) measured peak power between 700 and 900 W in elite oarsmen during rowing at racing speeds, while their female counterparts produced peak powers of about 500 W during ergometric rowing and also at racing speeds (Mason et al., 1988).

Thorstensson (1976) noted that subjects having a predominance of slow twitch fibers exhibited a high resistance to fatigue. This association may be a factor in the natural selection process that might influence an athlete in the choice of and continued participation in a specific sport. It is well known that most successful elite endurance athletes have very high proportions of oxidative muscle fibers and that subjects with an abundance of fast twitch fibers have the highest attrition rate in endurance training programs (Ingjer & Dahl, 1979).

Although the ability to maintain high muscular forces for a 5–6 min competitive effort is important, it appears that strength and muscle power are not as crucial to rowing performance as are the development of rowing technique for each crew member and the process of molding the performances of the individual crew members into a highly coordinated cohesive crew effort (Rodriquez et al., 1990).

Aerobic Metabolism

Maximal Aerobic Power. It has now been well established that the absolute maximal aerobic power of elite rowers is among the highest recorded (Celentano et al., 1974; Clark et al., 1983; DiPrampero et al., 1971; Hagerman, 1975, 1984; Hagerman & Hagerman, 1990; Hagerman et al.,

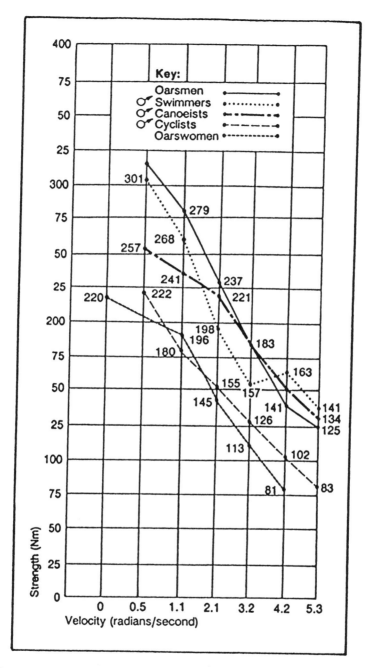

FIGURE 6-6. *Peak torque generated during knee extension at various isokinetic velocities for selected groups of athletes (n = 40/group).* Data from Hagerman, 1984.

1972, 1975a, 1975c, 1978, 1979; Jackson & Secher, 1973, 1976; Larsson and Forsberg, 1980; Nowacki et al., 1969, 1971a; Saltin & Åstrand, 1967; Secher, 1983, 1990, 1993; Secher et al., 1982b). We have measured absolute peak $\dot{V}O_2$max values exceeding 7 L/min in four elite oarsmen, the highest being 7.5 L/min, and more than 5.5 L/min in three female rowers. These results translate into relative values of more than 80 mL·kg^{-1}·min^{-1} for the men and over 70 mL·kg^{-1}·min^{-1} for the women. It is necessary for those who are most successful at the international level to achieve absolute peak $\dot{V}O_2$max levels in excess of 6 L/min for men and 4.5 L/min for women (Table 6-5).

Successful lightweights, as expected, attain absolute values that are 500 to 1000 mL/min less than their heavyweight counterparts, but, because of their significantly lower body weights, they tend to have higher relative $\dot{V}O_2$max values, with some as high as 85–88 mL·kg^{-1}·min^{-1}.

Absolute aerobic power may be more important than relative values in the assessment of a rower's aerobic power because body weight is supported in a seated position. Such objective criteria were used by scientists from the former German Democratic Republic to assist in identifying rowing athletes with outstanding physiological potential (Pohlentz, 1980). Rowers from the former DDR dominated international rowing during the 1980s.

Aerobic Power Testing. Although some limited research was conducted with oarsmen during the 1920s (Henderson & Haggard, 1925; Liljestrand & Lindhard, 1920), it was not until the late 1960s that physiological data for oarsmen and oarswomen began to appear more frequently in the literature (Åstrand, 1967; Åstrand & Rodahl, 1986; DePauw & Vrijens, 1971; Hamby & Thomas, 1969; Hay, 1968; Ishiko, 1967; Mader & Hollmann, 1977; Mellerowicz & Hansen, 1965; Niu et al., 1966; Nowacki et al., 1969, 1971a, 1971b; Saltin & Åstrand, 1967; Scharschmidt & Pieper, 1984; Secher et al., 1983; Steinacker et al., 1983; Strømme et al., 1977; Yamakawa & Ishiiko, 1966). However, $\dot{V}O_2$max was determined during cycling and running in these studies. Oxygen consumption was first measured during tank rowing by Hagerman and Lee (1971) and by DiPrampero et al. (1971), followed by a similar study from Asami et al. (1978). Rowing tanks are

TABLE 6-5. *Means (±SE) for peak power, heart rate (HR), minute ventilation ($\dot{V}_E$), oxygen uptake ($\dot{V}O_2$), and blood lactate concentration (LA) achieved by the 1992 U.S. Olympic Rowing Team during a simulated 2000-m competitive rowing effort on a Concept II rowing ergometer. Data from the author's laboratory.*

N	Power (W)	HR (beats/min)	$\dot{V}_E$ (L/min)	$\dot{V}O_2$ (L/min)	$\dot{V}O_2$ (mL·kg^{-1}·min^{-1})	LA (mmol/L)
♂ 35	467 (18.1)	189 (6.10)	212.7 (11.33)	6.25 (0.26)	70.9 (2.12)	17.4 (2.06)
♀ 25	310 (19.2)	190 (9.19)	153.1 (10.91)	4.31 (0.46)	58.6 (3.65)	13.1 (1.73)

special indoor training facilities, similar in many aspects to modern swimming flumes, where rowers may enhance skill and conditioning.

Measurements of $\dot{V}O_2$max were made on the water during actual rowing by DiPrampero et al. (1971); Hagerman et al. (1972, 1975a, 1975c); Jackson and Secher (1976); and Strømme et al. (1977). Hagerman and Howie (1971), Hagerman and Lee (1971), and Hagerman et al. (1972, 1975a, 1975c) introduced measurement of aerobic power during ergometric sweep rowing, and these investigations were followed by similar ergometric studies (Carey et al., 1974; Cunningham et al., 1975; Koutedakis, 1982; Mickelson & Hagerman, 1982; Roth et al., 1983; Secher et al., 1982b, 1983; Steinacker et al., 1983, 1984a, 1984b, 1986, 1991a, 1991b; Williams, 1978). Similar measurements have also been made during sculling (Hagerman et al., 1988; Hartmann et al., 1987).

The mechanically braked rowing ergometer (Gamut-Stanford ergometer) used in our earlier studies was described in 1978 (Hagerman et al., 1978), and its mechanical operation and task specificity value were discussed in earlier reports (Harrison, 1967, 1970) (Figure 6-7). It was appropriately designed for sweep rowing evaluation but was quite expensive. More recently, the mechanically-braked and fixed-resistance Gjessing-ErgoRow and variable resistance Concept II ergometers have been used more extensively to determine aerobic power among elite rowers. They both have advantages over the Gamut-Stanford ergometer because they are much less expensive and lighter in weight and thus more portable. According to coaches and athletes, they also offer more accurate simulations of rowing. They can be used interchangeably for testing sweep rowers or scullers.

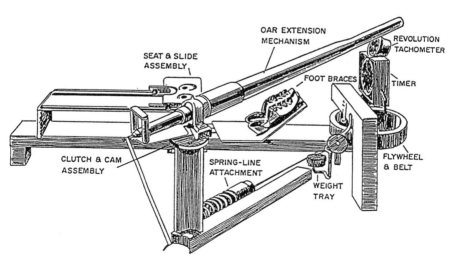

FIGURE 6-7. *Drawing of a Gamut-Stanford mechanical rowing ergometer.*

The Gjessing-ErgoRow, because of its relatively simple mechanical design (Figure 6-8), probably offers a more accurate means of determining power output, whereas the Concept II ergometer is designed as a variable wind-resistance device with power output controlled by the relative amount of air contacted by the fan blades mounted on the flywheel (Figure 6-9). Relative power output is determined by the amount of air admitted to the flywheel chamber, and this amount is regulated by an air vent leading into the chamber. This ergometer has been described previously (Hagerman et al., 1988), and the basic design has been modified by replacing the original bicycle wheel with an aluminum flywheel.

Although all three ergometers are equipped with flywheels, power measurement during rowing ergometry differs slightly from power measurement using a cycle ergometer. In cycle ergometry, power is determined based on resistance, flywheel circumference, and a fixed ratio of

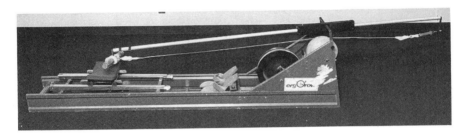

FIGURE 6- 8. *Gjessing Ergorow mechanical rowing ergometer.*

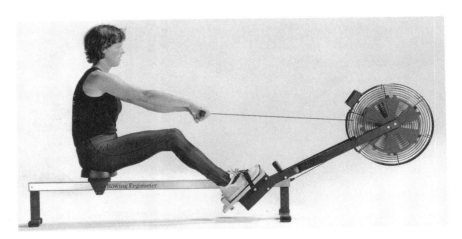

FIGURE 6-9. *Concept II variable resistance rowing ergometer.*

pedal revolutions to flywheel revolutions. In contrast, the rowing ergo-meter's measurement of power is a combination of resistance, circumfer-ence of flywheel, and a non-fixed ratio of strokes to revolutions in which flywheel revolutions can be increased by raising stroke frequency or by increasing tension (pull) on the oar handle, or by doing both.

Because our data on metabolic responses to ergometric rowing were to be applied to evaluations of training and team selection, we decided from the outset to make our testing as task specific as possible. Thus, it was decided to simulate a 2000-m competitive effort. Because a 6-min, all-out effort was about average for international caliber eight-oared crews to cover the 2000 m course, a 6-min time limit was chosen and used in our earlier studies (Hagerman, 1975; Hagerman & Howie, 1971; Hagerman et al., 1975a, 1975c, 1978). More recently, with the ability to measure more accurately the 2000-m distance on most rowing ergometers, a standard 2000-m simulated competitive effort has been utilized (Falkel et al., 1987; Hagerman, 1984; Hagerman & Hagerman, 1990; Hagerman & Korzeni-owski, 1989; Hagerman & Falkel, 1987; Korzeniowski & Hagerman, 1991).

Peak $\dot{V}O_2$ Versus $\dot{V}O_2$max. Instead of $\dot{V}O_2$max, we have often re-ferred to the highest O_2 consumption in our studies as peak $\dot{V}O_2$. This seems appropriate because $\dot{V}O_2$max is usually determined during a stan-dardized graded exercise rather than during a simulated competitive ef-fort such as we used. Although several studies have measured $\dot{V}O_2$max for rowers, these values are consistently lower than the peak $\dot{V}O_2$ mea-surements we have reported (Hagerman, 1974, 1975, 1984; Hagerman & Howie, 1971; Hagerman & Korzeniowski, 1989; Hagerman et al., 1972, 1975a, 1975c, 1978; Korzeniowski & Hagerman, 1991). Peak $\dot{V}O_2$ mea-sured during simulated maximal efforts is about 6–8% higher than $\dot{V}O_2$max recorded during a standard rowing ergometer exercise of increasing in-tensity; e.g., peak $\dot{V}O_2$ average for the 1976 U.S. Men's Olympic Team was 6.6 L/min, whereas the average $\dot{V}O_2$max was 6.2 L/min.

This difference between "peak" and "maximal" values for oxygen up-take is probably due to the fact that the test used to determine peak $\dot{V}O_2$ more closely resembles the specific competitive rowing task for which the rowers train on a daily basis than does the more restrictive incremental $\dot{V}O_2$max test. Finally, maximal values for $\dot{V}O_2$ do not seem to be affected by the model of rowing ergometer used for the tests (Carey et al., 1974; Cunningham et al., 1975; Falkel et al., 1987; Hagerman et al., 1987; Hahn et al., 1988; Kosinski, 1987; Mahler et al., 1984a; Mickelson & Hagerman, 1982; Roth et al., 1983; Secher, 1983, 1990, 1993; Steinacker et al., 1983, 1986, 1991a).

Although values for peak $\dot{V}O_2$ for elite rowers in all of our studies have always been higher than their $\dot{V}O_2$max scores recorded during stan-dard incremental rowing ergometer exercises, the results may be reversed for non-elite rowers. Less well-trained or less skilled rowers often achieve similar or higher values of $\dot{V}O_2$ during incremental $\dot{V}O_2$max tests than during simulated competitive efforts. This finding has recently been supported in other sports by Foster et al. (1993) during their experiments with elite speed skaters, cyclists, and triathletes.

Pacing Patterns. Rowers are accustomed to initiating a competitive effort with a vigorous start in which the highest power outputs and stroke ratings have been achieved. Stroke ratings may reach as high as 40–50 strokes/min and last for 30–40 s. After this initial sprint, power output is reduced and stroke cadence is decreased to 32–38 strokes/min. With the exception of brief strategical increases in power and stroke ratings to insure competitiveness, power output and stroke ratings remain relatively constant for about the next 4 min. The final 30–60 s of the race involve an all-out sprint to the finish during which power and stroke ratings (40 strokes/min or more) are increased dramatically. A typical 2000-m international race, if divided into four 500-m segments, would show that the first 500-m segment is the fastest phase, with each 500-m segment of the middle 1000-m being about 3–4 s slower than the first 500 m. Although the boat will not usually reach the speed of the first 500 m during the sprint to the finish because of rower fatigue, the final 500 m is usually the second fastest segment and is about 1–2 s slower than the first 500 m.

Because simulated competitive efforts on the ergometer mimic this pacing pattern, the $\dot{V}O_2$ responses reflect this somewhat unique pattern of racing strategy. If the curve representing oxygen uptake during a simulated competition for heavyweight rowers is examined carefully (Figure 6-10), the data indicate that, with the exception of the first minute of exercise, oarsmen perform near their peak aerobic power for the entire duration of the race and often reach that peak $\dot{V}O_2$ between the second and fifth minute of the simulated exercise and never during the final minute. Because of fatigue and the more prominent role of anaerobiosis, $\dot{V}O_2$ decreases significantly during the last minute of the ergometer exercise.

The $\dot{V}O_2$ curve for women (Figure 6-10) is slightly different from the men's because it takes women longer to row 2000 m. The more gradual increase in $\dot{V}O_2$ is probably a result of a lower power output due to lesser absolute aerobic power and muscle mass. With the exception of the first and last minutes of the 2000-m effort, when anaerobiosis is more important, the absolute aerobic power of male rowers is 45–50% higher than that of female rowers. Relative $\dot{V}O_2$, based on body weight only, results in lowering this difference to 21%, and, if lean body mass is considered, males have only a 12% higher aerobic power than their female counterparts. Maximal aerobic power measured during an incremental exercise shows a slightly smaller difference for both absolute and relative values. Therefore, the relative aerobic power of oarsmen is only slightly higher than that of oarswomen.

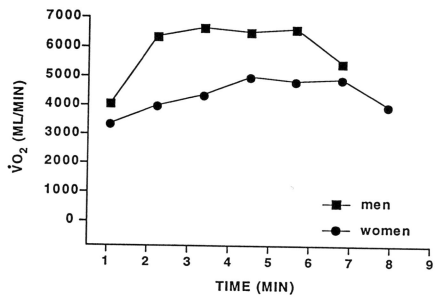

FIGURE 6-10. *Typical time course of oxygen uptake in heavyweight rowers during simulated 2000-m rowing on a rowing ergometer (n = 2000 for men, 500 for women).* Data from the author's laboratory.

Many of the earlier maximal metabolic studies conducted with rowers used treadmill running and cycle ergometry, so there is some question whether aerobic power measured in these studies accurately reflects $\dot{V}O_2$max. Some of these studies reported $\dot{V}O_2$max values for elite rowers that were similar to or slightly greater than those obtained during rowing ergometry (Bouckaert et al., 1983; Carey et al., 1974; Cunningham et al., 1975; Hagerman et al., 1975a, 1975b, 1988). These results are reversed in untrained subjects and unskilled rowers.

Average $\dot{V}O_2$. In most aerobic events, $\dot{V}O_2$max is often considered to be the most important limitation to performance. However, aerobic data accumulated over nearly a 30-y period have demonstrated that average $\dot{V}O_2$ measured during a simulated competitive effort is far more important. Correlations exceeding +0.95 have been calculated between average $\dot{V}O_2$ and competitive rowing performance, whereas correlations of less than +0.86 were obtained between peak $\dot{V}O_2$ and performance. The higher correlation for average $\dot{V}O_2$ as opposed to peak $\dot{V}O_2$ is probably due to the importance of sustaining such a high power output throughout the competitive effort in order to be successful. Although rowers have achieved outstanding absolute peak and maximal $\dot{V}O_2$ values, their single most impressive physiological attribute seems to be the ability to sustain an extremely high percentage of absolute peak $\dot{V}O_2$ even after they have exceeded their anaerobic threshold levels (Hagerman & Mickelson, 1981; Hagerman et al., 1978; Mickelson & Hagerman, 1982).

One of the major criteria used in predicting successful rowing performances at the international level is the ability of the rower to sustain an average $\dot{V}O_2$ that is very close (e.g., $> 98\%$) to peak $\dot{V}O_2$ measured during simulated rowing. This criterion is especially impressive because it demonstrates that exercise intensities eliciting $\dot{V}O_2$max values can be sustained for 7–10 min. Foster et al. (1993) obtained similar results during simulated competitive efforts of other elite aerobic athletes. It is, therefore, common practice for our laboratory to use average absolute $\dot{V}O_2$ data obtained during a simulated competitive effort as opposed to peak $\dot{V}O_2$ when a more desirable measure of aerobic power is needed. This criterion measure has become far more important than either peak $\dot{V}O_2$ or $\dot{V}O_2$max as a selector of potentially successful international rowers.

In many cases, the emphasis on the use of our data for the purposes of team selection and monitoring and modification of training programs has provided a strong incentive for the athletes to perform at their highest levels. The average absolute $\dot{V}O_2$ is determined by averaging all values for each minute of a simulated 2000-m effort, excluding the first minute of exercise, during which there is a time lag in the aerobic response.

The $\dot{V}O_2$ measurements made during ergometric tests tend to agree with estimates of oxygen cost during actual rowing (Droghetti et al., 1991; Hagerman et al., 1975b, 1975c; Jackson & Secher, 1976; Secher, 1983).

Anaerobic Metabolism

The relative contribution of anaerobic metabolism to rowing has been estimated using a variety of methods, including measurements of O_2 deficit, O_2 debt, and the energy equivalent of post-exercise blood lactate concentrations (Asami et al., 1978; Connors, 1974; DiPrampero et al., 1971; Hagerman, 1974, 1975; Hagerman et al., 1975b, 1975c, 1978, 1979; Hagerman, G.R., 1976; Polinski, 1976; Roth et al., 1983; Steinacker et al., 1986). A study of lightweight oarsmen showed no significant correlation between aerobic endurance measured by average aerobic-anaerobic thresholds and performances in the anaerobic tests (Lormes et al., 1991). It was concluded that use of anaerobic tests may be of little value for prediction of competitive performance.

Koutedakis and Sharp (1986) developed a modified Wingate test for measuring anaerobic performance in rowers and confirmed that, in addition to possessing unusually high aerobic capacities, rowers also exhibit outstanding anaerobic qualities.

O_2 **Deficit.** Although O_2 deficit would probably be the best estimate of anaerobic metabolism during maximal exercise, the difficulties involved with its accurate calculation discourage its use by most investigators. Unless a submaximal steady-state oxygen consumption can be achieved, it is not possible to calculate a valid representative value. Although oarsmen do maintain a relatively high steady-state during actual competition and during simulated rowing during ergometry testing, oxygen consumption does vary somewhat over the duration of the race (Figure 6-10). We utilized this high steady-state portion of the $\dot{V}O_2$ curve and the early rise of $\dot{V}O_2$ during exercise to estimate O_2 deficit. We estimated O_2 deficits ranging from 6 to 8 L for both oarsmen and oarswomen (Hagerman et al., 1979), but Secher et al. (1982a) reported slightly lower values. Roth et al. (1983) and Steinacker et al. (1986) also reported lower values that ranged between 300–400 mL/min for a 7–13 min ergometer exercise.

It has been suggested that maximal anaerobic power can be represented by calculating oxygen deficit during exercise of more than 2 min duration (Medbø et al., 1988). For rowers, relative oxygen deficits of 88–97 mL/kg have been determined (Hagerman et al., 1979; Polinski, 1976; Szögy & Cherebetiu, 1974) and this range compares with 52–90 mL/kg measured for runners during treadmill exercise (Medbø et al., 1988). Bangsbo et al. (1990) compared indirect O_2 deficit and debt measurements with anaerobic energy yield in an isolated human muscle during exhaustive exercise and found that the O_2 deficit measurement represented an accurate appraisal of anaerobic energy contribution to a specific exercise. The O_2 debt measurement, however, whether related to the active muscle or to the whole body, overestimated anaerobic energy release.

O_2 Debt. Oxygen debt has also been used to estimate anaerobic capacity of rowers, but because some of the excess oxygen consumed during recovery is used for functions not associated with anaerobiosis, oxygen debt probably cannot be a suitable estimate of anaerobic capacity. We have observed O_2 debts as high as 20 L measured over a 30-min recovery period, with an average of 13.5 L for international caliber oarsmen (Hagerman et al., 1978). Secher et al. (1982a) reported a maximum value of 33 L. The O_2 debts calculated for oarswomen and lightweight men were 10 L and 12 L, respectively (Hagerman, 1974; Hagerman et al., 1979).

Blood Lactate. Extremely high venous blood lactate responses are elicited by maximal actual and simulated rowing. Maximal lactate concentrations in elite oarsmen ranged from 14 to 18 mmol/L following a 6-min simulated rowing exercise (Hagerman et al., 1979). Vaage (1986) reported average team values of 11 mmol/L following races at a national regatta, 15 mmol/L after treadmill running, and 17 mmol/L after an international regatta. We have consistently measured lactates ranging from 10–20 mmol/L in rowers following simulated competitive 2000-m efforts on a rowing ergometer; women's competitive values were slightly lower than those recorded for men (Hagerman, 1984; Hagerman & Korzeniowski, 1989; Hagerman et al., 1989; Korzeniowski & Hagerman, 1991).

Lactic acid concentrations were measured immediately following competitions at World Rowing Championships (Hagerman et al., 1989), and values for men ranged between 16 and 28 mmol/L, the latter value being the highest our group has thus far recorded; women's values ranged from 10 to 20 mmol/L. It is clear that rowers show rather dramatic increases in blood lactate during exercise; furthermore, plasma bicarbonate tends to be lower after rowing than after running or arm cranking (Haber & Ferlitsch, 1979; Rasmussen et al., 1991; Secher et al., 1974). The excessive lactate values reported following maximal actual and simulated rowing indicate that the anaerobic capacities of these athletes are extremely high; when expressed as O_2 deficit, they may be equivalent to 97 mL O_2/kg body weight (Szögy & Cherebetiu, 1974).

In our earlier ergometric studies, the lactate levels we measured prompted us to determine the intensity and duration of exercise at which rowers produce the highest lactate levels. Since it is impossible to row at high intensities with an indwelling venous catheter in either an arm or a leg, we asked 33 U.S. Olympic Rowing Team candidates during the 1976 testing and selection process to repeat the 6-min simulated 2000-m competitive effort on the ergometer on a subsequent day. All candidates had been tested previously with a similar procedure at least 5 d prior to this repetitive effort, and the results of the initial effort were used as a basis for team selection. Prior to the repeated 6-min effort, each athlete was assured that he was rowing a second 6-min competitive effort and that the results would be used compatibly with initial test results as selection criteria. However, the rowers were stopped randomly at minute 1, 2, 3, 4, or 5 of the exercise, and venous blood was withdrawn after a 5-min recovery. All 33 subjects were naive to the random procedures and, after being requested not to reveal the specific procedures of the second test, they provided full cooperation.

When the lactate results of these interrupted tests were compared with lactate data analyzed for all subjects following the 6-min maximal exercise, the comparison revealed that 90% of the peak lactate value measured following the 6-min test was formed as a result of the first min of exercise. Lactate concentrations reached their highest levels at 2 min at values higher than those measured after the 6-min test. These lactate results are summarized in Figure 6-11 and clearly show that rowers, after producing significant lactate concentrations early in the exercise, must maintain a high tolerance to lactate throughout the remainder of the exercise period.

This protocol was repeated again in 1989 (Figure 6-12) for both men and women, and, with the exception of the first minute of exercise, the 1976 and 1989 curves for the men were similar. When one considers the pattern of energy expenditure of rowers during a 2000-m competitive effort, it may not seem surprising that these high lactate levels are observed in the first 2 min of exercise. The increase in lactate values for women is

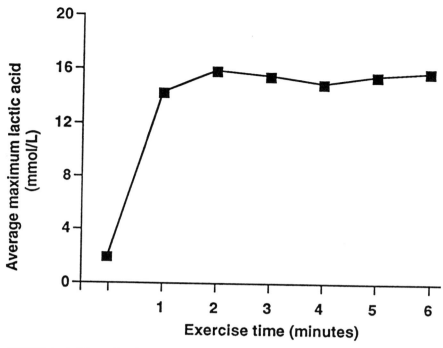

FIGURE 6-11. *Maximal blood lactic acid concentrations during a 6 min rowing ergometer test. Values shown are averages for 30 members of the 1976 US men's Olympic rowing team.* Data from the author's laboratory.

more gradual and reaches maximum during the final minutes of exercise (Figure 6-12). This response, in contrast to the men, probably reflects a difference in pacing, closely following the women's $\dot{V}O_2$ curve (Figure 6-10), and indicates a lower anaerobic capacity and power output for women than for men.

Measurement of lactates during recovery from exercise has been used extensively to characterize rowing training intensities and to monitor training programs (Hagerman & Korzeniowski, 1989; Hartmann et al., 1987, 1990; Korzeniowski & Hagerman, 1991; Mader & Hollmann, 1977). Some of the guesswork by coaches for planning and modification of training programs has been removed as a result of combining heart rate and lactate measurements recorded during specific training sessions (Koutedakis & Sharp, 1985). These measurements have been used to more accurately distinguish between relatively aerobic and relatively anaerobic training efforts.

Rowers have a greater than normal buffering capacity in skeletal muscle, especially in the critical vastus lateralis (Parkhouse et al., 1985). However, induced alkalosis via bicarbonate ingestion does not improve

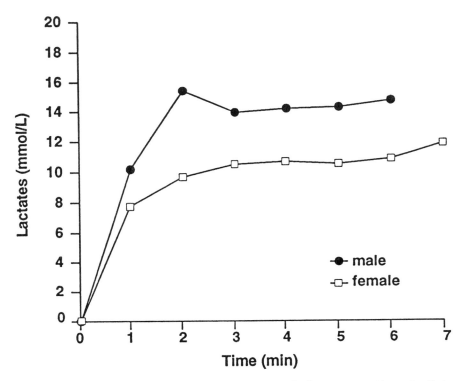

FIGURE 6-12. *Blood lactic acid concentrations during a 6 min simulated 2000-m competitive rowing effort. Values shown are averages for 30 members of the 1989 US men's and women's Olympic rowing teams. Data from the author's laboratory.*

rowing performance (Brien & McKenzie, 1989). As might be expected, the most successful rowers produce significantly less lactate at a given level of rowing intensity (Hagerman & Korzeniowski, 1989; Korzeniowski & Hagerman, 1991; Steinacker et al., 1985).

Energy Expenditure

It has been estimated from O_2 consumption and lactate data during rowing that the relative contributions of aerobic and anaerobic energy pathways are approximately 70–80% and 20–30%, respectively (Connors, 1974; Hagerman, 1984; Hagerman et al., 1978; Secher, 1990, 1993). These data were generated during simulated competitive conditions (rowing ergometry).

Connors (1974) attempted to estimate the relative energy contributions of the phosphagens (ATP-PCr system), anaerobic glycolysis (lactic acid system), and aerobic energy production (the O_2 system). The aerobic component was calculated from net exercise $\dot{V}O_2$ measured during rowing ergometry to be 77.8% of the total. Postexercise venous blood lactate concentrations were incorporated into Margaria's formula (Margaria et al., 1963, 1964), indicating that anaerobic glycolysis contributed 13.8% of the total energy expenditure. This value is comparable to the 14% attributed to glycolysis proposed by Secher (1983). The contribution of the phosphagens in this study, determined using Fox's equation (Hagerman, 1974), was 4%.

Roth et al. (1983) reported an alactic component of 10% during a simulated 2000-m effort. Hagerman et al. (1978), using $\dot{V}O_2$ and oxygen debt, estimated an aerobic to anaerobic ratio of 70%:30%, which is similar to that reported previously (Szögy & Cherebetiu, 1974) and in more recent studies in our laboratory (Hagerman & Hagerman, 1990). Telemetered data and post-competition lactate values seem to confirm these relative proportions (Hagerman & Hagerman, 1990). Because many of these earlier ergometric studies used a maximum of 6 min of exercise and some rowing events last slightly longer than 6 min, Secher suggested that the relative proportion of aerobic metabolism to actual rowing may be greater than that determined from the 6-min tests (Secher, 1990).

Each year, competitive times improve in all boat classes; over the last 30 y, races in the men's eight-oared event have become about 35 s faster (Secher, 1983). In fact, since 1968 the time for this event in the Olympic Regatta has become almost 40 s faster. Although the slowest times for the smaller boats are about 7 min, our recent determinations of relative metabolic proportions confirm a 70–80:20–30% ratio favoring aerobic metabolism, with the smaller slower boats tending to be at the upper end of the aerobic range (Hagerman, 1984; Hagerman & Hagerman, 1990). This ratio was also confirmed by Roth et al. (1983).

The metabolic cost during actual rowing is difficult to measure directly, but Secher (1983) estimated that it has probably increased by about 0.2 L/min per decade as racing times have improved. Our more recent metabolic and performance data suggest that this value of 0.2 L/min is an underestimation and should be doubled (Hagerman et al., 1989).

In addition to the improvement of rowers' metabolic capacities over the years, skill levels have also improved, and boat and oar designs have been enhanced. An oxygen cost of 5.1 L/min reported in 1919 had increased to 6.4 L/min by 1979 (Secher, 1983). As early as 1925, Henderson and Haggard (1925) had estimated the O_2 cost of rowing a competitive race to be about 6.1 L/min, i.e., approximately 30 kcal/min. Current estimations of O_2 cost recorded during ergometric rowing range from 6.7 to 7.0 L/min (Droghetti et al., 1991).

The metabolic cost of rowing is affected by the drag force on the boat, and at least three mathematical models have been described comparing the metabolic capacity of rowers and the energy cost of rowing (McMahon, 1971; Sanderson & Martindale, 1986; Secher & Vaage, 1983). Secher reported that race results from international regattas have been predicted with an $r = 0.99$ from these models. The body weight of rowers also influences metabolic cost, and the basis for these models has been the assumption that aerobic capacity and boat resistance increase with the size of the oarsmen to the second power. However, it is obvious that having bigger rowers in shorter races would be advantageous because of the importance of the largely anaerobic muscular power required for success in these races.

In addition to the work of Jackson and Secher (1973, 1976), the on-the-water metabolic cost of rowing was determined earlier from data on oxygen uptake and heart rate by DiPrampero et al. (1971). From the determination of O_2 consumption on the water, the metabolic cost of rowing increases with speed to the 2.4 power (Secher, 1983, 1990; Törner, 1959), which is less than the calculated 3.0 power required to overcome the drag force on the shell (Secher, 1983). These differences in actual versus theoretical metabolic cost could perhaps be attributed to the effects of rowers moving forward and backward on their sliding seats, thereby affecting boat acceleration and deceleration; unfortunately, the extent to which movement on the seat influences the metabolic cost is not known (Secher, 1990).

The relative contributions of aerobic and anaerobic metabolism to rowing performance over 2000 m are not unusual; other workers have reported similar contributions during other simulated sport activities of about the same time duration (Ekblom & Hermansen, 1968; Gollnick & Hermansen, 1973; Hansen, 1967; Lundin & Saltin, 1971). What is unusual is the manner in which the energy systems are recruited and the maximal capacities of these systems (Hagerman, 1974, 1984; Hagerman et al., 1978).

It has been mentioned previously that each crew begins a race with a vigorous sprint using the highest power output and stroke frequency that will be achieved during the 2000-m effort. The practice of having peak power occur in the first 30 s, followed by a high steady-state and finally an all-out sprint, seems a very uneconomical method of energy utilization or "pacing." However, one study reported that only 7 of 19 oarsmen were able to perform the same total work on a rowing ergometer for 6 min with constant power output as they could when an initial sprint was applied (Grujic, 1989).

There seem to be two possible reasons for the use of a sprint at the onset of rowing competition. One is the need to overcome the inertia of the boat to bring it to racing speed; another is that each crew, regardless of its potential speed, desires to keep close contact with the leading crews in the race.

It is difficult to accurately determine the energy expenditure in a sport by using simulated exercise or training efforts. This was emphasized recently when we measured lactate concentrations and heart rates of rowers during and following World Championships and Olympic competitions and discovered responses clearly different from those recorded during simulated competitive efforts or during actual competitions of lesser caliber and significance. We now know conclusively that what we measure as maximum or peak physiological responses are specific for the relative competitive conditions. Most elite endurance athletes, including rowers, seem to have another "gear" for very special or more important competitive efforts (Hagerman et al., 1989).

The accumulation of energy cost data over several years for elite athletes, especially rowers, has permitted us to build on the energy continuum originally developed by Åstrand and Rodahl (1986). Figure 6-13 represents energy cost comparisons at varying exercise intensities for several different endurance sports and clearly demonstrates that the power output and energy costs of rowing are at the upper limits of human capacity (Hagerman, 1992b).

Estimation of Power Output and Mechanical Efficiency

Assessment Techniques—Simulated versus Actual Rowing. Production of power in the rowing stroke dictates vigorous sequential extension of all joints of the lower limbs, beginning with the hips and ending with a forceful push of the toes against the foot-stretchers, with both legs working together. These actions are followed by a significant extension of the back, with only a minor contribution coming from the shoulders and

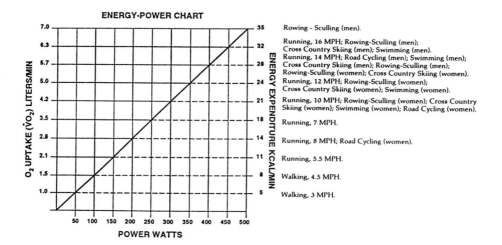

FIGURE 6-13. *Oxygen uptake and energy expenditure at exercise intensities from 0-500 W with examples shown for various sports events (Hagerman, 1992b).* Data are based on studies of more than 3000 athletes.

arms. Although ergometric rowing in many ways resembles actual sweep rowing, there is a slight difference in the biomechanical application of the upper limb segments (Lamb, 1989; Nolte, 1991). Although the legs are extending simultaneously during actual sweep rowing, the inside leg (closest to the oar) contributes less force than does the outside leg. This is due to a slight torquing action required of the trunk while the rower is manipulating one oar with both hands on one side of the boat (Asami et al., 1985). Most rowing ergometers do not account for this action and thus tend to more closely simulate sculling.

The peak force applied to the oar is dependent on a number of factors including technique, stroke frequency, and mass of the rower, but this force may approach a value of 1000 N (Ishiko, 1968). Power generated during normal rowing ergometry was compared with that on an ergometer mounted on wheels (Martindale & Robertson, 1984), and it was reported that oarsmen considered the ergometer on wheels to better simulate actual rowing. This finding suggested that the heavy parts of the body do little external movement on the wheeled ergometer.

Secher (1983) calculated the power generated at racing speed in the coxed pair boat at 386 W in the direction of the boat and, considering work done in a transverse direction because of the biomechanics of the rowing stroke, a total power output of 471 W was estimated. Using this power datum and a total metabolic cost of rowing at racing speed of about 6.4 L/min, he calculated a mechanical efficiency of approximately 22%.

We have measured peak power outputs that exceed 500 W and approach 0.80 horsepower during simulated rowing. The highest power output during a simulated 2000-m effort occurs early in the exercise. A typical power curve during a simulated 2000 m rowing effort is represented in Figure 6-14. It is interesting to note that the occurrence of peak power is concurrent with or followed immediately by peak lactate values and peak $\dot{V}O_2$ (Figures 6-10, 6-11, and 6-12). All three values appear to closely follow the energy demands and the time constraints placed on the energy systems during each major segment or phase of a 2000-m competitive effort; some men's small boat and women's power values extend slightly farther because of slower racing times. As expected, power data during simulated rowing follow the same pattern of pacing selected by rowers during actual racing, with the highest power outputs achieved during the vigorous start, followed by a slightly lower, almost steady-state output, and then ending with an increase in power output beginning with the sprint to the finish.

Average power outputs during simulated rowing for the 1992 U.S. Olympic Team were 457 W for men and 310 W for women. Average power output values for men in 1992 were significantly higher than the 390 W reported previously for elite oarsmen during 6 min of simulated

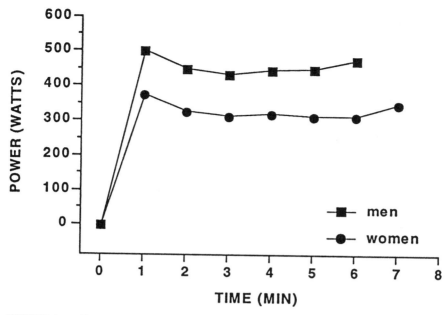

FIGURE 6-14. *Power production during a 6 min simulated competitive rowing effort. Values shown are averages for elite male (n = 2000) and female (n = 500) rowers.* Data from the author's laboratory.

rowing. This power output in 1992 was produced at an aerobic cost of approximately 30 kcal/min and at a calculated mechanical efficiency of 20%. Our power and efficiency measures compare favorably with those estimated by Secher (1983).

Mechanical efficiency measured during a maximal simulated rowing effort has ranged from 10% to 25% (Connors, 1974; Cunningham et al., 1975; DiPrampero et al., 1971; Fukunaga et al., 1986; Hagerman et al., 1978, 1979; Jackson & Secher, 1976; Roth et al., 1983; Secher, 1983; Steinacker et al., 1986). Our earlier work showed a mechanical efficiency of 14%. However, this rather low value was obtained using the Gamut-Stanford type ergometer, which provides an unusually heavy load compared with other contemporary ergometers and actual rowing. Roth et al. (1983) calculated mean efficiency values of 26% (ranging from 17% to 41%) during simulated rowing. Our more recent mechanical efficiency values for simulated rowing have ranged between 18% and 24%, and these data compare favorably with mechanical efficiencies estimated during actual rowing, (Cunningham et al., 1975; DiPrampero et al., 1971; Harrison, 1970; Secher, 1983). Because of the similarity of efficiency data between simulated and actual rowing, it may be concluded that a simulated 2000-m rowing effort may be used to adequately represent the task of rowing.

Anaerobic Threshold

Since its inception, the phenomenon of anaerobic threshold has been a controversial topic (Brooks, 1985; Davis, 1985). The anaerobic threshold (AT) has been defined as that intensity of exercise, expressed as power, pace, heart rate, or oxygen consumption, at which anaerobic metabolism in skeletal muscle is accelerated (Davis et al., 1976). The term "anaerobic threshold" was selected by Wasserman and McIlroy (1964) because it was assumed that an increase in blood lactate and the lactate/pyruvate ratio during incremental exercise was due to an O_2 lack in the exercising muscles (Wasserman et al., 1973).

Increased oxygen utilization by elite rowers could delay the possible deleterious side effects of increasing lactic acid during high-intensity exercise (Åstrand & Rodahl, 1986; Hagerman et al., 1978). The high anaerobic thresholds, coupled with unusually high values for $\dot{V}O_2$max and for average exercise $\dot{V}O_2$, may also be indicative of endurance athletes' ability to use lactic acid as a fuel during exercise (Orfeldt, 1970; Spitzer, 1974). The oxidation of lactic acid by skeletal and cardiac muscle during exercise could raise the AT of rowers. It may, therefore, seem reasonable that during the high steady-state phase of a 2000-m race, lactate clearance may be markedly elevated (Figures 6-11 and 6-12).

There is a linear relationship between $\dot{V}O_2$ and both $\dot{V}_E$ and $\dot{V}CO_2$ at low exercise intensities during an incremental exercise test on the rowing ergometer; the first departure of the curves for $\dot{V}_E$ and $\dot{V}CO_2$ away from that for $\dot{V}O_2$ as the rowing intensity increases has been designated the AT for rowing. This procedure has not only produced acceptable estimates of AT but has also elicited $\dot{V}O_2$max results similar to peak values of $\dot{V}O_2$ obtained during simulated competitive 2000-m efforts (Hagerman & Mickelson, 1981; Mahler et al., 1984a, 1984b; Mickelson & Hagerman, 1982; Steinacker et al., 1991a). Anaerobic thresholds of 85 to 95% of $\dot{V}O_2$max (Hagerman & Mickelson, 1981; Mahler et al., 1983; Mickelson & Hagerman, 1982) attest to the very high aerobic capacities of rowing athletes reported earlier in this chapter.

The high values for AT and $\dot{V}O_2$max in rowers can be attributed, at least in part, to the specific nature of their training programs. Because rowing for both men and women is primarily an aerobic event, 75–85% of training time is devoted to aerobic conditioning. Furthermore, rowing training induces increases in maximal cardiac output, minute ventilation, diffusing capacity for oxygen, and arteriovenous oxygen difference (a-v O_2 diff), and a decrease in the $\dot{V}_E$:$\dot{V}O_2$ ratio, suggesting that AT, too, most likely adapts to the rigors of training for rowing. A final piece of evidence consistent with the contention that AT adapts to rowing training is the fact that AT in rowers is only 70–75% of $\dot{V}O_2$max when recorded during the off-season but 85–95% of $\dot{V}O_2$max during the season (Hagerman &

Mickelson, 1981; Hagerman & Staron, 1983; Mickelson & Hagerman, 1982). Average data from these three studies are shown in Figure 6-15. Data on elite rowers confirm these results (Hagerman & Korzeniowski, 1989; Korzeniowski & Hagerman, 1991).

Ventilation

We have recorded several maximal or peak $\dot{V}_E$ values exceeding 240 L/min BTPS during simulated rowing, the highest being 263 L/min BTPS. Excluding the ventilatory adjustments during the first min of a 2000-m simulated exercise, most elite oarsmen average 200 L/min BTPS throughout exercise. We have also measured $\dot{V}_E$ values in excess of 200 L/min BTPS in some women rowers, and it is not unusual for oarswomen to maintain an average $\dot{V}_E$ greater than 170 L/min BTPS for an exhaustive 2000-m effort.

Peak minute ventilations in our simulated studies have always exceeded $\dot{V}_E$max recorded during standard incremental rowing protocols. Similar responses were also observed by Foster et al. (1990). These large ventilatory volumes are due, at least in part, to the large chests of elite rowers. They tend to have large vital capacities, sometimes exceeding 9 L (Hagerman et al., 1975b; Secher, 1983). Biersteker and Biersteker (1985) and Biersteker et al. (1986) measured normal pulmonary function in rowers and also suggested that the increases in intrathoracic pressure produced during rowing should limit lung elasticity. However, this phenomenon was found only in female rowers, and there seemed to be no clear explanation why male rowers do not exhibit this response since they apply a higher intrathoracic pressure during exercise.

The ventilatory response to exercise in rowers is usually characterized by a low ventilation equivalent ($\dot{V}_E/\dot{V}O_2$) (Mahler et al., 1991a, 1991b; Secher, 1983), presumably because the rower maintains a cramped body position during the initial or catch phase of the stroke, thus impairing normal excursion of the diaphragm (Cunningham et al., 1975). However, we have shown that ventilatory equivalents for rowers equal or exceed those for most other endurance athletes (Hagerman, 1975, 1984; Hagerman et al., 1972, 1975a, 1975b, 1975c).

Hyperventilation during rowing is more pronounced than during cycling and is accomplished with a higher breathing frequency accompanied by a relatively lower tidal volume (Szal & Schoene, 1989). Breathing frequencies in our studies have ranged from 60–88 breaths/min, and tidal volumes of greater than 3 L have been observed. A high breathing frequency during rowing at high intensity indicates that pulmonary ventilation is linked to the stroke rate (Mahler et al., 1991a, 1991b).

Steinacker et al. (1992) investigated ventilatory responses in elite rowers during an incremental simulated rowing exercise and observed

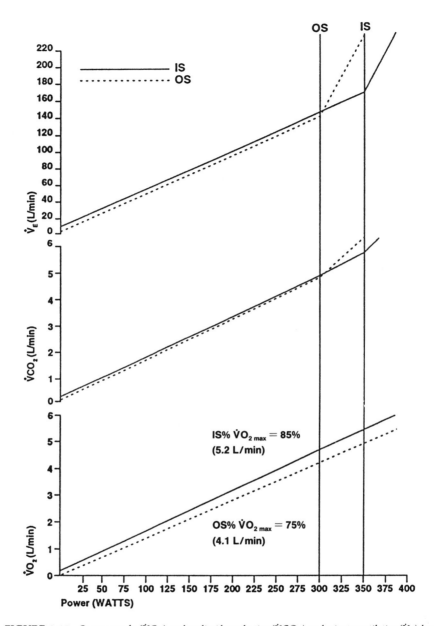

FIGURE 6-15. *Oxygen uptake (V̇O₂), carbon dioxide production (V̇CO₂), and minute ventilation (V̇E) during a graded performance test on a rowing ergometer both in-season (IS) and off-season (OS) (n = 150).* Anaerobic thresholds, indicated by vertical lines, occurred at 300 W off-season and increased to 350 W in-season. Composite data are from Hagerman & Mickelson (1981), Hagerman & Staron (1983), and Mickelson & Hagerman (1982).

two distinct breathing patterns—type 1, with one expiration per stroke and one inspiration during recovery, and type 2, with one complete breath during the stroke and one complete breath during recovery. All subjects entrained their breathing to stroke frequency. There is no evidence that ventilation is impaired during rowing (Hagerman, 1975; Hagerman et al., 1972, 1975a, 1978, 1979, 1988); ventilatory responses of elite rowers during continuous graded treadmill running were identical to those recorded during a competitive simulated rowing effort (Clark et al., 1983).

Exhaustive rowing has been associated with marked hypoxia. Despite a marked hyperventilation, arterial oxygen tension declines from a PO_2 of 105 mm Hg at rest to 88 mm Hg during the last minute of maximal simulated rowing (Clifford et al., 1990). Dempsey (personal communication, 1988) also noted extreme femoral artery hypoxia in elite oarsmen. Hemoglobin saturation was reported to decrease to 91%, and arterial pH to 6.8 (Rasmussen et al., 1991). This could be accompanied by a severe reduction in bicarbonate to the point where it may be temporarily eliminated from the blood. The decrease in arterial PO_2 during intense rowing may also indicate a diffusion limitation for oxygen through the alveolar membrane when cardiac outputs for rowers reach extraordinary levels.

Circulation

Heart Rate, Stroke Volume, and Cardiac Output. An increase in heart rate was probably the first physiological response to be observed during rowing (Fraser, 1868–1869); this same study also noted a marked increase in pulse pressure. Similar heart rates have been measured during high-intensity simulated and actual rowing (Cunningham et al., 1975; Droghetti et al., 1985; Hagerman, 1984; Hagerman & Hagerman, 1990; Hagerman & Howie, 1971; Hagerman & Lee, 1971; Hagerman et al., 1972, 1975a, 1978, 1979, 1987, 1988; Jackson & Secher, 1976; Korzeniowski & Hagerman, 1991; Niu et al., 1966; Secher, 1983, 1990, 1993; Secher et al., 1982a, 1982b; Steinacker et al., 1986; Williams, 1976). Figure 6-16 depicts a typical heart rate response to actual and simulated 2000-m efforts (Hagerman, 1984). In addition, the time course for heart rate changes parallels those for changes in $\dot{V}O_2$ and power output (Figures 6-10 and 6-14).

Maximal and peak heart rates for elite rowers range primarily between 180 and 200 beats/min with a limited number of responses as low as 170 beats/min and as high as 230 beats/min. Earlier studies measured heart rate via direct electrocardiography, but by the early 1970s, indirect biotelemetry was the diagnostic choice. The maximal heart rate for some rowers during ergometer rowing is similar to that measured for rowers during cycling (Bouckaert et al., 1983; Cunningham et al., 1975; Hamby & Thomas, 1969) but lower than that during treadmill running (Carey et al., 1974; Clark et al., 1983).

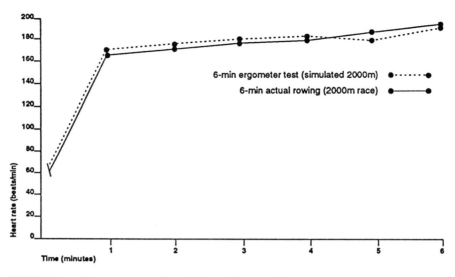

FIGURE 6-16. *Representative recordings of telemetered heart rates during a 6 min simulated 2000-m rowing competition compared to those during an actual 2000-m race (Hagerman, 1984).*

Measurement of cardiac output of rowers was first reported by Liljestrand and Lindhard (1920) during actual rowing, and they recorded a value of 17 L/min. Later, rowing ergometer exercise produced similar results, but cardiac output was measured at rather low exercise intensities ($\dot{V}O_2$ = 2.4 L/min) and in non-elite athletes (Rosiello et al., 1987). The slope of the line relating the increase in cardiac output to the increase in $\dot{V}O_2$ during rowing is 5.2–6.1, which is similar to that for other forms of aerobic exercise (Secher, 1983).

We measured cardiac output by the dye-dilution technique in U.S. Olympic oarsmen in 1968 and again in 1988 with doppler-echocardiography, both at rest and during an incremental cycle ergometer exercise test to exhaustion. Maximal cardiac outputs ranged from 29 to 40 L/min, with the highest values recorded for rowers whose heights and weights exceeded 203 cm and 90 kg, respectively, and who had achieved absolute maximal oxygen consumptions greater than 6.7 L/min. Similarly high values have been reported for other endurance athletes (Ekblom & Hermansen, 1968). Saltin (1969) suggested that maximal stroke volume is the most important distinguishing difference between elite endurance athletes and non-elite endurance-trained subjects; our cardiac output data tend to support this observation.

Several studies have reported large internal diameters and wall thicknesses of hearts of oarsmen (Chignon & Distel, 1981; Dickhuth et al., 1979; Jensen et al., 1986; Pelliccia et al., 1991; Weiling et al., 1981). Hearts of oarsmen are apparently similar to those of weightlifters, who routinely exhibit selective hypertrophy of the myocardial mass (Howald et al., 1977).

We have recorded resting heart rates of rowers in the sitting position as low as 26 beats/min. Such low rates seem to reflect extraordinary stroke volumes. The greatest value we have calculated for oxygen pulse in elite oarsmen during exhaustive rowing ergometry was 39.4 mL O_2/beat in a rower whose $\dot{V}O_2$max was 7.1 L/min and whose maximal heart rate was 180 beats/min (Hagerman, 1984).

Blood Volume and Blood Pressure. Blood volumes at rest of 95 mL/kg for rowers vs. 76 mL/kg for controls have been reported; pulmonary blood volume at similar resting cardiac outputs was 25% greater in the rowing athletes, suggesting that their intraventricular circulation time at rest was markedly greater than that of the controls (Falch & Strømme, 1979).

Blood pressure measurements during rowing are difficult to carry out because of constant arm movements. However, Hanel et al. (1990) noted dramatic changes in blood pressure during rowing. They recorded a pulse pressure (systolic minus diastolic pressure) of 100 mm Hg during the initial or catch phase of the stroke, where transient isometric actions of trunk and limb muscles take place and are associated with a simultaneous Valsalva maneuver. This is followed by an immediate decrease in blood pressure during the recovery phase of the stroke (Lassen et al., 1989). However, the net effect of these pulse pressure changes on mean arterial pressure during rowing is an insignificant slight increase.

CONTEMPORARY TRAINING PRACTICES

Influence of Science

There is a dearth of reports on scientific investigations of rowing training (Bloomfield & Roberts, 1972; Grujic et al., 1987; Hagerman & Falkel, 1987; Hagerman & Staron, 1983; Hagerman et al., 1989; Mahler et al., 1984b; Secher et al., 1982a; Steinacker, 1988; Strydom et al., 1967; Tumility et al., 1987; Wright et al., 1976), and few of these studies involved applied training programs.

Hagerman and Staron (1983) compared off-season and in-season physiological data for nine members of the U.S. Men's Olympic Rowing Team. No changes were noted for body composition or maximal heart rates, but values for $\dot{V}_E$max, $\dot{V}O_2$max and ergometer power increased from off-season to in-season. Isokinetic leg strength increased at six different velocities from in-season to off-season, especially at the lower velocities. Based on these comparisons, it might be inferred that oarsmen should attempt to maintain higher aerobic power during off-season so that there is less of a decrement to overcome as the season begins. Also, it appears that during the off-season, rowers should de-emphasize resistance training at low velocities and emphasize power development at greater velocities, i.e., train more specifically for the types of movements used in rowing competition.

Results of the 1983 study by Hagerman and Staron prompted a recent comparison of the effects of normal weight training and no weight training during the off-season on muscular strength and power, muscle fiber proportions, aerobic power, and ergometric power of elite men and women rowers (Hagerman et al., unpublished data, 1993). The rowers who performed off-season weight training significantly reduced their aerobic power and did not improve their ergometer performance; more importantly, the off-season weight training may actually have detracted from in-season rowing performance. Accordingly, it appears that elite rowers would benefit more from performing only simulated or actual rowing training during the off-season rather than including resistance training. Alternatively, the intensity and duration of resistance training should probably be restricted.

Mahler et al. (1984a) also reported effects of rowing training on $\dot{V}O_2$max and AT of elite athletes and showed a slower rate of increase in $\dot{V}O_2$max and a faster improvement in AT during a six-month period; this reflected a shift in training emphasis from primarily aerobic to more anaerobic training.

Since the early 1970s, competitive rowing has been dominated by Germany, first the German Democratic Republic, and now unified Germany. Between 1985 and 1988, approximately 40 elite German male rowers were studied during training with emphasis on heart rate and lactate measurements during and following training sessions of varying intensities and duration (Hartmann et al., 1990). The specific training intensities were divided into four categories based on post-exercise lactate response: Category I—greater than 8 mM, Category II—4–8 mM, Category III—2–4 mM, Category IV—less than 2 mM. These categories were determined as a result of careful observations of lactate responses during submaximal exercise (Hartmann, 1987; Heck et al., 1985a, 1985b; Hollmann & Hettinger, 1980; Jacobs et al., 1981; Mader & Heck, 1986; Mader et al., 1976). A lactate concentration of 8.0 mM is considered by these investigators to be the transition limit between exercises of moderate and high intensity, whereas a lactate concentration of 12 mM or more represents exhaustive exercise. Using the four intensity categories, the percentage of the different training intensities related to the total amount of training and to the training phase were determined, and these results are shown in Table 6-6.

Throughout the total training period, excluding competition, the duration of lower intensity aerobic training (categories III and IV) represents over 90% or more of training according to the scheme depicted in Table 6-6. Category IV decreased to 73.5% during the competitive period, where-

TABLE 6-6. *Percent of the different training intensities related to the total amount of training and to the training phase.*

| Training Period | Categories (% of the total amount of training) | | | | |
	IV	III	IV+III	II	I
Preparation Period					
—autumn/winter	90–94	8–5	98–99	1	1–0
—winter/spring	86–88	9–5	95–93	4	1–3
Competition Period	70–77	22–15	92–93	6	2

as category III increased to an average of 17.5%. The greater emphasis on low intensity aerobic training for rowing is somewhat surprising because other experts have recommended a greater proportion of high-intensity training (Fritsch, 1981, 1985, 1986; Marx & Steinacker, 1988; Nolte, 1986, 1988), especially during the competitive period.

Previous work suggested that endurance training is only effective if it is done at a lactate concentration between 2.5 mM and 3.5 mM (Lormes et al., 1988; Steinacker, 1988; Urhausen et al., 1986) or 4.0 mM (Hirsch, 1977). However, Hartmann et al. (1990) found that the athletes they observed subjectively chose training intensities so as to maintain steady-state exertion for long durations with low concentrations of blood lactate (Table 6-6). It was very difficult for the athletes to exercise for 45 min at an intensity corresponding to a lactate concentration of 3.5 mM; even higher intensities were found to be quickly exhausting (Hartman et al., 1990). Thus, it appears that training for endurance improvement in rowing at lactate levels of 4.0 mM or higher is not advisable.

Contrary to the results of the German investigators, our lactate measurements during training suggest that lactate values proposed by Hartmann et al. (1990) may underestimate an elite rower's lactate tolerance. We also developed a training intensity continuum that was modified from one originally proposed by Nilsen et al. (1987a, 1987b). Using several years of careful observation of training heart rates and lactates and the collation of national coaches' and rowers' training diaries, we have produced a more specific account of rowing training intensities (Table 6-7). The major categories of training intensities are: anaerobic, transportation, anaerobic threshold, and utilization. Anaerobic training emphasizes the phosphagen and glycolytic systems, whereas transportation training loads the cardiovascular and respiratory systems. The anaerobic threshold training represents a transition stimulus between aerobic and anaerobic training, and utilization training is designed to encourage the uptake of O_2 by the active muscles. Although not precise, the categories offer the coach and athlete a relatively easy continuum to understand and provide some useful data to more accurately monitor specific training sessions.

As indicated in Table 6-7, we have presented a wider range of lactate responses for each training intensity than did Hartmann et al. (1990),

TABLE 6-7. *Rowing training intensities. See text for details.*

Training Intensity	Optimal Time	% Max Effort	% HR* Max	HR* Range	Lactate Range (mM)	Energy Systems
Anaerobic 1 (AN$_1$)	10–30 s	≥ 100	100	190+	Small Amounts	ATP-PCr
Anaerobic 2 (AN$_2$)	30–90 s	95–100	95–100	180–190	Maximum Values (10–25)	LA
Transportation (TR)	90 s–10 min	90–95	90–95	170–180	6–10	LA (Most) O$_2$ (Some)
Anaerobic Threshold (AT)	10–20 min	85–90	85–90	160–170	4–6	LA-O$_2$ (About Equal)
Utilization 1 (U$_1$)	10–40 min	75–85	75–85	140–160	2–4	O$_2$ (Most) LA (Some)
Utilization 2 (U$_2$)	30–120 min	65–75	65–75	125–140	2 or less	O$_2$ (More than U$_1$) LA (Less than U$_1$)
Utilization 3 (U$_3$)	30–120 min	55–65	55–65	105–125	Small Amounts	O$_2$ (Almost All) LA (Little-None)

*Based on a maximum heart rate of 190 beats/min.
ATP-PC: energy derived primarily from adenosine triphosphate and phosphocreatine.
LA: energy derived primarily from anaerobic glycolysis.
O$_2$: energy derived primarily from oxidative sources.

with our upper limits being slightly higher. It has been our observation that rowers can train at relatively high exercise intensities before producing significant amounts of lactic acid, and, contrary to the observations of Hartmann et al. (1990), that rowers can tolerate lactate concentrations of 4 mM for long periods of rowing. Similar to the German program (Table 6-6), most of the training by U.S. rowers takes place at an intensity of utilization 2 (U_2); as the competition period begins, more training occurs at utilization 1 (U_1), anaerobic threshold, transportation, and anaerobic 2.

Serial testing of rowers demonstrated that prolonged training improves mechanical efficiency (Hagerman, 1984). Most of these observations were made between 1972 and 1980. Of all the test values measured and/or calculated for the 6-min simulated rowing exercise during this period, mechanical efficiency exhibited the most significant change (Figure 6-17). Maximal or peak values for $\dot{V}_E$, $\dot{V}O_2$, and heart rate increased only slightly over the same time period. The data in Figure 6-17 represent three of the many subjects who were studied consecutively over an 8-y period; they were able to serially produce higher power outputs with gradually decreasing total O_2 cost.

Although probably favored genetically, these athletes gradually improved important physiological responses necessary to increase mechanical efficiency. Consistent, specific, and prolonged training; better coaching; and rowing with more skilled and highly conditioned teammates resulted in increases in cardiac output, intramuscular oxidative enzyme activities, a-v O_2 differences, and anaerobic thresholds (Chance, et al., 1992; Hagerman, 1984).

The three examples shown in Figure 6-16 were outstanding college oarsmen during the first two to three years of their candidacies for the U.S. National and Olympic teams, but they did not become successful candidates until they were able to achieve mechanical efficiencies at or near 20%. Because of these consistent dramatic changes in efficiency by successful elite oarsmen, this measurement is an excellent criterion for predicting performance.

Applied Training

A complete discussion of training for competitive rowing is beyond the scope of this chapter. In order to understand specific training requirements for this sport, certain general and specific training principles will be presented.

Although competitive rowing efforts only last from 5–8 min, the elite rower generally trains twice daily with each training session usually lasting 60–120 min. Total training time thus seems extraordinary, considering the duration of the races. However, success at the international level dictates such an imbalance between training time and competition time. Because the sport of rowing requires a unique mixture of skill, aerobic

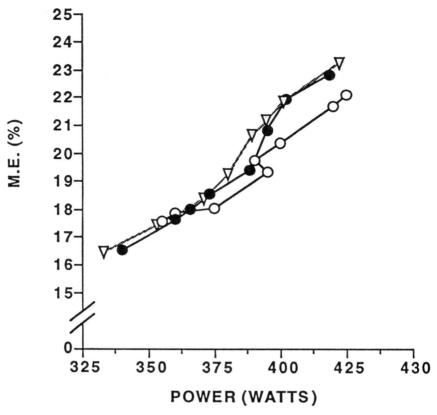

FIGURE 6-17. *Mechanical efficiency (M.E.) and average power maintained during a 6 min simulated 2000-m competitive rowing effort on a rowing ergometer.* The eight points on each of the three curves shown represent results of annual tests over eight successive years for three representive elite rowers. The data demonstrate substantial improvements in both power and efficiency over the 8 y for each rower (Hagerman, 1984).

and anaerobic endurance, and muscular power, each of these factors must be given special attention; the optimal extent and timing of that attention during off-season or in-season are difficult to assess.

The majority of competitive rowers train throughout the year, usually concentrating on low-intensity aerobic conditioning, limited anaerobic exercise, and high-resistance, low-repetition weight training early in the off-season (September through December). Consulting Table 6-7; about 95% of training during this period would be conducted at U₁ and U₂ intensities, with only 5% of training conducted at high intensities, mostly at TR. In locations where inclement weather prevents rowing, cross-training, including cycling, swimming, running, and cross-country skiing, is used extensively.

Higher intensity aerobic conditioning, increased anaerobic exercise, and lower resistance, higher repetition resistance training usually follows during the remainder of the off-season (January–April). During this period, the proportion of U1 training is gradually increased as total aerobic training decreases from about 95% in the previous four months to 85–90%. Transportation training increases to about 10%, and AT and AN_2 training are gradually increased. These eight months represent the preparation period in some training programs.

During the competitive season (May–August), a mixture of high- and low-intensity aerobic and anaerobic conditioning sessions are employed, with only limited use of weight training. Aerobic training will now account for about 80 to 85% of total training time, but more attention is given to U_1 training. The contributions of AT, T_R, and AN_2 training all increase, using higher intensity interval training, with T_R and AN_2 training being very critical 4–6 weeks prior to competition.

The month of September in the northern hemisphere represents a transition period, in which physical and mental relaxation, abstinence from systematic rowing training, and the introduction of cross-training usually occur.

The Fédération Internationale des Sociétés d'Aviron Coaches' Development Program (Nilsen et al., 1987a, 1987b) and Hagerman and Falkel (1987) have emphasized the importance of training the aerobic metabolic system, because this system provides about 70–80% of the energy during a rowing race. The following training recommendations have been presented by these authors.

1. To improve oxygen utilization in the muscle, long distance training should be employed at a heart rate of 130–160 beats/min, below the anaerobic threshold.
2. To increase oxygen delivery to the exercising muscle, interval training should be used at a heart rate of 180–190 beats/min, above the anaerobic threshold.

Two major objectives of training are to improve a rower's ability to compete at a greater percentage of maximal oxygen consumption without producing significant lactate accumulation and to improve the rower's ability to tolerate lactate that does accumulate. The type of training that most effectively addresses the first objective is training at or near the AT; interval training at high intensities with sufficient rest periods to remove all or most of the accumulated lactate improves the athlete's ability to tolerate accumulated lactate.

Maximal aerobic power decreases quite rapidly in the elite endurance athlete who discontinues regular training; for example, inability to train for one week results in a decline in aerobic power by 10–50% (Costill et al., 1985). Similarly, aerobic power in elite rowers declines during the off-season or early preparation period when more emphasis is placed on resistance training and less on endurance training (Hagerman & Staron, 1983). These earlier observations were consistent with a 5 y summary of data on U.S. National and Olympic Team oarsmen (Table 6-8); these data show that all metabolic responses and power output increased from the early preparation period (December) to the early (May) and middle (July) competitive periods. The inability to sustain high aerobic power during the off-season reflects emphasis on strength-power training during this period, whereas the elevation in AT and AT-related responses during the competitive periods demonstrates the important effects of training at ever-increasing intensities (Table 6-8).

Evaluation of Training

Anaerobic threshold and $\dot{V}O_2$max can be determined during an incremental rowing ergometer test, usually beginning at a power output of 100 W and increasing in power by 50 W every 2 min until exhaustion. Peak ATs under these incremental test conditions range from 80–85% $\dot{V}O_2$max during the competitive season and often drop to 65–70% $\dot{V}O_2$max during the off-season.

The most common test sequence we now use for evaluation of elite rowers is a test protocol first used in 1989 (Korzeniowski & Hagerman, 1991) to determine both peak physiological capacity and to monitor and

TABLE 6-8. *Mean (±SE) responses during maximal ergometric rowing (2000-m simulated competition) (5-year average).*

Response	Dec.	Feb.	May	July
Peak Power	345	380°	393*~	457**
(W)	(18.6)	(17.1)	(16.8)	(18.3)
Peak $\dot{V}O_2$	5.61	5.65	6.16*	6.35*
(L/min)	(0.59)	(0.63)	(0.36)	(0.29)
Peak $\dot{V}O_2$	61.4	62.0	68.4*	71.3**
($mL \cdot kg^{-1} \cdot min^{-1}$)	(2.11)	(1.88)	(1.97)	(1.91)
$\dot{V}O_2$ @ AT	4.04	4.26	5.14***	5.46***
(L/min)	(0.73)	(0.69)	(0.81)	(0.77)
AT	72	75	83*	86*
(% Peak $\dot{V}O_2$)	(1.01)	(1.31)	(1.11)	(1.21)

° Significant difference (p<0.05) between Feb. and July data.
~ Significant difference (p<0.05) between May and July data.
* Significant difference (p<0.05) between Dec. and May data and between Dec. and July data.
** Significant difference (p<0.01) between Dec. and July data.
***Significant difference (p<0.01) between Dec. and May data; Dec. and July data; between Feb. and May data and Feb. and July data.
All other comparisons are statistically nonsignificant.

regulate training. It is generally agreed that most training for rowing should be devoted to improving oxygen utilization and transport (Nilsen et al., 1987a, 1987b). With the exception of measuring $\dot{V}O_2$ during and following actual rowing or rowing ergometry (Hagerman, 1974, 1984; Hagerman et al., 1972, 1978, 1979; Jackson & Secher, 1973, 1976; Secher, 1983) or applying the Conconi test to determine anaerobic threshold (Droghetti, 1986; Droghetti et al., 1985) or lactate analysis (Mader & Heck, 1986), most of the current fitness tests are not specific enough to adequately measure rowing fitness, and the others are logistically inappropriate in a field setting.

With this in mind, we developed a test that: 1) permits team testing over a 1–2 d period, i.e., the time available during a test weekend for elite rowers; 2) assesses $\dot{V}O_2$max and other physiological responses at AT and below AT; 3) provides useful information to coaches and athletes concerning the relative development of and effects of training on oxygen utilization and transport systems; and 4) is easily administered and reproduced in any boathouse (Korzeniowski & Hagerman, 1991). We have routinely conducted the testing described above over a 2-d period. On the first day, each subject rows a 2000-m simulated competitive effort on a rowing ergometer. If possible, ventilatory, cardiovascular, metabolic, and hematological responses are noted continuously during and following this effort. On the second day of testing, the athlete performs three consecutive 5-min ergometer efforts, the first at 60% of maximal power for the simulated 2000-m exercise, the second at 70% of maximal power, and the third at 80% of maximal power. Heart rate is telemetered and recorded at the end of each minute of exercise. Fingertip blood samples are withdrawn after 5 min of recovery from each 5 min rowing effort for lactate analysis, and heart rate is recorded during each minute of the 5-min recovery period. We have now standardized all elite rowing testing with the Concept II variable resistance ergometer (Hagerman & Korzeniowski, 1989) by closing the speed ring vents and placing the chain on the small sprocket.

Optimally, the test conducted at 60% of maximal power should elicit a heart rate range of 120–140 beats/min and postexercise lactates ranging from 1–2 mM. The expected heart rate and lactate values for the 70% and 80% efforts are 140–160 beats/min and 2–4 mM, and 160–180 beats/min and 4–6 mM, respectively. The initial maximal power test serves as the baseline, and the submaximal tests relative to this baseline can then be performed periodically during the training season to determine the effects of that training.

Since an abundance of oxygen utilization training is used in rowing, periodic submaximal testing will provide an excellent means of charting training responses. As training progresses, the heart rate and lactate values should gradually decrease for the standard exercise. The characteristic shift downward and to the right for the 60, 70, and 80% plots is shown in a typical training response graph in Figure 6-18. Because the 80% effort is an approximation of the optimal anaerobic threshold stimulus for most rowers, a shift in this value will permit estimation of the effects of training on anaerobic threshold.

Weight Training

The use of non-specific resistance or weight training to improve rowing performance has long been a controversial topic. There is no doubt that muscular strength and power are important to this sport, but it is difficult to determine their precise contributions. Rowing coaches adopted supplemental resistance training programs for their athletes at about the same time as coaches of other aerobic sports and have continued to use weight training primarily during the preparation period (Hagerman & Mickelson, 1979a, 1979b, 1979c). In the early years of use, it was common to employ a program of high-resistance, low-repetition training during

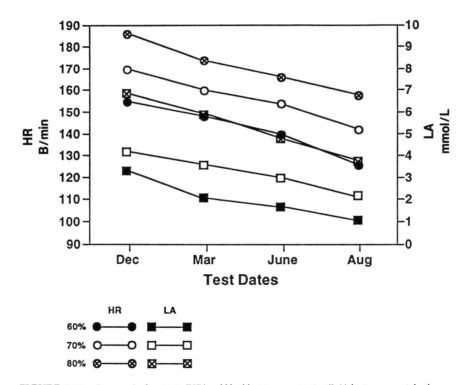

FIGURE 6-18. *Averages for heart rate (HR) and blood lactate concentration (LA) during sequential submaximal rowing ergometer tests for 40 elite rowers in an Olympic year.* The rowing intensities were 60%, 70%, and 80% of the maximal power exerted during a simulated 2000-m competitive rowing effort on a rowing ergometer (Hagerman & Korzeniowski, 1989).

the early preparation period, followed by a gradual transition to lower resistance, higher repetition local muscular endurance work during the later preparation period, and only a small amount of resistance training during the competitive period. More recently, emphasis has shifted to a greater volume of local muscular endurance training during the preparation period, especially using exercises that simulate the rowing motion, and there has been a significant reduction of or a cessation of any resistance training during the competitive period.

Table 6-9 was developed by Kris Korzeniowski, technical director and team coach of the United States Rowing Association in 1992, and published in *Stroke*, a newsletter to athlete members of the United States Rowing Association, 1991–1992. It prescribes resistance and metabolic-specific training for prospective 1992 Olympic rowers. As indicated in both the early (September, October, November, December) and late (January, February, March, April) preparation periods, the emphasis was on local, muscular endurance resistance training with little or no resistance training during the competitive period. Recommendations for rowing training or cross-training emphasized activity at oxygen utilization intensities during the early preparation period and then gradually shifted to intensities emphasizing the oxygen transportation system as the preparation period ended; anaerobic threshold and anaerobic training were introduced in the competitive period.

ENVIRONMENTAL EFFECTS ON ROWING PERFORMANCE

Altitude

The importance of aerobic power to rowing performance was accentuated during acute and chronic hypoxic exposure (Hagerman, 1969; Hagerman et al., 1975b). There were more dyspneic-hypoxia-related physical collapses recorded during the rowing competition at the 1968 Olympic Games in Mexico City than for any other aerobic-type event or sport. In Mexico City, rowing officials reported more than 80 incidents of physical exhaustion during races in the first 2 d of competition, and several more were recorded during subsequent racing (Hagerman, 1969).

The complete cessation of rowing by a crew during competition very rarely occurs at an international regatta; if so, it is usually due to mechanical difficulty. However, several crews stopped frequently and some failed to finish races at the 1968 Olympic Regatta. Not once in any episode of collapse or exhaustion was either the stroke member of the crew or a single sculler involved. In other words, those athletes responsible for dictating the intensity of exercise were never affected. These episodes reinforce the fact that any multiple-oared crew is only as effective as its weakest link.

TABLE 6-9. *A recommended training program for prospective 1992 Olympic rowers* (K. Korzeniowski, *Stroke*, USRowing 1992; reproduced with permission)

SEPTEMBER AND OCTOBER TRAINING PROGRAM

In 1992, the major goal for the openweights will be the Olympics in Barcelona July 25–August 2. For the lightweights the goal will be the World Championships in Montreal August 8–12. The starting date of both events is unusually early, and the training program has to take this into consideration. Athletes who think seriously about making the National Teams should start to train much earlier than usual.

September should be a month of "introduction." The goal is to prepare the body for the next period, which will be the very intensive general preparation period. The athletes should try to improve technical skills, maintain aerobic level and start to work on general fitness (body circuits and light weight circuits).

Training Program for September 1991

Day	Training Model	Stroke rate	Heart rate
Mon.	2 × body circuit 2–3 × general circuit		
Tues.	Rowing 2 × 40 min. of steady state	18–20	140–150
Wed.	see Monday		
Thurs.	Rowing 70 min steady state alternate (4′ + 3′ + 2′ + 1′)	18/20/22/24	140–150
Fri.	see Monday		
Sat.	Rowing steady state 2 × 40 min	18–20	130–150
Sun.	Off		

A consistent and systematic approach will determine the effectiveness of a given training program.

Body Circuit

Stress correct execution of each exercise. A maximum number of repetitions should be done in each 30 second period, followed by a 15 second rest. The rest period between each circuit is three minutes. Do not let the heart rate drop below 140.

30 seconds on/15 seconds rest

Exercises
 1. push-ups
 2. one leg squats (right leg)
 3. one leg squats (left leg)
 4. leg circles
 5. bench jumps
 6. pull-ups
 7. squat jumps with push-ups
 8. sit-ups (feet elevated)
 9. jumpies
10. sit-ups (sculling motion)

General Circuit

20 reps of each exercise at 40% maximum load.

Exercises
 1. clean
 2. bench pulls
 3. squats
 4. sit-ups
 5. snatch
 6. bench press
 7. back extension
 8. lat pulls
 9. squat jumps
10. arm curls
11. bend overs (good mornings)

In October, despite the very attractive head races, athletes should not forget about their major goals and compromise their training in order to do well in the fun races. The month of October should be the first month of general preparation (heavy lifting, *i.e.*, maximum strength, and basic aerobic, *i.e.*, long distance running and rowing).

Training Program for October 1991

Day	Training Model	Rest	Heart rate	Stroke rate	Effect
Mon.	Weights— Program A or B				Max. Strength
Tues.	40 min. steady state + 20 min of 20 on/10 off		140–150 160–170	18–20 26–28	Utilization AT
Wed.	Weights— Program A or B				Max. Strength
Thurs.	2 × 40 min. steady state	5'–7'	130–150	18–20	Utilization
Fri.	Weights— Program A or B				Max. Strength
Sat.	Head race or "AT" 2 × 20 min.	5'	160–175	28–30	AT
Sun.	Off				

Weight Program A

(for athletes who need to increase maximum strength without increasing muscle mass)

8 sets of 3 reps increasing to 4 sets of 6 reps

Exercises
1. a. clean
   b. stand—biceps curl

2. a. bench pulls
   b. bench press

3. a. squats
   b. thigh biceps curls

4. a. sit-ups 3 × 30
   b. back extension
      3 × 15 per set then add weight

Weight Program B

(for athletes trying to increase muscle mass)

5 sets of 8–12 reps

Exercises
1. a. clean
   b. stand—biceps curl

2. a. bench pulls
   b. bench press

3. a. squats
   b. thigh biceps curls

4. a. sit-ups 3 × 30
   b. back extension

Weight program A & B—Alternate between each numbered pair of exercises (a & b) until all sets are completed. Then move to the next numbered pair of exercises.

NOVEMBER/DECEMBER TRAINING PROGRAM

Day		Training Model	Rest	Heart Rate	Stroke Rate	Effect
Monday		Rowing/Ergometer—Long Interval 4 × 10 minutes or Running 6 × 6 minutes	6 minutes	max—10	26–28	Transport
Tuesday	a.m.	Rowing/Ergometer or Running or all of above Total 80 minutes (steady state)		140–150	18–22	Utilization
	p.m.	Weights "D1"				Muscular Endurance
Wednesday		Rowing/Ergometer or Running (4 × 20') 100 minutes (steady state) = 5 × 20' 1st 10 minutes (4' + 3' + 2 + 1') 2nd 10 minutes (same)	3 minutes	140–160	18/20/22/24 20/22/24/26	Utilization
Thursday	a.m.	Rowing/Ergometer Short Interval 3 sets of 7" × (1' on/1' off) or running stadium stairs	6–8 minutes	max—10	28–32	Transportation
	p.m.	Weights "D2"				Musc. Endurance
Friday		See Wednesday Workout				Utilization
Saturday	a.m.	Ergometer 3 × 2500 m Competitive!!	8 minutes	max	28	Transportation
	p.m.	Weights "D3"				Musc. Endurance
Sunday		See Wednesday Workout Every Second Sunday Off				Utilization

Training Program

The major emphasis for the next two months should be aerobic base (utilization & transportation workout) and specific muscular endurance (weights—workout)

Weights—D1

"Back"

	Load
1. Back Extensions	20–40 lbs
2. Sit-ups	20–40 lb
3. Leg Raise	20–40 lbs
4. Bench Press	50–60%
5. Clean	50%
6. Squat Jumps	—

In November 6 sets of 40 reps at each exercise
In December 4 sets of 60 reps at each exercise

Weights—D2

Focus "Legs"

	Load
1. Squats	40–60%
2. Back Extensions	20 lbs
3. Squat Jumps	—
4. Sit-ups	20 lbs
5. Rabbit Jumps	—
6. Bench Pulls	50–60%

Weights—D3

Focus "Arms"

	Load
1. Bench Pulls (Free feet)	50–60%
2. Back Extensions	20–40 lbs.
3. Bench Pulls (Legs hold)	50–60%
4. Sit-ups	20–40 lbs

JANUARY TRAINING PROGRAM

Day		Training Model	Rest	Heart Rate	Stroke Rate	Effect
Monday		4 × 10 minutes (running, rowing tank or ergometer)	5'–7'	Max–Max–10'	26–28	Transportation
Tuesday	a.m.	45' steady state running	—	140–150	18–22	Utilization
	p.m.	Weights—E1				Explosive Strength
Wednesday		80–90 minutes steady state of: —cross-country skiiing —ergometer + running —rowing tank + running	—	140–160	18–22	Utilization
Thursday	a.m.	Running/Fast 4 + 5 minutes	5'	Max	18–22	Transportation
	p.m.	Weights—E1				Explosive Strength
Friday		80–90 minutes steady state of: —cross-country skiiing —ergometer + running —rowing tank + running	—	140–160	18–22	Utilization

Day						
Saturday	a.m.	Short interval (running stadium stairs, ergometer, rowing tank) 3 × 15 min. of 45″ on/15″ off	8′	Max—10′	28	Transportation
	p.m.	+ 20 minute warm-up ergometer Weights—E2	—	140–150	18–22	Muscular Endurance
Sunday		80–90 minutes steady state of: —cross-country skiing —ergometer + running —rowing tank + running	—	140–150	18–22	Utilization

The January Training Program is for the four-week period from January 6 to February 3. The last week should be easier (reduce weight volume by 30%) with an ergometer test of 10,000 meter at the end.

Weights—Explosive strength at 60% of maximum. To find your maximum see how much weight you can lift in 16 repetitions.

Exercises (E1)
3 sets of 12 reps
1. Back Extensions
2. Leg Press
3. Bench Pulls
4. Jumps (knee high)
5. Sit-ups

Exercises (E2)
Same exercise as (E1) only 7 sets of 45 seconds on and 15 seconds off. You will complete one exercise in 7 minutes and then continue to the next.

FEBRUARY TRAINING PROGRAM

Day		Training Model	Rest	Heart Rate	Stroke Rate	Effect
Monday		Rowing/tank or erg 4 × 10' (4' + 3' + 2' + 1')	6–7'	Max–10	24/26/28/30	Transportation
Tuesday	a.m.	45–60 min. continuous steady state activities (running, rowing, erg) every 10 min. acceleration of 20 st max. power at 38–40		140–160	16–20	Utilization
	p.m.	erg—20 min. steady state weights (Program D1)		140–150	16–18	Utilization Musc. Endurance
Wednesday		3 × 25 mins. steady state* with some stretching between (1' + 2' + 3' + 4' + 5' + 4' + 3' + 2' + 1')	5'	140–160	14/16..22..14	Utilization
Thursday	a.m.	Erg/Rowing 4 × 5'	5'	Max—10	28	Transportation
	p.m.	erg—20 min. easy steady state + weights (Program D2)		140–150	16–18	Utilization Musc. Endurance
Friday		See Wednesday				
Saturday	a.m.	Rowing/Erg/Running 3 × 20 mins.	5'	160–175	26–28	Anaerobic Threshold
	p.m.	Weights (Program D3)				Musc. Endurance
Sunday		See Wednesday		140–160	16–18	Utilization

FEBRUARY TRAINING PROGRAM

February is a first month of specific preparation period. The main goal will be to develop a good aerobic foundation so important to the results late in the season. The weight workouts also should be specifically directed toward muscular endurance.

Note: Warm-ups (even on the erg)

[only catch × 3 strokes / regular strokes × 5 strokes] × 5

[½ slide/straight arms × 5 strokes / ½ slide/bend arms × 5 strokes] × 5

[pick swing/straight arms × 5 strokes / pick swing/bend arms × 5 strokes] × 5

[full slide/straight arms × 5 strokes / full slide/bend arms × 5 strokes] × 5

Obey Heart Rate Intensity for all Workouts!

Weight Program	Exercise	# Series	# Reps	Load	Frequency
Program D1 Focus "Back"	back extension	4–3	60–80	40–60%	slow
	sit-ups	4–3	30–40	20 lbs.	20/min.
	leg raises	4–3	60–80	20–40	continuous
	bench pulls	1	60–80	50%–60%	30/min.
	squats	1	60–80	50%	30/min.
Program D2 Focus "Legs"	squats	4–3	60–80	50%	30/min.
	sit-ups	1	60–80	20–40%	—
	squats on one leg	4–3	60–80	—	correct execution
	squats on another leg	4–3	60–80	—	correct execution
	back extensions	1	80	20 lbs.	—
Program D3 Focus "Arms"	bench pulls (free feet)	4–3	60–80	50%–60%	30/min.
	sit-ups	1	80	—	fluid
	bench pulls (legs hold)	4–3	60–80	50%–60%	30/min.

MARCH TRAINING PROGRAM

March is the second month of specific rowing preparation with a major goal to improve aerobic capacities and to develop higher muscular endurance with weight training. It also prepares the athlete for their first test on the water (transportation workouts).

Weights—Circuit G1
Build up from 5 to 7 circuits.

Exercise	Load	#Reps
1. Clean	@ 50%	30 reps
2. Squat	@ 50%	40 reps
3. Back extensions	20–40 lbs.	30 reps
4. Pulleys (full stroke)	@ 50%	30 reps
5. Sit-ups	20–40 lbs.	40 reps
6. Upright row	@ 50%	30 reps

Weights—G2

Exercise	Load	#Reps
1. Clean	@ 50–60%	7 mins (45" on/15" off)
2. Pulleys (full stroke)	@ 50–60%	7 mins (45" on/15" off)
3. Squat jumps	@ 50–60%	7 mins (45" on/15" off)
4. Bench pulls	@ 50–60%	7 mins (45" on/15" off)

MARCH TRAINING PROGRAM

Day		Training Model	Rest	Heart Rate	Stroke Rate	Effect
Monday		Long intervals—competitive 4 × 10'	5'–6'	Max—10	26–28	Transportation
Tuesday	a.m.	80 min. steady state of:	—			Utilization
		1. 20' alternate 2'/2'		140–160	16/18	
		2. 20' alternate 3'/2'/1		140–160	20/22/24	
		3. 20' alternate 2'/2'		160–180	16/18	
		4. 20' of 30" on/10" off		160–180	30/32	
	p.m.	Weights (G1)				Muscular Endurance
Wednesday		"AT" 3 × 20 min.	5'	160–175	26–28	Anaerobic Threshold
Thursday	a.m.	See Tuesday a.m.				Utilization
	p.m.	Weights (G1)				Muscular Endurance
Friday	a.m.	Long interval—competitive can be seat racing 4–5 × 5 min.	6'–7'	Max	28–30	Transportation
Saturday	a.m.	See Tuesday a.m.				Utilization
	p.m.	Weights (G2)				
Sunday	a.m.	3 × 2000 meters	10'–15'	Max	28–30	Transportation

APRIL TRAINING PROGRAM

Day		Training Model	Rest	Heart Rate	Stroke Rate	Effect
Monday		3 × 30 mins. steady state	5'	140–160	20–22	Utilization
Tuesday	a.m.	Long Interval 4 × 8 mins.	6–8'	Above 175	28–30	Transportation
	p.m.	Weights (Maintenance)				Muscular Endurance
Wednesday		"AT" 3 × 20 min.	5'	160–175	26–28	Anaerobic Threshold
Thursday	a.m.	60 min. st. st.	—	140–155	16–20	Utilization
	p.m.	Power pyramid (1' + 2' + 3') × 4 Maximum Power	6–8'	160–180	14/16/18 16/18/20 18/20/22 20/22/24	Specific Rowing Power
Friday		Short Interval 3 × 20 mins. of 25 st. on/5 st. off	10'	Above 175	30–34	Transportation
Saturday	a.m.	80–90 min. steady state/	—	140–155	16–20	Utilization
	p.m.	Weights (Maintenance E)				Muscular Endurance
Sunday		Long intervals—Test 3 × 2000 m Racing	10'–15'	Max	28–32	Transportation

This is a month of pre-competition period. We still are working on aerobic base but stroke rates for transportation workouts are getting very close to the racing cadence.

Weights (Maintenance)
6 × 45" on/15" off each exercise and then switch to the next exercise.

Exercises
1. Clean
2. Squats
3. Bench Pulls
4. Back Extensions

MAY TRAINING PROGRAM

Day		Training Model	Rest	Heart Rate	Stroke Rate	Effect
Monday	a.m.	60–80 mins. steady state	—	130–150	18–22	Utilization
Tuesday	a.m.	Long Interval 1 × 7 mins. 2 × 5 mins. 2 × 3 mins.	5′	Max—10	28–30 30–32 32–34	Transportation
	p.m.	Weights (Program E)				Muscular Endurance
Wednesday		"AT" 3 × 20 min.	4′–6′	Max—15	28–30	Anaerobic Threshold
Thursday	a.m.	60 min. steady state		150–160	18–22	Utilization
	p.m.	Power pyramid. 4 × (1′ + 2′ + 3′)			14/16/18 16/18/20 18/20/22 20/22/24	Specific Rowing Power
Friday	a.m.	Long Interval 5 × 5 mins. competitive	6′–7′	Max—10	32–34	Transportation
	p.m.	60 mins. steady state	—	140–150	18–20	Utilization
Saturday	a.m.	Short Interval 3 × 15 mins. of 25 on/5 off	10′	Above 175	32–36	Transportation
	p.m.	Weights (Program E)				Muscular Endurance
Sunday		Racing: 3 × 2000m	12′–15′	Max	32–34	Transportation

This is the first month of the competition period. There should be a gradual increase of intensity and an introduction of some racing pieces. Pieces at low cadence should be rowed with square blades.

Weight Program E

6 × 45″ on/15″ off to 50% of maximum weight each exercise. Then switch to next exercise.

1. clean
2. squat
3. bench pulls
4. back extensions

JUNE–JULY–AUGUST TRAINING PROGRAM

Day		Training Model	Rest	Heart Rate	Stroke Rate	Effect
Monday		60 min. steady state + Fartlek 10 strokes at max/20 off + 20 strokes at 36 spm × 5	4'–5'	150–160 Max	22–26 36	Utilization
Tuesday	a.m.	Long interval—competitive 4 × 8 min	6'–8'	Max—10	28–30	Transportation
	p.m.	60 mins. steady state + Fartlek (see Monday)		150–160	20–22	Utilization
Wednesday		"AT" 3 × 20 mins.	5'	Max—15	28–30	Anaerobic Threshold
Thursday	a.m.	Lactate Tolerance 3 series of 3 × 2' on/1' off 1st: 2 min.—with start 2nd: 2 min.—race pace 3rd: 2 min.—with sprint	10'–12'	Max	36–40	Lactate Tolerance
	p.m.	60 mins. very easy/regeneration steady state		140–150	16–20	Utilization
Friday	a.m.	Power pyramid 5 × (4' + 3' + 2' + 1')	4'–6'	Max	18/20/26/30	Transportation
	p.m.	45 mins. easy steady state		140–150	18–20	Utilization
Saturday	a.m.	5 × 5 min. racing	5'–6'	Max	34–36	Transportation
	p.m.	45 mins. easy/steady state		140–150	18–20	Utilization
Sunday		Racing: 2 × 2000m	12'–15'	Max	34–36	Transportation

June/July/August Training Program

These are the months of the competition which allow for peak performances at the USRowing Nationals June 25–28 and other key regattas. Athletes who have trials or important selection races in early June should follow the June program during May.

TRAINING PROGRAM 10 DAYS BEFORE COMPETITIONS

Day		Training Model	Rest	Heart Rate	Stroke Rate
Saturday	a.m.	(4–6) × 500 meters	3′	Max	Max
	p.m.	2 × 1000 meters, 1 × 1500 meters	5–6′	Max	Max
Sunday	a.m.	1 × 500 meters, 1 × 1000 meters, 1 × 500 meters flat out	3′–5′		Max
	p.m.	45 mins. steady state	—	150–160	20–24
Monday	a.m.	60 mins. steady state	—	150–160	20–24
	p.m.	off	—		
Tuesday	a.m.	Fartlek 3 × (20 on/20 off + 30 steady state)		varying	36
	p.m.	with start paddle 40 mins.		140–160	20–24
Wednesday	a.m.	1 × 1000 meters, 1 × 500 meters	3′–5′	Max	Max
	p.m.	Steady state 45 mins.		150–160	20–24
Thursday	a.m.	45 mins. easy steady state		150–160	20–24
	p.m.	off			
Friday	a.m.	40 mins. steady state + ten starts @ 30% power		150–160 varying	20–24
	p.m.	Steady state 40 minutes		140–160	20–24
Saturday		Regattas			
Sunday		Regattas			

It has been estimated that for every 300 m of ascent above 1500 m elevation, aerobic power decreases about 1% (Billings et al., 1971). In addition, the high intensity of exercise at the start of the race under hypoxic conditions exacerbates a serious oxygen deficit that eventually catches up with the rower at some point early in the 2000-m effort. This was especially true in 1968 when crews insisted on using the same race strategies they had used successfully at sea level. Significant effects on ventilatory adaptation were also noted for oarsmen following acute and chronic exposure to moderate altitude (Hagerman et al., 1975a).

Training at altitude or under hypoxic conditions seems logical if rowers are to compete in this environment. Training and competitive performances at altitude will improve as adaptation occurs, but there is no conclusive evidence that hypoxic training will improve sea level performance (Hagerman et al, 1975a). No effect on $\dot{V}O_2$max or work capacity was reported in oarsmen after altitude training (Secher et al., 1992). This observation is supported by results of other altitude training studies (Adams et al., 1975; Buskirk et al., 1967). However, altitude training is frequently used by elite rowers and other athletes competing in aerobic events. With the exception of only a few teams, successful national rowing teams train periodically at altitude (Hagerman et al., 1975a; Hartmann, 1987; Nowacki et al., 1971b).

After careful analysis of various altitude training programs, the consensus seems to indicate that the training site should be about 1800–2000 m above sea level, the duration of altitude training should be 3–5 wk, training intensity and duration should be reduced significantly early in the adaptive process, and under no circumstances should an athlete expect to achieve performances comparable to sea level efforts (Nilsen et al., 1987a, 1987b). Also, fluid intake should be consciously increased because the decreased humidity at high altitude increases body water loss by evaporation, potentially causing a decrease in plasma volume, and because the maintenance of adequate body fluids is important to aid in the buffering of acid by the kidneys.

For the elite athlete, training at altitudes between 2000–2300 m for as little as 14 d proved to have a detraining effect (Billings et al., 1968). The rowers were not able to train as intensely as at sea level, so aerobic and anaerobic capabilities gradually deteriorated. Training at altitude is therefore not recommended when the goal is to train at either transportation or anaerobic intensities; on the other hand, altitude training during the preparation or competitive periods when oxygen utilization is emphasized may be of benefit.

The altitude training routine used by many teams involves perhaps as many as three brief visits to altitude, with the rationale being that multiple and timely hypoxic exposures will compound the benefits.

Positive adaptations in elite rowers seem to occur very early upon hypoxic exposure. In a study conducted with elite rowers from 10 different countries training at 2300 m, we found significant increases in resting hemoglobin levels and significant decreases in heart rate and $\dot{V}O_2$ for standard ergometer efforts of 70% and 80% of maximal power generated at sea level. Similar decreases were noted for lactate concentrations. What was most surprising about these results was that the changes were noted after only 10 d of training. A third test after 20 d of exposure to altitude revealed no significant effect of the second 10 d of exposure.

In an earlier study by Adams et al. (1975), no beneficial effects of altitude training on $\dot{V}O_2$max of elite rowers were indicated. Although $\dot{V}O_2$max is enhanced in untrained subjects training at altitude, a similar change is not seen in highly trained athletes. This was supported in an extensive hypoxic study conducted in the mid-1960s (Bason et al., 1973; Billings et al., 1968, 1971) showing that a hypoxic environment caused an aerobic training effect in untrained subjects without exercise intervention, whereas their highly trained counterparts showed clear evidence of detraining, despite their efforts to continue aerobic training at altitude. In addition, endurance at sea level appears to increase more after training at sea level than after altitude training (Levine et al., 1992).

Currently, our advice to rowers who must compete at altitudes above 1500 m is one of two extremes: 1) if time, financial assistance, and a suitable training venue are available, spend 8–12 wk training at this site or 2) arrive at the competitive site 24–48 h before competition, compete over the next 48 to 72 h, and then depart before the hypoxic environment exacts deleterious effects on performance.

Hyperthermia

Rowing competition usually lasts 5–8 min. Thus, even under the most severe heat and humidity conditions, there is seldom a heat-related injury during a single race. Heat injury may be more likely in international lightweight rowers, many of whom acutely dehydrate themselves to attain appropriate body weights and remain dehydrated while racing.

Although lightweight rowers (59 kg maximum for women and 72.5 kg for men) have been encouraged to lose weight gradually over several months, to maintain at least 10% (women) or 5% body fat (men), and to be no more than 2 kg over their weight limits on January 1 of the competitive year, this advice is ignored by many of these rowers. They resort to such extreme practices as fasting, bulimia, water deprivation, and use of diuretics to lose weight quickly.

Failure to adequately rehydrate or to heed the warning signs of potential heat injury are of more concern when athletes are training twice daily for 2 h or more each session in hot, humid conditions, especially when sunlight reflected from the water increases radiative heat gain (Hagerman & Hagerman, 1977; Sawyer & Hagerman, 1974).

We first became aware of possible dehydration in open class oarsmen in 1981 when we performed a series of muscle biopsies on national team oarsmen over the course of the summer training period in preparation for the World Championship Regatta. Periodic muscle samples showed gradual dehydration from June through August, when temperature and humidity registered extremes. Measurement of plasma volumes indicated that the extracellular fluid compartments were also chronically and seriously compromised. Based on these findings suggestive of chronic dehydration, we recommended alterations in diet and fluid intake of the rowers; although we were unable to obtain subsequent biopsies and plasma samples on these athletes because of the impending World Championships, they all achieved medal performances at this regatta. Still, rowers and their coaches typically do not consider dehydration a problem of high priority. Bauer (1990) provided an excellent discussion of this problem from an athlete's perspective.

Hypothermia

Cold weather rowing, especially in the northern hemisphere during late phases of the preparation period (March and April), could cause significant hypothermia. Wearing appropriate clothing, avoiding rowing on days that are excessively windy or cold, and adhering to acceptable safety standards can prevent serious hypothermic problems or drowning. It is, of course, necessary to increase water and energy intake during prolonged periods of cold exposure.

Many rowers believe water consumption can be decreased in cold weather, thereby ignoring the effects of drying winds, excessive clothing, and dry, warm indoor environments on overall body fluid losses. We recommend that rowers be just as conscious of the need for adequate rehydration during colder temperatures as they are during hot weather training and competition.

MEDICAL CONSIDERATIONS

Overtraining

A failure to adapt to imposed training demands is often termed overtraining, and its consequences for the elite rower, including a gradual deterioration in performance, can be extensive (Beall, 1986; Hagerman, 1992a; Lehmann et al., 1993; Levin, 1991). It is difficult to distinguish between the serious condition of overtraining and the less serious but more common day-to-day variations in fatigue that are often experienced during intense training. The latter condition has been labeled "overreaching" or "short-term overtraining" and can be relieved within a few days by easy training, no competition, and/or a carbohydrate-rich diet (Lehmann et al., 1993). The remainder of this discussion focuses on the more serious, long-term type of overtraining.

At present there are no universally accepted clear early warning signs of overtraining. As a result, before it is recognized, the overtraining syndrome often has progressed too far to be easily reversed. Common symptoms of overtraining are listed in Table 6-10. In one investigation of immune system function, 6 rowers were among 40 elite athletes observed in an attempt to correlate impairment of immune function with the overtraining syndrome (Parry-Billings et al., 1992). Results suggested that a decrease in plasma glutamine concentration in overtrained rowers and other endurance athletes may contribute to impaired immune function. Subsequently, dietary glutamine supplementation has been employed by rowers and other athletes during periods of hard training in an attempt to forestall potential overtraining.

Although the causes for deterioration in performance as a result of overtraining are not clear, it appears that excessive intensity of training is more likely to be a principal causal factor than are either the duration or frequency of training. Furthermore, problems totally unrelated to training, including those associated with academic performance, job performance, economic factors, or social relationships, may be partly or entirely

---

TABLE 6-10. *Common symptoms of overtraining.*

Physical and Functional Symptoms

- Excessive and unusual loss of body weight
- Decrease in body fat
- Decreased appetite
- Localized muscular tiredness, heaviness, soreness, and/or stiffness
- Sleep disturbances
- Elevated resting heart rate, blood pressure, and core temperature
- Decreased markers of immunity
- Decreased plasma concentrations of testosterone or estradiol

Psychological Symptoms

- Frustration
- Loss of confidence
- Wide swings of mood
- Uncertainty and tentativeness
- Irritability
- Withdrawal
- Self-pity
- Tardiness and absenteeism
- Failure to assume responsibility for actions
- Depression
- Anxiety
- Trying too hard
- Inability to relax

to blame for the overtraining syndrome. Finally, it is also possible that overtraining may be related to Chronic Fatigue Syndrome (CFS).

There is no universally effective remedy for treating overtraining, although decreasing training intensity and increasing rest are obvious first steps in addressing the problem (Koutedakis et al., 1990). A recent review of overtraining in endurance athletes (Lehmann et al., 1993) would be an excellent resource for rowing athletes and coaches.

Rowing Injuries

The most common injuries directly related to rowing are those associated with overuse syndromes and affect primarily muscle and connective tissue. The anatomical areas most injured are the lower back, knee joint, wrist, shoulder, and sternum-ribs. About half of the injuries to rowers occur during off-season resistance training, and probably the most frequent maladies in rowers during the competitive season are upper respiratory infections. An injury questionnaire study sponsored by the United States Rowing Association revealed that, out of 931 responses of competitive rowers, 59 injuries were reported (Strayer, 1990a). Injuries were defined as any debilitating condition that prevented the athlete from training or competing for one or more days.

Of the 59 injuries reported, 26 athletes (44%) suffered from chronic low back pain. There seems to be an unusually large number of vertebral disk and vertebral surgeries among rowers (three competed in the 1992 Olympic Regatta following back surgery). These injuries are probably due to a combination of extreme rower height, body position during rowing, and high-intensity exercise.

The next most frequently occurring injury was chronic knee pain, which represented 19% of the injuries reported. This was followed by "rower's wrist" or extensor tenosynovitis, which represented 15% of the injuries. Shoulder injuries accounted for 5% of the injuries; other less frequent injuries, including muscle strains, joint sprains, and severe blistering of the hands, accounted for the remainder of the injuries. In the 1987 World Championships, only 40 injuries were reported for 880 rowers competing (Secher, 1990).

Competitive rowing appears to have a rather low incidence of injuries and this seems reflected in the scarcity of injury studies. Knee problems were described by Hagerman (1978) and Stallard (1980), and low back pain was discussed by Williams (1973). Frequent stress fractures of the ribs have been reported in rowers (Holden & Jackson, 1985); Strayer, 1990b). Although these stress fractures were often formerly diagnosed as intercostal muscle damage, such muscle damage apparently is less common than the actual rib fractures.

Rowers often experience dry pharynxes and coughs following racing, perhaps because mild pulmonary edema develops due to the heavy vascular load and high pulmonary capillary pressure that occur during exhaustive exercise.

Because of excessive dehydration and fasting and the nature of their body structures, lightweight rowers, especially women, tend to be more susceptible to injury than are their open class counterparts (Howell, 1984).

Strenuous endurance training combined with weight loss increases a woman's risk of anovulation, irregular menses, and amenorrhea. In a study comparing two groups of trained elite oarswomen, one group showing disruption of the normal menstrual cycle during heavy training and the other exhibiting no such disruption, regardless of the intensity of training, it was observed that the two groups lost weight and fat equally during high-intensity training. However, the disrupted women had an elevated activity of estradiol 2-hydroxylase (Snow et al., 1989). Thus, significant body fat loss and gonadotropic disturbances among elite oarswomen are associated with menstrual irregularities during high-intensity training.

It is well known that chronic dehydration and energy deficit, both of which lead to a loss of body weight, can cause muscular fatigue that can lead to injuries. Therefore, adequate hydration and nutrition should be emphasized in an attempt to minimize rowing injuries. Rowers are also encouraged to perform extensive warm-up and cool-down exercises during training and competition (Mickelson & Hagerman, 1978). Warm-up exercises should include stretching of the leg and back muscles prior to disembarking, followed by a 10–30 min rowing warm-up at low power outputs before participating in high-intensity training or competition. Cool-down usually consists of rowing for 10–20 min at low power before docking. It is also important that training intensity be increased gradually (no more than 1% per week) because an extreme increase in intensity is often associated with onset of injury.

NUTRITIONAL CONSIDERATIONS

Energy Intake

As might be expected, the high power outputs generated during competition and training by rowers require extraordinary amounts of energy. It has been estimated that a 2000-m race costs between 25 and 40 kcal/min (Hagerman et al., 1978; Hagerman & Hagerman, 1990) (Figure 6-13). During the preparation and competitive phases of training, rowers train for 1–2 h/d, and, although a rower will expend about 200–250 kcal during a competitive effort, this is small compared with the range of 1000–2000 kcal that is often the cost of a single training session.

Many rowers have difficulty maintaining adequate energy intake and thus may lose body mass, especially lean body mass. Although several studies have investigated the effects of diet on exercise performance, controlled nutrition studies of elite endurance athletes are scarce; only recently have we been able to confidently combine our knowledge of energy input and output of rowing to propose dietary recommendations (Hagerman & Hagerman, 1990).

We studied 28 elite female and 16 elite male rowers, all candidates for the U.S. National Team (Hagerman & Hagerman, 1990). Daily energy expenditure was estimated for each athlete by measuring peak $\dot{V}O_2$ and heart rate during rest and exhaustive simulated rowing and calculating the energy output during typical training sessions. Average daily energy output for our subjects is displayed in Table 6-11.

Dietary computer analysis and individual counseling were conducted over 8 wk during training, with special reference to identification of foods, food selection, food preparation, accurate dietary record keeping (including use of a food scale), and the application of nutrition to enhancing training and competitive performances. Food records were completed during the first and eighth weeks, with each record including two weekdays and one weekend day. Although there was only a small difference between energy output and input (Table 6-11), if this imbalance were permitted to continue, rowers would have difficulty maintaining weight.

In addition to discovering how little elite rowing athletes knew about the food they were eating and that their diets contained somewhat too little energy, we found that many of the rowers' diets were far too low in carbohydrates and too high in fats. We thought that these elite athletes were aware of the importance of maintaining high levels of ingested carbohydrates, especially during training, when glycogen depletion could be a problem. However, many of the athletes confessed that they seldom consciously selected foods high in carbohydrates, other than the obvious choices such as pasta and pancakes. The beneficial effects of these foods were often compromised by large supplements of cheese and butter.

Although glycogen depletion is significant during 2000-m simulated competitive efforts, this does not seem to be a major concern for the 5–7 min exercise. Based on our previous glycogen depletion studies, Type I fibers were about 85% depleted and Type IIA fibers were 75% depleted following high-intensity ergometer exercise. Because IIB fibers were not present in most subjects, no attempt was made to analyze glycogen con-

TABLE 6-11. *Summary of mean (±SE) energy expenditure and dietary data. See text for details.*

	Energy Output (kcal/d)	Energy Input (kcal/d)	CHO (%kcal)	Fat (%kcal)	Protein (%kcal)	Alcohol (%kcal)
Women n=28	3177 (103.9)	3169 (167.7)	52.0 (1.30)	34.6 (1.13)	13.0 (0.45)	0.40 (0.17)
Men n=16	4710 (98.7)	4688 (321.7)	49.6 (3.57)	34.3 (3.57)	15.1 (0.93)	1.00 (0.54)

tent in these fibers. Many rowers and coaches think that "carbohydrate-loading" is necessary prior to competition to insure success. However, we believe it is more important to keep glycogen levels high during training than to be concerned about glycogen depletion during the shorter duration competition, assuming, of course, that daily carbohydrate intake is maintained at or near 60% of total calories consumed.

Simonsen et al. (1991) compared the effects of a high-carbohydrate diet (10 g CHO·kg body mass^{-1}·d^{-1} or 70% of energy) and a moderate carbohydrate diet (5 g CHO·kg body mass^{-1}·d^{-1} or 42% of energy) on vastus lateralis glycogen content and power output on the rowing ergometer in 22 male and female collegiate rowers during 4 wk of intense twice-daily training. They reported that the high-CHO diet promoted greater muscle glycogen content and a slightly higher power output on the 26th day of training than did the moderate CHO diet. Still, the moderate CHO diet maintained steady glycogen concentrations and did not impair power output when compared to initial baseline values. It appeared that both diets were sufficient to maintain normal blood glucose, and no sign of hypoglycemia was detected in either group.

The differences in power output between the two diet groups were smaller than expected, but the fact that this difference only became significant during the fourth and last week of the study may be important; it supports the concept that dietary effects on performance become more evident the longer the diets and training are continued. This concept is especially applicable to national team training that is often conducted continuously for several months leading up to an important championship regatta.

In summary, it is evident that during training, rowers have marked deficiencies in carbohydrate intake and consume slightly fewer calories than they burn (Hagerman & Hagerman, 1990). These conditions could have deleterious effects on both the quality and quantity of training. Although Simonsen et al. (1991) did not find large differences in glycogen content and power output when comparing training diets high and moderate in carbohydrate content, even small differences in power output could be crucial in a race. Furthermore, previous non-rowing studies have demonstrated the importance of maintaining carbohydrate levels at 60% of daily caloric intake if high values for muscle glycogen content and superior performance efforts are to be realized (Costill & Miller, 1980; Coyle et al., 1983, 1986; Evans & Hughes, 1985; Hagerman, 1992b; Sherman & Wimer, 1991). However, Table 6-11 shows that the average 3-d intake of calories from carbohydrates for women sampled periodically over the 8-wk test period was 52% and for men, only 49.6%. One of the male rowers was consuming only 34% of his energy as carbohydrate, whereas one woman consumed only 36% of her calories as carbohydrate. Both of these subjects were finding it difficult to train, even at low intensities; the woman rower thought she might be anemic. Fat consumption was 34.6% of energy for women and 34.3% for men, higher than the recommended range of 25–30%.

Based on the protein intake data for rowers shown in Table 6-11 and an estimated protein requirement of 1.4 g/kg body weight, nearly 40% of the women consumed insufficient protein; protein intake for the men was deemed adequate.

There have been other nutrition studies (Steele, 1970; de Wijn et al., 1979) conducted with rowers, and the results tend to support our findings, e.g., rowers were reported to consume 43% of their total energy as fat and only 43% as carbohydrate; protein represented 13% of energy intake or about 1.6 g/kg body weight daily.

Dietary Supplementation

Elite rowers are similar to other elite athletes in their fascination and obsession with dietary supplements. However, such supplementation has often not been advised because it was assumed that an adequate diet could account for any possible dietary deficiency (Hagerman & Hagerman, 1990). Telford et al. (1992) could not detect any effects from 7–8 months of vitamin/mineral supplementation on the performances of a small number of rowers.

In another study that included rowers among a group of several Dutch elite athletes participating in a national sports nutrition study (van Erp-Baart et al., 1989), it was concluded that intakes of calcium and iron were positively related to energy intake; i.e., if energy intake is low, calcium and iron intake may be compromised. Thus, women rowers and all lightweight rowers could potentially be vulnerable to deficiencies in dietary calcium and iron.

Table 6-12 shows the percentage of men and women rowers who were able to meet the recommended dietary allowances for selected vitamins and minerals through diet alone; to assume that elite athletes are always eating adequate diets is a gross misconception (Hagerman & Hag-

TABLE 6-12. *Percent of rowers who met recommended dietary allowances for vitamins and minerals by food consumption. Recommended daily dietary allowances are shown below table.*

	Vit C	Vit B1	Vit B2	Niacin	Calcium	Iron	Potassium	Magnesium
Women n=28	43	96	89	86	86	64	57	54
Men n=16	40	90	90	90	100	100	70	70

Recommended daily dietary allowances: Vitamin C—3 mg/kg body weight; Vitamin B1—0.5 mg/1000 kcal energy intake; Vitamin B2—0.6 mg/1000 kcal energy intake; Niacin—6.6 mg/1000 kcal energy intake; Calcium—800 mg; Iron—10 mg for men, 18 mg for women; Potassium—4 g; Magnesium—5 mg/kg body weight.

erman, 1990). All of the women and all but one of the men received more than 60 mg of vitamin C per day, but only 43% of the women and 40% of the men were ingesting enough vitamin C to meet the standard of 3 mg/kg body weight. This standard is based on Van Huss's (1980) review of the literature, in which he concluded that it would be prudent for athletes in training to consume daily 3–5 mg vitamin C/kg body weight. Accordingly, the subjects in the study reported by Hagerman and Hagerman (1990) were advised to eat more fruits and vegetables high in vitamin C and to select foods that would increase their dietary intakes of potassium and magnesium, which were low. Intake of the B vitamins was adequate for most rowers.

The recommended dietary allowance for calcium was 800 mg/d, but oarswomen were urged to consume 1000 mg/d in view of the role of calcium in decreasing the risk of osteoporosis. This is especially important for any female athlete who is amenorrheic, a common problem among elite oarswomen. Many of the women had diets that were too low in iron, a finding consistent with data from the non-athletic population as well. The men had no difficulty meeting their basic needs for iron. RDA standards of 10 mg iron for men and 18 mg for women were used as baselines.

Lightweight rowers present special nutritional problems because of their routine practices of fasting and dehydrating. Body composition and resting and exercise metabolism have been measured for female lightweight rowers during training (Koutedakis et al., 1991, 1992a, 1992b, 1992c), and the findings showed higher resting metabolic rates among these athletes than predicted, perhaps because of the residual effects of great energy expenditures during strenuous daily training. Voluntary weight reductions coupled with high energy expenditures over a period of 6–8 wk adversely affect $\dot{V}O_2$ max, peak anaerobic power, and ergometric power output. However, 6 months of caloric restrictions did not prevent reductions in resting energy expenditures, and 6–7% losses of initial body weights did not affect muscle force outputs.

SUGGESTIONS FOR FUTURE RESEARCH

1. To confirm indirect estimates of the anaerobic energy contribution to rowing, O_2 deficit should be compared to direct analyses of anaerobic metabolism in muscle, using biopsy sampling or MRI analysis.
2. Cardiac output, shifts in regional blood flow, and femoral a-v O_2 differences should be measured during simulated rowing.
3. Considering the magnitude of lactic acidosis in competitive rowing, the effects of bicarbonate ingestion on acid-base balance and on performance should be investigated in rowers.
4. The overtraining syndrome should be studied more thoroughly

in rowers, with an emphasis on immunosuppression, chronic dehydration, and abnormal endocrine function.

5. It would be important to determine if rowers can train and compete successfully on what appears to be less than adequate dietary carbohydrate.
6. A detailed study of the effects of various off-season weight training programs should be conducted.
7. The effects of rowing training on possible morphometric and biochemical factors that could contribute to improved performance should be studied with MRI and infrared spectroscopy measurements.
8. A detailed survey of common rowing injuries, including diagnostic, preventive, and rehabilitative procedures, should be conducted.
9. Because pacing in competitive rowing seems grossly uneconomical, a comparative metabolic study of traditional versus non-traditional pacing is recommended.
10. A careful analysis of the nutritional practices of lightweight rowers should be undertaken.
11. To better understand the influence of rowing training on menstrual function, the effect of rowing on endocrine function should be better categorized.
12. Because of inconsistencies in results reported for altitude training studies conducted with rowers, a more definitive study over several months should be carried out with multiple altitude exposures.
13. A comparison of various training "periodicity" schemes should be conducted.
14. Because most rowing efficiency studies lack sufficiently accurate data on energy output and input, a more thorough and accurate assessment of mechanical or physiological efficiency should be carried out.
15. Although several physiological criteria have been projected as possible predictors of performance in rowing, further work is needed to verify these criteria and to explore other possible factors that might predict performance and assist in the team selection process.

SUMMARY

Rowers are tall, lean athletes who train for long durations and compete at extremely high intensities. Ventilatory, metabolic, and cardiovascular responses to exercise in elite rowers are at the upper limits of human capacity, as is the power they can generate in the rowing task. It is rather extraordinary that aerobic metabolism contributes 70–80% of the energy for a 2000-m racing effort, because rowing competition is of such short duration compared to most aerobic events. Rowers possess an abundance of oxidative muscle fibers in the principal muscles used in rowing and exhibit exceedingly high aerobic and anaerobic potential. Rowers also use a racing pace that seems uneconomical and counterproductive; the high-intensity initial sprint creates a significant O_2 deficit and associated lactacidemia that is unparalleled in other aerobic sports. Elite rowers often are subject to overtraining in attempts to achieve successful competitive performances. Despite overtraining, injuries are minimal; upper respiratory infections are more frequent than orthopedic problems. Despite attempts at maintaining high-carbohydrate diets, a lack of basic nutritional knowledge and a failure to focus on sensible eating causes rowers to fall well short of the recommended intake of carbohydrates in their daily diets.

ACKNOWLEDGEMENTS

Our rowing studies have been supported by the United States Rowing Association, United States Olympic Committee, the New Zealand Amateur Rowing Association, Fédération Internationale des Sociétés d'Aviron (International Rowing Federation), and the Ohio University Foundation. I am especially grateful to Randall Jablonic, Kris Korzeniowski, Harry Parker, and the coaches of past U.S. National and Olympic teams for their encouragement and cooperation. I also thank all of those oarsmen and oarswomen who participated in our studies from 1966 to the present. The wealth of data we have gathered over the years would not have been possible without the extraordinary efforts and excellent science of Janice Gault, Marjorie Hagerman, and Thomas Murray, and Drs. Gary Dudley, Jeffrey Falkel, Topper Hagerman, Robert Hikida, Timothy Mickelson, William Polinski, Kerry Ragg, and Robert Staron. I also appreciate the work of the many graduate and undergraduate students from Ohio University, who over the years provided valuable input to our rowing studies.

BIBLIOGRAPHY

Adams, W.C., E.M. Bernauer, O.B. Dill, and J.B. Bomar (1975). Effect of equivalent sea-level and altitude training on VO_2max and running performance. *J. Appl. Physiol.* 39:262–266.

Anderson, P. (1975). Capillary density in skeletal muscle of man. *Acta Physiol. Scand.* 95:203–205.

Asami, T., N. Aduchi, K. Yamamoto, K. Ikuta, and K. Takahashi (1978). Biomechanical analysis of rowing skill. In: E. Assmussen and K. Jorgensen (eds.) *Biomechanics VI-B.* Baltimore: University Park Press, pp. 109–114.

Asami, T., K. Yamamoto, A. Matsuo, and T. Fukunaga (1985). Some biomechanical factors of rowing performance. In: L. Winter et al. (eds.) *Biomechanics IX.* Champaign: Human Kinetics Publishers, pp. 477–480.

Åstrand, P-.O. (1967). Work tests with the bicycle ergometer. Vorberg, Sweden: Br. Carlssons Baktr. AB.

Åstrand, P.O., and K. Rodahl (1986). *Textbook of Work Physiology, 3rd ed.* New York: McGraw-Hill.

Bangsbo, J., P.D. Gollnick, T.E. Graham, C. Juel, B. Kiens, M. Mizuno, and B. Saltin (1990). Anaerobic energy production and O_2 deficit-debt relationship during exhaustive exercise in humans. *J. Physiol.* (London) 422:539–559.

Bason, R., E. Fox, C. Billings, J. Klinzing, K. Ragg, and E. Chaloupka (1973). Maintenance of physical training effects by intermittent exposure to hypoxia. *Aerospace Med.* 44:1097–1100.

Bauer, S. (1990). Some like it light. *Am. Rowing* 22:26–29.

Beall, B.G. (1986). The overtraining syndrome. *Am. Rowing* 18:40–42.

Bell, G.J., S.R. Petersen, H.A. Quinney, and H.A. Wenger (1989). The effect of velocity-specific strength training on peak torque and anaerobic rowing power. *J. Sports Sci.* 7:205–214.

Bergh, U., A. Thorstensson, B. Sjödin, B. Hulten, K. Riehl, and J. Karlsson (1975). Maximal oxygen uptake and muscle fiber types in trained and untrained humans. *Med. Sci. Sports* 7:37–43.

Biersteker, M.W.A., and P.A. Biersteker (1985). Vital capacity in trained and untrained healthy young adults in the Netherlands. *Eur. J. Appl. Phys.* 54:46–53.

Biersteker, M.W.A., P.A. Biersteker, and A.J.M. Schreurs (1986). Reduction of lung elasticity due to training and expiratory flow limitation during exercise in competitive female rowers. *Int. J. Sports Med.* 7:73–79.

Billings, C., D. Mathews, R. Bartels, E. Fox, R. Bason, and D. Tanze (1968). The effects of physical conditioning and partial acclimatization to hypoxia on work tolerance at high altitude. Columbus, OH: *The Ohio State University Research Foundation*, Report RF:2002-2004.

Billings, C., R. Bason, D. Mathews, and E. Fox (1971). Cost of submaximal and maximal work during chronic exposure at 3800 m. *J. Appl. Physiol.* 30:406–408.

Bloomfield, J., and A.D. Roberts (1972). A correlation and trend analysis of strength and aerobic power and scores in the prediction of rowing performance. *Austral. J. Sports Med.* 4:25–36.

Bompa, T.O., and W.A. Roaf (1977). Some characteristics of strength development for rowing. *Can. J. Appl. Sports Sci.* 2:142–148.

Bonde-Peterson, F., P.D. Gollnick, T.I. Hansen, N. Kristensen, N.H. Secher, and O. Secher (1975). Glycogen depletion pattern in human muscle fiber during work under curarization (d-tubocurarine). In: H. Howald and J. Poortmans (eds.) *Metabolic Adaptation to Prolonged Physical Exercise.* Basel: Birkhauser Verlag, pp. 422–430.

Bouckaert, J., J.L. Pannier, and J. Vrijens (1983). Cardiorespiratory responses to bicycle and rowing ergometer exercise in oarsmen. *Eur. J. Appl. Physiol.* 51:51–59.

Brien, D.M., and D.C. McKenzie (1989). The effect of induced alkalosis and acidosis on plasma lactate and work output in elite oarsmen. *Eur. J. Appl. Physiol.* 58:797–802.

Brooks, G.A. (1985). Anaerobic threshold: review of the concept and directions for future research. *Med. Sci. Sports Exerc.* 17:22–31.

Buskirk, E., J. Kollias, R. Akers, E. Prokop, and E. Picon-Reátegui (1967). Maximal performance at altitude and on return from altitude in conditioned runners. *J. Appl. Physiol.* 23:259–266.

Carey, P., M. Stensland, and L.H. Hartley (1974). Comparison of oxygen uptake during maximal work on the treadmill and the rowing ergometer. *Med. Sci. Sports* 6:101–103.

Celentano, F., G. Cortili, P.E. DiPrampero, and P. Cerretelli (1974). Mechanical aspects of rowing. *J. Appl. Physiol.* 36:642–647.

Chance, B., S. Nioka, J. Kent, K. McCully, M. Fountain, R. Greenfeld, and G. Holtom (1988). Time-resolved spectroscopy of hemoglobin and myoglobin in resting and ischemic muscle. *Anal. Biochem.* 174:698–707.

Chance, B., M.T. Dait, C. Zhang, T. Hamaoka, and F.C. Hagerman (1992). Recovery from exercise-induced desaturation in the quadriceps muscles of elite competitive rowers. *Am. J. Physiol.* 262:C766–C775.

Chignon, J.C., and R. Distel (1981). Vector cardiographic criteria of ventricular hypertrophy in a population of athletes. *Archiv. de Mollades de Ceur* 74:1099–1105.

Clark, J.M., F.C. Hagerman, and R. Gelfand (1983). Breathing patterns during submaximal and maximal exercise in elite oarsmen. *J. Appl. Physiol.* 55:440–446.

Clarkson, P.M., J. Graves, A.M. Melchionda, and J. Johnson (1984). Isokinetic strength and endurance and muscle fiber type of elite oarswomen. *Can. J. Appl. Sports Sci.* 9:127–132.

Cleaver, H. (1957). *A History of Rowing.* London: H. Jenkins.

Clifford, P.S., B. Hanel, and N.H. Secher (1990). Arterial blood gases during exhaustive exercise. *Med. Sci. Sports Exerc.* 22:S99.

Connors, M.C. (1974). An energetic analysis of rowing. (Unpublished Doctoral Dissertation). Ohio University, Athens, Ohio.

Costill, D.L., W.J. Fink, and M. Pollock (1976). Muscle fiber composition and enzyme activities of elite distance runners. *Med. Sci. Sports* 8:96–100.

Costill, D.L., W.J. Fink, M. Hargreaves, D.S. King, R. Thomas, and R. Fielding (1985). Metabolic characteristics of skeletal muscle during detraining from competitive swimming. *Med. Sci. Sports Exerc.* 17:339–343.

Costill, D.L., and J. Miller (1980). Nutrition for endurance sport: Carbohydrate and fluid balance. *Int. J. Sports Med.* 1:2–14.

Coyle, E.F., J.M. Hagberg, B.F. Hurley, W.H. Martin III, A.A. Ehsani, and J.O. Halloszy (1983). Carbohydrate feeding during prolonged strenuous exercise can delay fatigue. *J. Appl. Physiol.* 55:230–235.

Coyle, E.F., A.R. Coggan, M.K. Hemmert, and J.L. Ivy (1986). Muscle glycogen utilization during prolonged strenuous exercise when fed carbohydrate. *J. Appl. Physiol.* 61:165–172.

Cunningham, D.A., P.B. Goode, and J.B. Critz (1975). Cardiorespiratory response to exercise on a rowing and bicycle ergometer. *Med. Sci. Sports* 7:37–43.

Davis, J.A. (1985). Anaerobic threshold: review of the concept and directions for future research. *Med. Sci. Sports Exerc.* 17:6–18.

Davis, J.A., P. Vodak, J.H. Wilmore, J. Vodak, and P. Kurtz (1976). Anaerobic threshold and maximal aerobic power for three modes of exercise. *J. Appl. Physiol.* 41:544–550.

deGaray, A.L., L. Levine, and J.E.L. Carter (1974). *Genetic and Anthropological Studies of Olympic Athletes.* New York: Academic Press.

DePauw, D., and J. Vrijens (1971). Untersuchungen bei Elite-Ruderern in Belgien. *Sportsarzt Sportsmed.* 22:176–179.

DeRose, E.H., S.M. Crawford, D.A. Kerr, R. Ward, and W.D. Ross (1989). Physique characteristics of Pan American Games lightweight rowers. *Intl. J. Sports Med.* 10:292–297.

de Wijn, J.F., J. Leusink, and G.B. Post (1979). Diet, body composition and physical condition of champion rowers during periods of training and out of training. *Biblthca Nutr. Dieta* 27:143–148.

Dickhuth, H.-H., G. Simon, W. Kindermann, A. Wildenberg, and J. Keul (1979). Echocardiographic studies on athletes of various sports types and non-athletic persons. *Z. Kardiol.* 68:449–453.

DiPrampero, P.E., G. Cortilli, F. Celentano, and P. Cerretelli (1971). Physiological aspects of rowing. *J. Appl. Physiol.* 31:853–857.

Dodd, C. (1983). *The Oxford and Cambridge Boat Race.* London: S. Paul.

Droghetti, P. (1986). Determination of the anaerobic threshold on a rowing ergometer by the relationship between work output and the heart rate. *Scand. J. Sports Sci.* 8:59–62.

Droghetti, P., C. Borsetto, I. Casoni, M. Cellini, M. Ferrari, A.R. Paolini, P.G. Ziglio, and F. Conconi (1985). Noninvasive determination of the anaerobic threshold in canoeing, cross-country skiing, cycling, roller- and ice-skating, rowing, and walking. *Eur. J. Appl. Physiol.* 53:299–303.

Droghetti, P., K. Jensen, and T.S. Nielsen (1991). The total estimated metabolic cost of rowing. *FISA Coach* (2):1–4

Ekblom, B., and L. Hermansen (1968). Cardiac output in athletes. *J. Appl. Physiol.* 25:619–625.

Evans, W., and V. Hughes (1985). Dietary carbohydrates and endurance exercise. *Am. J. Clin. Nutr.* 41:1146–1154.

Falch, D.K., and S.B. Strømme (1979). Pulmonary blood volume and intraventricular circulation time in physically trained and untrained subjects. *Eur. J. Appl. Physiol.* 40:211–218.

Falkel, J.E., F.C. Hagerman, T.F. Murray, K. Green, K. Korzeniowski, and L. O'Leary (1987). Comparison of cardiorespiratory and metabolic responses between incremental and competitive simulated rowing (abstract). *Med. Sci. Sports Exerc.* 19:549.

Foster, C., M.A. Green, A.C. Snyder, and N.N. Thompson (1993). Physiological responses during simulated competition. *Med. Sci. Sports Exerc.* 25:877–882.

Fountain, M.R., and R.R. McCully (1988). A new approach to exercise testing and training evaluation. *Am. Rowing* 20:42–43.

Fraser, T.R. (1868–1869). The effect on the circulation as shown by examination with the sphygmograph. *J. Anat. Physiol.* 3:127–130.

Fritsch, W. (1981). Zur entwicklung der speziellen Ausdauer in Rudern. In: DSB (eds.) *Information zun Training: Rudern.* Frankfort: DSB, Bundesausschuss Teistung sport (Suppl. 26).

Fritsch, W. (1985). Trainingssteuerung im Rudern. *Rudersport* 35(10): Trainerjournal No. 80.

Fritsch, W. (1986). Die letzten wochen vor dem Finale. *Rudersport* 36(32): Trainerjournal No. 82.

Fukunaga, T., A. Matsuo, K. Yamamoto, and T. Asami (1986). Mechanical efficiency in rowing. *Eur. J. Appl. Physiol.* 55:471–475.

Gardner, E.N. (1965). *Athletics of the Ancient World.* Oxford, O.B.: Oxford University Press.

Gollnick, P.D., and L. Hermansen (1973). Biochemical adaptations to exercise: Anaerobic metabolism. In: Wilmore, J. (ed.) *Exercise and Sport Sciences Reviews, Vol. 1.* New York: Academic Press, pp. 1–43.

Grujic, N. (1989). The long-term follow up of the physical working capacity of rowers. In: M.J. Karvonen (ed.) *The Physiological Follow Up Methods of Sports Training.* Helsinki: Varala, pp. 20–37.

Grujic, N., M. Bajic, B. Vukovic, and D. Jakovijevic (1987). Energy demand of competitive rowing (abstract). *Seventh Balkan Congress of Sports Medicine.* 112.

Haber, P., and A. Ferlitsch (1979). Vergleichende Einschätzung des Trainingszustandes mittels Spiroergometrischer Untersuchungen am Ruder-und Fahrradergometer bei Ruderern. *Schweiz. Z. Sportsmed.* 27:53–59.

Hagerman, F.C. (1969). Respiratory distress among oarsmen during competition at the 1968 Summer Olympic Games. *Med. Tribune* May, pp. 12–15.

Hagerman, F.C. (1974). Metabolic responses of women rowers during ergometric rowing (abstract). *Med. Sci. Sports* 6:87.

Hagerman, F.C. (1975). Teamwork in the hardest pull in sports. *Physician Sportsmed.* 3:39–44.

Hagerman, F.C. (1984). Applied physiology of rowing. *Sports Med.* 1:303–326.

Hagerman, F.C. (1978). Knee pain. *The Oarsman* 10:34–42.

Hagerman, F.C. (1992a). Failing to adapt to training. *FISA Coach* 3:1–4.

Hagerman, F.C. (1992b). Energy metabolism and fuel utilization. *Med. Sci. Sports Exerc.* 24:S309–S314.

Hagerman, F.C., W.W. Addington, and E.A. Gaensler (1975a). Severe steady state exercise at sea level and altitude in Olympic oarsmen. *Med. Sci. Sports* 7:275–279.

Hagerman, F.C., W.W. Addington, and E.A. Gaensler (1972). A comparison of selected physiological variables among outstanding competitive oarsmen. *J. Sports Med. Phys. Fit.* 12:12–22.

Hagerman, F.C., M.C. Connors, J.A. Gault, G.R. Hagerman, and W.J. Polinski (1978). Energy expenditure during simulated rowing. *J. Appl. Physiol.* 45:87–93.

Hagerman, F.C., and J.E. Falkel (1987). Training the energy systems. *Am. Rowing* 18:40–43.

Hagerman, F.C., J.E. Falkel, K. Korzeniowski, L. O'Leary, and D. Proctor (1989). Lactic acid responses of elite rowers following heavy training, tapering, competitive and simulated rowing. Proceedings of *Seoul Olympic Scientific Congress* 1:13–16.

Hagerman, F.C., J.E. Falkel, T.F. Murray, K. Korzeniowski, L. O'Leary, and D. Proctor (1987). A comparison of maximal absolute and relative metabolic responses between elite men and women rowers (abstract). *Med. Sci. Sports Exerc.* 19:549.

Hagerman, F.C., J.A. Gault, M.F. Connors, and G.R. Hagerman (1975b). A summary of physiological testing at the 1974 U.S. National Rowing Camp. *The Oarsman* 7:34–37.

Hagerman, F.C., and G. Hagerman (1977). Weight loss in the non-obese athlete—an impossible task? *The Oarsman* 7:24–49.

Hagerman, F.C., and M.T. Hagerman (1990). A comparison of energy output and input among elite rowers. *FISA Coach* 1:5–8.

Hagerman, F.C., G.R. Hagerman, and T.C. Mickelson (1979). Physiological profiles of elite rowers. *Physician Sportsmed.* 7:74–81.

Hagerman, F.C., and G.A. Howie (1971). Use of certain physiological variables in the selection of the 1967 New Zealand crew. *Res. Quart.* 42:264–273.

Hagerman, F.C., and K. Korzeniowski (1989). Applied rowing ergometer testing. *FISA Colloque des Entraineurs.* 19:115–133.

Hagerman, F.C., R.A. Lawrence, and M.C. Mansfield (1988). A comparison of energy expenditure during rowing and cycling ergometry. *Med. Sci. Sports Exerc.* 20:479–488.

Hagerman, F.C., and W.D. Lee (1971). Measurement of oxygen consumption, heart rate, and work output during rowing. *Med. Sci. Sports* 3:155–160.

Hagerman, F.C., M.D. McKirnan, and J.A. Pompei (1975c). Maximal oxygen consumption of conditioned and unconditioned oarsmen. *J. Sports Med.* 15:43–48.

Hagerman, F.C., and T.C. Mickelson (1979a). An introduction to weight training. *Oarsman* 11:12–14.

Hagerman, F.C., and T.C. Mickelson (1979b). Functional anatomy of the rowing stroke. *Oarsman* 11:6–9.

Hagerman, F.C., and T.C. Mickelson (1979c). Weight training for rowing. *Oarsman* 11:40–41.

Hagerman, F.C., and T.C. Mickelson (1981). A task specificity comparison of anaerobic thresholds among competitive oarsmen (abstract). *Med. Sci. Sports Exerc.* 13:17–20.

Hagerman, F.C., and R.S. Staron (1983). Seasonal variations among physiological variables in elite rowers. *Can. J. Appl. Sport Sci.* 8–3:143–148.

Hagerman, G.R. (1976). Metabolic evaluation of international caliber lightweight oarsmen. (Unpublished Doctoral Dissertation). The Ohio State University, Columbus, Ohio.

Hahn, A.G., D. Tumility, P. Shaekespear, and R.D. Telford (1988). Physiological testing of oarswomen on Gjessing and Concept II rowing ergometers. *Excel* 5:19–25.

Hamby, E.J., and V. Thomas (1969). Comparison of rowing and cycling work capacity tests using heart rate as the parameter (abstract). *J. Physiol.* 203:80P–81P.

Hanel, B., N.H. Secher, and P.S. Clifford (1990). Arterial blood pressure response to rowing (abstract). *Med. Sci. Sports Exerc.* 22:S26.

Hansen, G. (1967). Vergleichende Untersuchungen über dem Verhältnis der aeroben zur anaeroben Kapazität bei maximaler ergometrischen Belstung. *Schweiz. Z. Sportsmed.* 15:68–75.

Harrison, J.Y. (1967). A constant torque-brake for use in bicycle and other ergometers. *J. Appl. Physiol.* 23:482–483.

Harrison, J.Y. (1970). Maximizing human power output by suitable selection of motion cycle and load. *Human Factors* 12:315–329.

Hartmann, U. (1987). Querschnittuntersuchungen an Leistungsruderern in Flackland und Längschnittuntersuchungen an Elite-rudern in der Höhe mittels eines zwistufigen Tests auf einem Gjessing-Ruderergometer. Konstanz: Hartung-Gorre Verlag.

Hartmann, U., A. Mader, and W. Hollmann (1987). Querschnittuntersuchungen an Leistungs-ruderern mit einem zweisterfigen Test auf einem Gjessing-Ruderergometer. In: H. Riechert (ed.). *Sportsmedizine-Kursbestimmung.* Berlin-Heidelberg: Springer Velag.

Hartmann, U., A. Mader, and W. Hollmann (1990). Heart rate and lactate during endurance training programs in rowing and its relation to the duration of exercise by top flight rowers. *FISA Coach* 1:1–4.

Hay, J.G. (1968). Rowing: An analysis of the New Zealand Olympic selection tests. *New Zealand J. Health, Phys. Ed. Rec.* 1:83–90.

Haymes, E.M., and A.L. Dickinson (1980). Characteristics of elite male and female ski racers. *Med. Sci. Sports Exerc.* 12:153–158.

Hebbelinck, M., W.D. Ross, J.E.L. Carter, and J. Boems. (1980). Anthropometric characteristics of female Olympic rowers. *Can. J. Appl. Sports Sci.* 5:255–262.

Heck, H., G. Hess, and A. Mader (1985a). Vergleichende Untersuchungen zu verschiedenen Lakat-Schwellenkonzepten. *Deutsche Z. Sportmed.* 36: No. 1, 2.

Heck, H., A. Mader, G. Hess, S. Muecke, R. Muller, and W. Hollmann (1985b). Justification of the 4 mmol/L lactate threshold. *J. Sports Med.* 6:117.

Henderson, J.Y., and H.W. Haggard (1925). The maximum of human power and its fuel. *Am. J. Physiol.* 72:264–282.

Hirsch, L. (1977). Trainingsformen zur Verbesserung der aeroben Kapazitaet. In: DSB (eds.) Information zum Training: Ausdauertraining, Staffwechselgrundlegen und Steuerungsansatze. Frankfurt: DSB, *Bunderausschuss Leistungssport* (Suppl. 9).

Holden, D.L., and D.W. Jackson (1985). Stress fracture of the ribs in female rowers. *Am. J. Sports Med.* 13:342–348.

Hollmann, W., and T. Hettinger (1980). *Sportmedizin-arbeits-und Trainingsgrundlagen.* Stuttgart: Schattauer.

Howald, H., R. Marie, B. Heierli, and F. Follath (1977). Echokardiographische Befunde bei trainierten Sportlern. *Schweiz. Med. Woch.* 107:1662–1666.

Howell, D.W. (1984). Musculoskeletal profile and incidence of musculoskeletal injuries in lightweight women rowers. *Am. J. Sports Med.* 12:278–282.

Ingjer, F. (1979). Effects of endurance training on muscle fibre ATP–ase activity, capillary supply and mitochondrial content in man. *J. Physiol.* 294:419–432.

Ingjer, F., and H.A. Dahl (1979). Dropouts from an endurance training program. *Scand J. Sports Sci.* 1:21–22.

Ishiko, T. (1967). Aerobic capacity and external criteria of performance. *J. Can. Med. Assoc.* 26:746–749.

Ishiko, T. (1968). Application of telemetry to sports activities. In: J. Wartenweiler et al. (eds.) *Biomechanics I.* Basal: Karger, pp. 138–145.

Jackson, R.C., and N.H. Secher (1973). The metabolic cost of rowing and physiological characteristics of world class oarsmen (Abstract). *Med. Sci. Sports* 5:65.

Jackson, R.C. and N.H. Secher (1976). The aerobic demands of rowing in two Olympic rowers. *Med. Sci. Sports* 8:168–170.

Jacobs, I., B. Sjoedin, P. Kaiser, and J. Karlsson (1981). Onset of blood lactate exercise accumulation after prolonged exercise. *Acta Physiol. Scand.* 114:461.

Jensen, K., N.H. Secher, Ä. Fiskestrand, N.J. Christensen, and J.O. Lund (1986). Influence of body weight on physiologic variables measured during maximal dynamic exercise (abstract). *Acta Physiol. Scand.* 121:39A.

Khosla, T. (1983). Sports for tall. *Brit. Med. J.* 287:736–738.

Körner, T., and P. Schwanitz (1985). *Rudern.* Berlin: Sports Verlag.

Korzeniowski, K., and F.C. Hagerman (1991). Monitoring training of elite rowers (abstract). *Med. Sci. Sports Exerc.* 23:632.

Korzeniowski, K. (1991–1992). Training Programs. *Stroke* Sept. 1991–Aug. 1992.

Kosinski, A. (1987). Comparison of mechanical efficiency of untrained rowers on three different rowing ergometers. (Unpublished Masters Thesis). Ohio University, Athens, Ohio.

Koutedakis, Y. (1982). The role of physiological assessment in team selection with special reference to rowing. *Brit. J. Sports Med.* 23:51–55.

Koutedakis, Y., R. Budgett, and L. Faulmann (1990). Rest in underperforming elite competitors. *Brit. J. Sports Med.* 24:248–252.

Koutedakis, Y., P.J. Pacy, R.M. Quevado, N.C.C. Sharp, R. Hesp, and K. Fuecher (1992c). The effect of changes in body composition on resting energy expenditure and force levels in elite lightweight oarswomen. *J. Sports Sci.* (in press).

Koutedakis, Y., R.M. Quevado, P.J. Pacy, D. Millward, R. Hesp, and N.C.C. Sharp (1991). Resting energy expenditure in elite female rowers. *J. Sports Sci.* 9(4):421–422.

Koutedakis, Y., and N.C.C. Sharp (1985). Lactic acid removal and heart rate frequencies during recovery after strenuous rowing exercise. *Brit. J. Sports Med.* 19:199–202.

Koutedakis, Y., and N.C.C. Sharp (1986). A modified Wingate test for measuring anaerobic work of the upper body in junior rowers. *Brit. J. Sports Med.* 20:153–156.

Koutedakis, Y., N.C.C. Sharp, P.J. Pacy, R.M. Quevado, and C. Boreham (1992a). The effect of two different weight-reduction periods on selected physiological parameters in elite light-weight oarswomen. PHY-25 Proceedings, *Olympic Scientific Congress*, Malaga, Spain.

Koutedakis, Y., N.C.C. Sharp, R.M. Quevado, P.J. Pacy, J. Millward, and R. Hesp (1992b). The effect of changes in body composition on selected physiological parameters in light-weight oarswomen. PHY-26 Proceedings, *Olympic Scientific Congress*, Malaga, Spain.

Kramer, J.F., A. Leger, and A. Morrow (1991). Oarside and nonoarside knee extensor strength measures and their relationship to rowing ergometer performance. *J. Orthop. Sports Phys. Ther.* 14:213–219.

Lamb, D.H. (1989). A kinematic comparison of ergometer and on-water rowing. *Am. J. Sports Med.* 17:367–373.

Larsson, L., and A. Forsberg (1980). Morphological muscle characteristics in rowers. *Can. J. Appl. Sports Sci.* 5:239–244.

Lassen, A., J.H. Mitchell, D.R. Reeves, Jr., H.B. Rogers, and N.H. Secher (1989). Cardiovascular responses to static exercise in man with topical nervous blockade. *J. Physiol.* 409:333–341.

Lehmann, M., C. Foster, and J. Keul (1993). Overtraining in endurance athletes: a brief review. *Med. Sci. Sports Exerc.* 25:854–862.

Levin, S. (1991). Overtraining causes Olympic-sized problems. *Physician Sportsmed.* 19:112–118.

Levine, B.D., D.B. Friedman, K. Engfred, B. Hanel, M. Kjar et al. (1992). The effect of normoxic or hyperbaric endurance training on the hypoxic ventilatory response. *Med. Sci. Sports Exerc.* 24:769–775.

Liljestrand, G., and J. Lindhard (1920). Zur physiologie des ruderns. *Skand. Archiv Physiol.* 39:215–235.

Lormes, W., H.J. Debatin, M. Grünert-Fuchs, T. Müller, J.M. Steinacker, and M. Stauch (1991). Anaerobic rowing tests—test design, application, and interpretation. In: W. Backl, T.E. Graham, and H. Löllgen (eds.) *Advances in Ergometry.* Berlin: Springer Verlag, s. 477–482.

Lormes, W., R.J.W. Michalsky, M. Gruenert-Fuchs, and J.M. Steinacker (1988). Belastung und Beanspruchungsempfinden in Rudern. In: J.M. Steinacker (ed.) *Rudern.* Berlin: Springer Verlag, pp.332–336.

Lundin, A., and B. Saltin (1971). Oxygen demands of swimming. *II Medico-Scientific Conference of FINA.* Dublin, Ireland.

Mader, A., and H. Heck (1986). A theory of the metabolic origin of "anaerobic threshold." *Int. J. Sports. Med.* 7:45.

Mader, A., and W. Hollmann (1977). Zur Bedeutung der Stoffwechselleistungsfähigkeit des Eliteruderers in Training and Welt kampf. *Beiheft zum Leistungssport* 9:8–62.

Mader, A., H. Liesen, H. Heck, H. Phillipe, P.M. Schuerch, and W. Hollmann (1976). Zur Beurteilung der sportartspezifischen Ausdauerleistungsfaehigkeit im Tabor. *Sportarzt Sportmed.* 27(4):80; 27(5):109.

Mahler, D.A., B.E. Andrea, and D.C. Andresen (1984a). Comparison of six-minute "all-out" and incremental exercise tests in elite oarsmen. *Med. Sci. Sports Exerc.* 16:567–571.

Mahler, D.A., D.C. Andresen, H.W. Parker, W.S. Mitchell, and F.C. Hagerman (1983). Physiological comparison of rowing performance between national and collegiate women rowers (abstract). *Med. Sci. Sport Exerc.* 15:157.

Mahler, D.A., B. Hunter, T. Lentine, and J. Ward (1991b). Locomotor-respiratory coupling develops in novice female rowers with training. *Med. Sci. Sports Exerc.* 23:1362–1366.

Mahler, D.A., W.N. Nelson, and F.C. Hagerman (1984b). Mechanical and physiological evaluation of exercise performance in elite national rowers. *J.A.M.A.* 252:496–499.

Mahler, D.A., C.R. Shuhart, E. Brew, and T.A. Stukel (1991a). Ventilatory responses and entrainment of breathing during rowing. *Med. Sci. Sports Exerc.* 23:186–192.

Margaria, R., P. Cerretelli, P.E. DiPrampero, P.E. Massari, and G. Torelli (1963). Kinetics and mechanisms of oxygen debt contraction in men. *J. Appl. Physiol.* 18:371–377.

Margaria, R., P. Cerretelli, and F. Mangili (1964). Balance and kinetics of anaerobic energy release during strenuous exercise in man. *J. Appl.Physiol.* 19:623–628.

Mason, B.R., P. Shakespear, and P. Doherty (1988). The use of biomechanical analysis in rowing to monitor the effect of training. *Excel* 4:7–11.

Martindale, W.O., and D.G.E. Robertson (1984). Mechanical energy in sculling and in rowing an ergometer. *Can. J. Appl. Sports Sci.* 153–163.

Marx, U., and J.M. Steinacker (1988). Ruderspiroergometrische Längsschnittuntersuchungen über 2 Jahre bei zwei Weltmeisterschaftsteilnehmern. In: J.M. Steinacker (ed.) *Rudern* Berlin: Springer Verlag, pp. 83–89.

McCully, K.K., B.P. Boden, M. Tuchler, M.R. Fountain, and B. Chance (1989). Wrist flexor muscles of elite rowers measured with magnetic resonance spectroscopy. *J. Appl. Physiol.* 67:926–932.

McMahon, T.A. (1971). Rowing: A similarity analysis. *Science* 173:349–351.

Medbø, J.I., A.-C. Mohn, I. Tabata, R. Bahr, O. Vaage, and O.M. Sejersted (1988). Anaerobic capacity determined by maximal accumulated O_2 deficit. *J. Appl. Physiol.* 64:50–60.

Mellerowicz, H., and G. Hansen (1965). Sauerstaff Kapazität und andere spiro-ergometrische maximal werte der Ruder-Olympiasieger im viser mit st. vom Berliner Ruderclub. *Sportarzt Sportmed.* 5:188.

Mendenhall, T.C. (1980). *A Short History of American Rowing.* Boston: Charles River Books.

Mickelson, T.C., and F.C. Hagerman (1978). The warm-up, warm-down. *Oarsman* 10:15–19.

Mickelson, T.C., and F.C. Hagerman (1982). Anaerobic threshold measurements of elite oarsmen. *Med. Sci. Sports Exerc.* 14:440–444.

Nilsen, T., T. Daigneault, and M. Smith (eds.) (1987a). The FISA Coaching Development Programme Course, *Level 1 Handbook* Oberhoffen, Switzerland: International Rowing Federation.

Nilsen, T., T. Daigneault, and M. Smith (eds.) (1987b). The FISA Coaching Development Programme Course, *Level 2 Handbook* Oberhoffen, Switzerland: International Rowing Federation.

Niu, H., K. Ito, K. Takagi, and M. Ito (1966). A study of the development of cardio-respiratory function of the oarsmen. In: K. Kato (ed.) *Proceedings of 1964 International Congress of Sport Sciences.* Tokyo: Japanese Union of Sport Sciences, pp. 360–361.

Nolte, V. (1986). Traingssteuerung-Woraussetzungen, Anwendung, Grenzen. *Leistungssport* 16:39.

Nolte, V. (1988). Trainingsprotokollierung-Fuer wen? Und wie? Welche Konsequenzen werden daraus gezogen? In: J.M. Steinacker (ed.) *Rudern* Berlin: Springer Verlag, pp. 218–222.

Nolte, V. (1991). Introduction to the biomechanics of rowing. *FISA Coach* 2:1–6.

Nowacki, P.E., R. Krause, and K. Adam (1969). Maximal oxygen uptake by the rowing crew winning the Olympic gold medal 1968. *Pflügers Archiv* 312:R66–R67.

Nowacki, P.E., R. Krause, K. Adam, and M. Rulieffs (1971a). Über die cardiopulmonale Leistungsfäkigkeit des Deutschland—Achters vor seinein Olympiasieg 1968. *Sportarzt d.* 10:227–229.

Nowacki, P.E., K. Adam, R. Krause, and V. Ritter (1971b). Die Spiroergometrie in neuen Untersuchungs-System für den Spitzensport. *Trainer-Journal Rudersport* 26:I–VI.

Orfeldt, L. (1970). Metabolism of 1(+)–lactate in human skeletal muscle during exercise. *Acta Physiol. Scand.* 338(Suppl):1–66.

Parkhouse, W.S., D.C. McKenzie, P.W. Hochachka, and W.K. Ovalle (1985). Buffering capacity of deproteinized human vastus lateralis muscle. *J. Appl. Physiol.* 58:14–17.

Parry-Billings, M., R. Budgett, Y. Koutedakis, E. Blomstrand, S. Brooks, C. Williams, P.C. Calder, S. Pilling, R. Baigrie, and E.A. Newsholme (1992). Plasma amino acid concentrations in the overtraining syndrome: Possible effects on the immune system. *Med. Sci. Sports Exerc.* 24:1353-1358.

Pelliccia, A., B.J. Maron, A. Spataro, M. Proschan, and P. Spirito (1991). Cardiac hypertrophy in highly trained athletes. *N. Eng. J. Med.* 324:295-301.

Pohlentz, H. (1980). Physiological evaluation of rowers in the German Democratic Republic (abstract). *FISA Coach's Conference*; Rome, Italy. 4:5-8.

Polinski, W.J. (1976). Indirect determination of oxygen deficit during maximal ergometric rowing. (Unpublished Masters Thesis). Ohio University, Athens, Ohio.

Prince, R.P., R.S. Hikida, and F.C. Hagerman (1976). Human muscle fiber types in power lifters, distance runners, and untrained subjects. *Pflügers Archiv* 363:19-26.

Pyke, F.S., B.R. Minikin, L.R. Woodman, A.D. Roberts, and T.G. Wright (1979). Isokinetic strength and maximal oxygen uptake. *Can. J. Appl. Sports Sci.* 4:277-279.

Rasmussen, J., B. Hanel, B. Diamant, and N.H. Secher (1991). Muscle mass effect on arterial desaturation after maximal exercise. *Med. Sci. Sports Exerc.* 23:1349-1352.

Rodriquez, R.J., R.P. Rodriguez, S.D. Cook, and P.M. Sandbom (1990). Electromyographic analysis of rowing stroke biomechanics. *J. Sports Med. Phys. Fit.* 30:103-108.

Rosiello, R.A., D.A. Mahler, and J.L. Ward (1987). Cardiovascular responses to rowing. *Med. Sci. Sports Exerc.* 19:239-245.

Roth, W., E. Hasart, W. Wolf, and B. Pansold (1983). Untersuchungen zur synamik der Energiebereitstellung während maximaler Mittel zeitausdauerbelastung. *Med. Sport* 23:107-114.

Saltin, B., and P.O. Åstrand (1967). Maximal oxygen uptake in athletes. *J. Appl. Physiol.* 23:353-358.

Saltin, B. (1969). Physiological effects of physical conditioning. *Med. Sci. Sports* 1:50-59.

Saltin, B., J. Henriksson, E. Nygaard, P. Anderson, and E. Jansson (1977). Fiber types and metabolic potentials of skeletal muscle in sedentary man and endurance runners. *Ann. NY Acad. Sci.* 302:3-29.

Sanderson, B., and W. Martindale (1986). Towards optimizing rowing technique. *Med. Sci. Sports Exerc.* 18:454-468.

Sawyer, R.N., and F.C. Hagerman (1974). Rapid weight loss by light-weight oarsmen. *The Oarsman* 6:10-11.

Scharschmidt, F., and K.S. Pieper (1984). Die aerobe Leistungsfähigkeit junger Rudersportler beiderlei Geschlechts. *Med. Sport* 24:43-48.

Schwanitz, P. (1991). Applying biomechanics to improve rowing performance. *FISA Coach* 2:1-7.

Secher, N.H. (1973). Development of results in international rowing championships, 1893-1971. *Med. Sci. Sports* 5:195-199.

Secher, N.H. (1975). Isometric rowing strength of experienced and inexperienced oarsmen. *Med. Sci. Sports* 7:280-283.

Secher, N.H. (1983). The physiology of rowing. *J. Sports Sci.* 1:23-53.

Secher, N.H. (1990). Rowing. In: T. Reilly, N. Secher, P. Snell, and C. Williams (eds.) *Physiology of Sports*. London: E.& F.N. Spon, pp. 259-285.

Secher, N.H. (1993). Physiological and biomechanical aspects of rowing. *Sports Med.* 15:24-42.

Secher, N.H., M. Espersen, R.A. Brinkhorst, P.A. Andersen, and N. Rube (1982a). Aerobic power at the onset of maximal exercise. *Scand J. Sports Sci.* 4:12.

Secher, N.H., K. Jensen, and B. Serup (1992). Højdetræning (in Danish). In: Jensen, Lammert (eds.) *Roneng Team Danmark* (in press).

Secher, N.H., N. Rube, and J. Elers (1988). Strength of two and one leg extension in man. *Acta Physiol. Scand.* 134:333-339.

Secher, N.H., N. Rube, and S. Molbech (1981). The voluntary muscle contraction pattern in man. In: J.C. DePotter (ed.) *Adapted Physical Activities*. Bruxelles: Editions de L'Universite de Bruxelles, pp. 225-236.

Secher, N.H., N. Ruberg-Larsen, R.A. Brinkhorst, and F. Bonde-Peterson (1974). Maximum oxygen uptake during arm cranking and combined arm plus leg exercise. *J. Appl. Physiol.* 36:515-518.

Secher, N.H., O. Vaage, and R.C. Jackson (1982b). Rowing performance and maximal aerobic power in oarsmen. *Scand. J. Sports Sci.* 4:9-11.

Secher, N.H., and O. Vaage (1983). Rowing performance, a mathematical model based on body dimensions as exemplified by body weight. *Eur. J. Appl. Physiol.* 52:88-93.

Secher, N.H., O. Vaage, K. Jensen, and R.C. Jackson (1983). Maximal aerobic power in oarsmen. *Eur. J. Appl. Physiol.* 51:155-162.

Sherman, W.M., and G.S. Wimer (1991). Insufficient dietary carbohydrate during training: Does it impair athletic performance? *Int. J. Sport Nutr.* 1:284-4.

Simonsen, J.C., W.M. Sherman, D.R. Lamb, A.R. Dernback, J.A. Doyle, and R. Strauss (1991). Dietary carbohydrate, muscle glycogen, and power output during rowing training. *J. Appl. Physiol.* 70:1500-1505.

Snow, R.C., R.L. Barbieri, and R.E. Frish (1989). Estrogen 2-hydroxylase oxidation and menstrual function among elite oarswomen. *J. Clin. Endocrinol. Metab.* 69:369-376.

Spitzer, J.J. (1974). Effect of lactate infusion on canine myocardial free fatty acid metabolism *in vivo*. *Am. J. Physiol.* 226:213-217.

Stallard, M.C. (1980). Backache in oarsmen. *Brit. J. Sports Med.* 14:105-108.

Staron, R.S., M.J. Leonardi, D.L. Karapondo, E.S. Malicky, J.E. Falkel, F.C. Hagerman, and R.S. Hikida (1991). Strength and skeletal muscle adaptations in heavy-resistance-trained women after detraining and retraining. *J. Appl. Physiol.* 70:631–640.

Staron, R.S., E.S. Malicky, M.J. Leonardi, J.E. Falkel, F.C. Hagerman, and G.A. Dudley (1989). Muscle hypertrophy and fast fiber type conversions in heavy resistance-trained women. *Eur. J. Appl. Physiol.* 60:71–79.

Steele, J.E. (1970). Nutritional study of Australian Olympic athletes. *Med. J. Australia* 2:119–123.

Steinacker, J.M. (ed.) (1987). *Rudern: Sportmedizinische und sportwissenschaftliche Aspehte.* Berlin: Springer Verlag.

Steinacker, J.M. (1988). Methoden für die leistungsdiagnostik und trainingssteuerung im Rudern und ihre Anwendung. In: J.M. Steinacker (ed.) *Rudern.* Berlin: Springer Verlag, pp. 39–54.

Steinacker, J.M., M. Both, and B.J. Whipp (1992). Pulmonary mechanics and the entrainment of respiratory and stroke frequencies during rowing (abstract). *Med. Sci. Sports Exerc.* 24:S165.

Steinacker, J.M., C. Hübner, A. Berger, K. Röcker, and M. Stauch (1991a). Modified rowing ergometry in upper body exercise testing compared to supine bicycle ergometry in surgical patients (abstract). *Int. J. Sports Med.* 12:131.

Steinacker, J.M., W. Lormes, and M. Stauch (1991b). Sport specific testing in rowing. In: N. Bachl, T.E. Graham, and H. Löllgen (eds.) *Advances in Ergometry.* Berlin: Springer Verlag, S443–454.

Steinacker, J.M., T.R. Marx, F.A. Fiegenbaum, and R.E. Wodick (1983). Die Rudenspiroergometrie als eine Methode der sportartspezifischen Leistungsdiagnostik. *Deutsch Z. Sportmed.* 34:333–342.

Steinacker, J.M., U. Marx, M. Grünert, W. Lormes, and E. Wodick (1985). Vergleichsuntersuchungen über den Zweistufentest und den Mehrstufentest bei der Ruderergometrie. *Leistungssport* 6:47–51.

Steinacker, J.M., T.R. Marx, U. Marx, and W. Lormes (1986). Oxygen consumption and metabolic strain in rowing ergometer exercise. *Eur. J. Appl. Physiol.* 55:240–247.

Steinacker, J.M., T.R. Marx, and U. Thiel (1984a). A rowing ergometer test with stepwise increased workloads. In: N. Bachl, L. Prokop, and R. Suckert (eds.) *Current Topics in Sports Medicine.* München: Urban and Schwarzenberg, pp. 175–187.

Steinacker, J.M., T.R. Marx, and R.E. Wodich (1984b). The oxygen consumption for rowing. *Pflügers Archiv* 400 (Suppl) 1R61.

Strayer, L.M. (1990a). Common rowing injuries. *FISA Sports Medicine Symposium,* Lauceston, Tasmania, Australia.

Strayer, L.M. (1990b). The myth of the intercostal muscle pull. *Am. Rowing* 22:42–45.

Strømme, S.B., F. Ingjer, and H.D. Meen (1977). Assessment of maximal aerobic power in specifically trained athletes. *J. Appl. Physiol.* 42;933–837.

Strydom, N.B., C.H. Wyndham, and J.S. Greyson (1967). A scientific approach to the selection and training of oarsmen. *So. African Med. J.* 41:1100–1102.

Szal, S.E., and R.B. Schoene (1989). Ventilatory response to rowing and cycling in elite oarsmen. *J. Appl. Physiol.* 67:264–269.

Szögy, A., and G. Cherebetiu (1974). Physical work capacity testing in male performance rowers with practical conclusions for their training process. *J. Sports Med.* 14:218–223.

Telford, R.D., E.A. Catthpole, V. Deakin, A.G. Hahn, and A.W. Plank (1992). The effect of 7 to 8 months of vitamin/mineral supplementation on athletic performance. *Int. J. Sport Nutr.* 2:135–153.

Thorstensson, A. (1976). Muscle strength, fibre types and enzymatic activities in man. *Acta Physiol. Scand.* 443(Suppl.).

Törner, W. (1959). *Biologische Grundlagen den Leiberziehung.* Bonn: Dummer, p. 459.

Tumility, D., A. Hahn, and R. Telford (1987). Effect of test protocol, ergometer type and state of training on peak oxygen uptake in rowers. *Excel* 3:12–14.

Urhausen, A., M. Mueller, H.J. Foerester, B. Weiler, and W. Kindermann (1986). Trainingssteuerung im Rudern. *Deutsch Z. Sportmed.* 37:340.

Vaage, O. (1986). Table 14-2. In Åstrand, P.O., and K. Rodahl, *Textbook of Work Physiology,* 3rd ed. New York: McGraw-Hill, p. 673.

van Erp-Baart, A.M.J., W.M.H. Saris, R.A. Binkhorst, J.A. Vos, and J.W.H. Elvers (1989). Nationwide survey on nutritional habits in elite athletes. *J. Sports Med.* 10:S11–S16.

Van Huss, W. (1980). Vitamin C and physical performance. In: Still, G. (ed.) *Encyclopedia of Physical Education, Fitness and Sports.* Salt Lake City: Brighton.

Wasserman, K., and M.B. McIlroy (1964). Detecting the threshold of anaerobic metabolism in cardiac patients during exercise. *Am. J. Cardiol.* 14:844–852.

Wasserman, K., B.J. Whipp, R. Casaburi, M. Golden, and W.L. Beaver (1973). Anaerobic threshold and respiratory gas exchange during exercise. *J. Appl. Physiol.* 35:236–243.

Weiling, W., E.A. Borghols, A.P. Hollander, S.A. Darner, and A.J. Dunning. (1981). Echocardiographic dimensions and maximal oxygen uptake in oarsmen during training. *Br. Heart J.* 46:190–195.

Williams, J. (1973). Injuries in rowing. *Rowing* 1–4.

Williams, L.R.T. (1976). Work output and heart rate response of top level New Zealand oarsmen. *Res. Q.* 47:506–512.

Williams, L.R.T. (1978). Prediction of high-level rowing ability. *J. Sports Med.* 18:11–17.

Wilmore, J.H. (1974). Alterations in strength, body composition, and anthropometric measurements consequent to a 10-week weight training program. *Med. Sci. Sports* 6:133–138.

Wright, G.R., T. Bompa, and R.J. Shephard (1976). Physiological evaluation of a winter training programme for oarsmen. *J. Sports Med. Phys. Fit.* 15:22–37.

Yamakawa, J., and T. Ishiko (1966). Standardization of physical fitness test for oarsmen. In: K. Kato (ed.) *Proceedings of 1964 International Congress of Sports Sciences.* Tokyo: Japanese Union of Sports Sciences, pp. 435–436.

Zsidegh, M. (1981). A survey of the physiological and biomechanical investigations made into kayaking, canoeing, and rowing. *Hungar. Rev. Sports Med.* 22:97–116.

DISCUSSION

CLARKSON: According to your data, the typical rower's carbohydrate intake was obviously low. When you improved their diets, did their performances improve?

HAGERMAN: We have no data to demonstrate that their performances improved.

EKBLOM: I am concerned about the expression of dietary carbohydrate as a percent of energy intake. Because they consume so much energy, even 50% carbohydrate would provide the rowers with 400–500 g of carbohydrate each day.

HAGERMAN: The average weight of the women was about 77 kg and that of the men, 88 kg. At 49% carbohydrate, the women consumed 5.3 g/kg and the men, 6.6 g/kg. At 60% carbohydrate, the women consumed 6 g/kg and the men, 7.9 g/kg. At 65% carbohydrate, the values were 6.7 and 8.6 g/kg for the women and men, respectively. Thus, even at 65% carbohydrate, which is almost impossible for most athletes to consume regularly, the women rowers would not have reached the 8–10 g/kg recommended carbohydrate intake, and the men would have been at the low end of that recommendation. As far as the widely accepted recommendations are concerned, our rowers weren't eating enough carbohydrates.

EKBLOM: But when you got them to eat more carbohydrate, you didn't see any direct evidence that their performances improved.

HAGERMAN: That's true. It seems unrealistic to recommend 8–10 g/kg when a) most rowers can't consume that much carbohydrate, and b) we don't see any great beneficial effect on competitive performance of having that much carbohydrate in the diet. On the other hand, it makes sense to have the rowers eat high-carbohydrate diets during training, when the exercise duration is sufficient to substantially deplete muscle glycogen.

LAMB: There is very little evidence that high-carbohydrate diets lasting more than a few days have any major effect on athletic performance. However, they certainly don't hurt performance, and they are recommended to minimize the risk of cardiovascular disease and obesity.

SPRIET: Some of the confusion on this issue is related to the duration of the performance being tested. In humans, the initial concentration of muscle glycogen does not affect the maximal rate of muscle glycogenolysis during exercise. It is only in long duration events that one might expect an effect of differential initial glycogen stores.

COYLE: I agree; for 2,000-m rowing events that last only 6 min, we shouldn't expect much of a beneficial effect of a high-carbohydrate diet. I think the importance of carbohydrate in the diet is more for training intensely on a daily basis.

LAMB: In our study of rowers (Simonsen et al., 1991), there was no evidence of a beneficial effect of the high-carbohydrate diet on the quality of daily training. Similarly, we found no effect of chronic manipulations of dietary carbohydrate on the quality of daily intense swim training (*Amer. J. Clin. Nutr.* 52:1058–1063, 1990) or on running or cycling performance (*Amer. J. Clin. Nutr.* 57:27–31, 1993).

TERJUNG: You have shown that elite rowers improved their power output over 8 y of training without any increase in $\dot{V}O_2$. What factors might explain this apparent improvement in efficiency?

HAGERMAN: I think it is probably explained by improved rowing technique as the years of training accumulate.

TERJUNG: Is there evidence from biomechanical studies to confirm that improvement in motor skills is important?

HAGERMAN: I believe that both Schneider and Nolte have demonstrated that this is the case.

BAR-OR: Could there be a greater use of anaerobic energy sources so that greater power can be generated without greater $\dot{V}O_2$?

HAGERMAN: That is certainly possible, especially over the shorter duration races. It may be that the type of training they are doing today might improve that anaerobic capacity a bit more. Unfortunately, because it is such an illusive variable to measure, we do not have a firm handle on anaerobic capacity changes.

BAR-OR: If anaerobic capacity is increased over the years, the estimate of mechanical efficiency in Figure 6-17 may be too high.

HAGERMAN: That may be true, but the relative quantity of energy produced by anaerobic metabolism is very small, so the effect on mechanical efficiency would presumably be slight. Ed Coyle suggested that, rather than calling it mechanical efficiency, which it technically is not, I should simply plot the $\dot{V}O_2$ responses over time in relation to power.

COYLE: Figure 6-17 shows changes in efficiency from 16.5% up to 23%; i.e., at the same $\dot{V}O_2$, power output over 2,000 m goes up nearly 40%.

HAGERMAN: I agree that it seems like an awfully large improvement; perhaps increases in anaerobic capacity explain some of the change.

COYLE: In the cyclists we have been studying on a cross-sectional basis, by far the most important factor in distinguishing their performances is the wide range of differences in their mechanical efficiencies.

HAGERMAN: We see a large range of mechanical efficiencies in rowers too, i.e., 14–24%. Rowing technique involves repeated acceleration and deceleration of the boat; it is not a very efficient sport. Part of the rowers' emphasis on pacing is to overcome the inertia of the boat. They are off at 40/50 strokes/min for about 30–40 s; then they settle to about 36–38/min for 4–5 min; and for the last 40–50 s they are up again to 40–50 strokes/min. And believe me, when they finish, they are almost comatose; many have to be pulled out of the boat. Two of them could not attend the medal ceremonies after finishing because they could not stand up.

COYLE: In rowing, the technique is clearly important—much more so than in cycling.

HAGERMAN: Well, everybody has been on a bicycle, but few have found their way into a rowing shell.

COYLE: In cyclists there is a direct relationship between mechanical efficiency and percent slow twitch fibers in the vastus lateralis muscles. Can fiber type be changed with years of training to contribute to improved efficiency?

HAGERMAN: We improved efficiency and did not change fiber types, so I think improvements in technique are more important than changes in fiber type in rowers.

EKBLOM: May I suggest another explanation for changes in efficiency? Rowers perform arm and leg exercise simultaneously. It seems likely that there is an optimal balance between the arm and leg exercise that provides the maximal overall rowing efficiency. With years of training, one may approach that optimal balance between arms and legs, thereby making large improvements in overall efficiency.

HAGERMAN: I think that could explain much of the improvement, but I do not know of any research that has confirmed this concept.

TERJUNG: Could you describe for us the factors that you believe account for the differences in performance between elite male and female competitors?

HAGERMAN: I do not know of any one factor that explains the gender effect on rowing performance. The women tend to have smaller proportions of Type IIA muscle fibers, and I think their maximal cardiac outputs are relatively lower than those of the men, but I am sure there are other important factors, too.

SPRIET: The Canadian coaches believe the most important factor in recently improving the performances of the Canadian women rowers is a dramatic increase in the intensity of the rowing training. There is a widespread misconception that women can not train as hard as the men. I suspect that many of the gender differences in performance would be abolished if both sexes trained with equal intensity, duration, and frequency.

HAGERMAN: Although what you suggest about differential training between the sexes was true several years ago, both sexes have undergone similar training regimens over the last few years in most countries with good rowing teams. However, I do think the personality of the coach is important, because a good coach can motivate both sexes to train at progressively higher levels.

TERJUNG: While it is clear that the power output over the 6-min rowing period is absolutely enormous, is there any evidence that there might be a specific muscle or muscle group that accounts for the eventual fatigue? For example, I noticed that there is some asymmetry in muscle use across the trunk, at least at the initiation of the stroke with a single oar.

HAGERMAN: That is an interesting observation, but I do not know of any data that would answer that question.

MAUGHAN: It was interesting to note that the lactates on the rowers in 1989 were much lower than those in 1968. How do you explain that?

HAGERMAN: They peaked earlier, but they were comparatively lower, perhaps because the training program became more intense, e.g., with lactate tolerance training, over the years.

MAUGHAN: What was the difference in power output between 1968 and 1989?

HAGERMAN: The power was greater in 1989, i.e., 450–500 W vs. 350–400 W.

COYLE: You mentioned studies that claimed that the training intensity should not go above 3.5–4.0 mM for blood lactates. I think it is ludicrous to suggest that an athlete should not train at an intensity greater than 4.0 mM when blood lactate during the competitive event reaches 15–20 mM.

HAGERMAN: I agree 100%.

DAVIS: Do you think overtraining in rowers is related to inadequate dietary carbohydrate, resulting in inadequate muscle glycogen stores?

HAGERMAN: That is one possibility. Another possibility is that the rowers may be chronically dehydrated, resulting in reduced plasma volume and a concomitant fall in maximal cardiac output. Unfortunately, I do not have any hard evidence from rowers to support this idea.

GREGG: I think it is important to reinforce the point that it is potentially dangerous for rowers (as well as wrestlers, boxers, and other athletes) to fast and dehydrate themselves in order to make weight for rowing competitions.

HAGERMAN: We are very concerned about that issue. Lightweight rowing is no longer an event for genuine lightweights; it is an event for heavyweights who can reduce their weight and still row at a much higher power level than those people who are true lightweights. We have people who normally weigh 80–85 kg who go down to 72.5 kg in order to compete. They look like concentration camp prisoners when they row.

7

Road and Track Cycling

EDMUND R. BURKE, Ph.D.

INTRODUCTION

Competitive cycling races range from a 200-m match sprint lasting 10-12 s to the 5000-km Tour de France lasting 23 d. Between these extremes there are many other individual and team events. For example, in a 50-km points race that lasts about 60 min there are sprints every few kilometers, during which the cyclists accumulate points; the cyclist with

303

the most points wins the race. Different types of races obviously have different metabolic requirements, and cyclists have learned to specialize in those events best suited to their physiological attributes.

Match sprinting places demands on adenosine triphosphate (ATP) and phosphocreatine (PC) stores and on the anaerobic glycolytic system (Burke et al., 1981; Jacobs et al., 1983; Jones et al., 1985). The cyclist must sustain high velocity and power for the duration of the sprint. If the cyclist is in second place, the goals are to gain momentum by being pulled through the draft and to burst ahead in the last few meters. If leading the sprint, the cyclist hopes to have enough power to hold off the cyclist in second place. Sprint cyclists generate about 20% more power during the first 40 s of an all-out cycling test than do pursuit riders (Davies, 1992), and in the first 5 s of such a test, sprint-trained cyclists can generate four times more power than they can at $\dot{V}O_2$max (Capelli & di Prampero, 1991). This illustrates the large contribution that anaerobic energy sources can make to sprint cycling performance.

Pursuit and kilometer races place high demands upon both the glycolytic and aerobic energy systems, with the anaerobic glycolytic system playing the dominant role. The individual 4000 m pursuit race is a 4–5 min event and has the same energy demands as the mile run in track and field, whereas the kilometer race lasts about 65–75 s and requires the cyclist to generate as much power as possible from the start to the finish. This race begins from a standing rest position and requires maximal acceleration from 0 rpm to more than 120 rpm in a fixed gear.

Van Ingen Schenau et al. (1992) developed a power equation to show the optimal distribution of anaerobic energy during a kilometer cycling event and during a 4000-m pursuit race. Their simulations show that performance in the kilometer race depends to a great extent on a large power output at the onset of the race. Moreover, they demonstrated that the kilometer event should be cycled in an all-out fashion, not at a uniform velocity after the start, despite the greater air drag that accompanies the all-out technique. In contrast, in the 4000-m pursuit race, performance is optimal if the cyclist has a short but powerful start and then continues the race with a constant or slightly decreasing power output.

Little is known about the optimal strategy for expending effort during events such as the 1-km and 4-km time trials, but it is clear that high velocity at the end of the race represents wasted kinetic energy (Foster et al., 1993a; 1993b). Still, a rapid deceleration toward the end of the race as a consequence of premature fatigue can also be detrimental to performance.

To be successful in road racing, the cyclist must generate aerobic power ($\dot{V}O_2$max) sufficient to sustain a high mechanical power output for long durations with little relatively little reliance on anaerobic glycolysis. However, a great potential for generating energy through anaerobic glycolysis is also imperative for powering breakaways, hill climbing, and maximal sprints at the end of the race.

Many sprint and pursuit cyclists do not adhere to the principle of specificity in their training procedures; they spend most of their training sessions riding long distances at power outputs far slower than those required for sprint and pursuit cycling. Attempts to emulate the non-specific training regimens of champion cyclists are often misguided because each cyclist possesses unique physical and physiological potentials that must be developed. It is likely that the typical sprint or pursuit cyclist spends too little time training at high power outputs fueled by anaerobic metabolism.

The nutritional considerations of the cyclist center around proper energy, nutrient, and fluid intake during both training and competition. Energy needs of the road and track cyclist vary greatly; the long-distance road cyclist is more concerned about adequate intake of energy from carbohydrate and fat because of the great fuel requirements of road cycling. Both sprint and distance cyclists must monitor their carbohydrate and fluid intakes to ensure they have adequate stores of glycogen in their muscles and livers and that they are sufficiently hydrated; satisfying these nutritional requirements is a prerequisite to achieving high quality training sessions and peak competitive performances.

PHYSIOLOGY OF CYCLING

Anthropometric Characteristics and Body Composition of Cyclists

Anthropometric Characteristics. Carter (1982) described the somatotype of the typical competitive male cyclist at the Montreal Olympics as 1.7, 4.8, and 3.1 on the endomorphy, mesomorphy, and ectomorphy scales, respectively. This group of cyclists included a silver medalist sprinter and two members of a 100-km team that finished sixth. In a similar study of Olympic athletes directed by de Caray et al. (1974), athletes from various cycling events displayed minimal differences in body type, but certain characteristics were evident. There was a general decrease in mesomorphy and an increase in ectomorphy as the duration of the event increased. The average somatotypes (endomorphy/mesomorphy/ectomorphy) were 1.8/5.2/2.4 for sprinters, 1.8/5.1/2.6 for pursuit racers, and 1.8/4.9/2.7 for road cyclists (de Caray et al., 1974). Similar patterns were found by White et al. (1982a, 1982b), who reported mean somatotypes of 2.4/5.1/2.4 for sprinters and 2.0/4.3/2.7 for road cyclists.

Foley et al. (1989) conducted a study on amateur and professional sprint, pursuit, road, and time-trial cyclists who, on average, had been competing for 8.2 y. The sprint cyclists were significantly shorter and more muscular than the other three groups. Average height for the sprinters was 169.2 cm, body weight was 71.1 kg, and somatotype was 2.2/6.9/

1.4. The time-trial cyclists were the tallest (186.3 cm) and most ectomorphic group (somatotype: 2.9/3.9/3.7). They had the longest legs and the highest leg length/height ratio (47.6% versus 44.8% for the sprinters). The physiques of the pursuit racers and road cyclists were similar to one another and intermediate between the sprinters and time-trial cyclists.

Body Composition. Excess body fat does not contribute to power output in cycling. A high ratio of muscle mass to total body weight is essential for hill climbing efficiency; thus, a lean cyclist will have an advantage on hilly terrain. The estimated percent body fat for elite cyclists ranges from 6–9% for U.S. male road racers and from 12–15% for elite U.S. female cyclists (Burke, 1980). Ten members of the Czechoslovakian National Men's Sprint Team had an average body fat percentage of 6.8%. (Mackova et al., 1986).

White et al. (1982a) reported periodic changes in the body compositions of cyclists over a season of competitive cycling lasting from January to July. With the male road cyclists, there was a clear trend towards body weight reduction during the racing season due to a decrease in body fat accompanied by a reduction in endomorphy; no changes were noted in mesomorphy or ectomorphy. Percent body fat fell from 10.6% in January to 8.5% in July. There was a trend for the sprint cyclists to gain a small amount of body weight and reduce their body fat percentages (12.2 to 10.8%) during the racing season (White et al., 1982b) . The sprinters also became less endomorphic and exhibited trends toward being more mesomorphic and less ectomorphic.

Muscle Fiber Type Distribution

Elite road cyclists generally possess a high proportion of Type I fibers in their quadriceps muscles (Burke, 1980; Burke et al., 1977; Sjögaard et al., 1982). Coyle et al. (1991) reported that elite road cyclists who were good time-trial racers had 66% Type I fibers. Somewhat surprisingly, Czechoslovakian sprint cyclists had a rather high average proportion (58%) of Type I fibers (Mackova et al., 1986). However, these sprinters also exhibited Type II fibers with large diameters and high activities of glycolytic enzymes in their vastus lateralis muscles. Mackova et al. (1986) hypothesized that the muscle changes in this group of sprint cyclists were evidence of adaptations to sprint and resistance training. Consistent with this hypothesis are the data of Ahlquist et al. (1992), who showed that more Type II muscle fibers are recruited when great pedal forces are produced, such as those occurring during starts and jumps on the velodrome.

Coyle et al. (1992) showed that both gross mechanical efficiency and changes in mechanical efficiency while cycling at a cadence of 80 rpm are highly correlated ($r = 0.75-0.85$) with the proportion of Type I muscle fibers within the vastus lateralis muscles of well-trained endurance cyclists. This observation in endurance-trained cyclists indicates that at 80 rpm, Type I fibers are the preferred fibers for efficiently converting chemical energy into mechanical work.

Motor Unit Recruitment

Gregor and colleagues (1986, 1991) used surface electromyography (EMG) electrodes to record leg muscle activity patterns during cycling. Figure 7-1 demonstrates EMG patterns typically reported for a complete pedal revolution. There are, however, variations among riders in both the timing and the magnitude of EMG activity. Studies by Gregor et al. (1991) indicate that the one-joint knee extensors, i.e., the vastus medialis, vastus lateralis, and gluteus maximus, are active simultaneously and quite consistently among subjects at a constant power production of 250 W and at

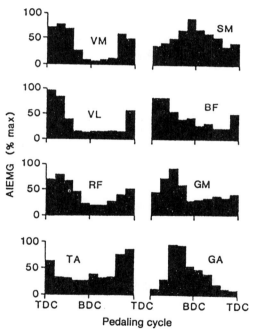

FIGURE 7-1. *Mean of normalized EMG recordings from 8 muscles of 10 subjects during cycling.* AIEMG = average integrated electromyogram; VM = vastus medialis; VL = vastus lateralis; RF = rectus femoris; TA = tibialis anterior; SM = semitendinosus; BF = biceps femoris; GM = gluteus maximus; GA = gastrocnemius; TDC = top dead center of pedaling cycle; BDC = bottom dead center of pedaling cycle. From R.J. Gregor, D. Green, and J.J. Garhammer (1982). An electromyographic analysis of selected muscle activity in elite competitive cyclists. In: A. Morecki, K. Fidelus, K. Kedzior, and A. Wit (eds.) *Biomechanics VII.* Baltimore: University Park Press, pp. 537–541. Reprinted with permission.

a constant pedaling cadence of 90 rpm. The two-joint rectus femoris muscle exhibits activation patterns similar to the vastus lateralis and vastus medialis during the early power phase (0 to 120 degrees) but displays an earlier onset of activity during the recovery phase of the pedaling cycle. The EMG patterns for the biceps femoris, semitendinosus, and semimembranosus display more variability among subjects, with the biceps femoris being the most variable. The EMG activity during cycling for the gastrocnemius and soleus displays consistent temporal patterns among riders, with activity in the soleus consistently beginning just prior to that in the gastrocnemius. The single-joint tibialis anterior is usually active just prior the pedal crank reaching its highest point, i.e., top dead center; however, secondary bursts of activity can occur in the first three quadrants (0 to 270°) of the pedaling cycle.

Saddle height also affects motor unit recruitment during cycling. Desipres (1974) studied EMG patterns in the leg muscles of three male cyclists who rode at three different loads with two different saddle heights. The general conclusions were that as the saddle heights increased, the leg muscles were activated earlier in the pedal cycle and stayed active longer. The amplitude of the EMG recordings was not affected by saddle height; EMG activity was simply sustained for a longer duration. Thorough reviews of biomechanics and pedaling technique in cycling have been published by Gregor et al. (1991) and Kautz et al. (1991).

Oxygen Uptake

The average values for $\dot{V}O_2$max of elite cyclists, i.e., 61 mL·kg^{-1}·min^{-1} for women and 67 to 77 mL·kg^{-1}·min^{-1} for men, are among the highest recorded. Some elite men and women cyclists at the U.S. Olympic Training Center have achieved $\dot{V}O_2$max values greater than 80 and 70 mL·kg^{-1}·min^{-1}, respectively (unpublished observations). Such values suggest that a high $\dot{V}O_2$max may be important for success in cycling, but Krebs et al. (1983) reported that neither $\dot{V}O_2$max nor body composition were significant predictors of road cycling performance by 35 cyclists in a 40-km time trial; competitive experience was the single best predictor.

In contrast, Coyle (1991) and Coyle et al. (1991) reported that U.S. national caliber time-trial cyclists (Group 1) had greater $\dot{V}O_2$max values, greater percentages of Type I fibers, and greater capillary densities in their quadriceps muscles than did regional caliber cyclists (Group 2) (Tables 7-1, 7-2). In addition, simulated 40-km time-trial performance on a bicycle ergometer was highly correlated with average absolute power output during a 1-h laboratory performance test, which in turn was highly related (r = 0.93) to $\dot{V}O_2$ at lactate threshold. Coyle et al. (1992) suggested that cyclists with a high percentage of Type I fibers have a distinct advantage because the Type I fibers are able to produce more power for

TABLE 7-1. *Power output and physiological data for national caliber time-trial cyclists (Group #1) and regional caliber cyclists (Group #2) (Coyle, 1991).*

	Laboratory 1-h Cycling Test			Progressive Cycling Test	
	Power (W)	$\dot{V}O_2$ (L/min)	Load (% $\dot{V}O_2$max)	Blood Lactate Threshold $\dot{V}O_2$ (L/min)	%$\dot{V}O_2$max
Group #1	346±7*	4.54±0.1*	90±1*	4.0±0.1*	79.1±1*
Group #2	311±12	4.18±0.1	86±1	3.7±0.2	75.1±1
#1–#2	11%*	9%*	5%*	9%*	5%*

*P < 0.05 versus Group #2

TABLE 7-2. *Properties of vastus lateralis muscles in national caliber time-trail cyclists (Group #1) and regional caliber cyclists (Group #2) (Coyle, 1991).*

	Type I Fibers (%)	Relative Oxidative Capacity	Capillary Density (Capillaries/mm² fiber area)
Group #1	67±5*	10*	464*
Group #2	53±6	8	377
#1–#2	26%*	20%*	5%*

*P < 0.05 versus Group #2

the same energy expenditure than are Type II fibers. Furthermore, Type I fibers are less vulnerable to fatigue and, coupled with a greater capillary density, allow the cyclist to better sustain a high percentage of $\dot{V}O_2$max throughout the race (Tables 7-1 and 7-2).

In many endurance sports, successful performance is associated with the ability to sustain power production at a high percentage of $\dot{V}O_2$max. Thus, years of training, a high $\dot{V}O_2$max, a high percentage of Type I muscle fibers, and the ability to perform at a high percentage of $\dot{V}O_2$max before lactic acid accumulates rapidly in the blood are several factors that may contribute to success in road and time-trial cycling.

Cardiovascular Adaptations

Fagard et al. (1983) reported an association between a season of cycling training and increased left ventricular diameter at end-diastole, due primarily to greater septal and posterior wall thickness. Internal heart diameter remained unchanged. These results are similar to those of Fananapazir et al. (1982), who showed increased left ventricular mass as well as an increased mass:volume ratio in both young and mature cyclists who underwent a season of cycling training.

White et al. (1982a) showed that peak $\dot{V}O_2$ increased by about 5% during the pre-season to peak-season period in elite cyclists. These results were corroborated by those of Fagard et al. (1983), who reported a 6% increase in peak $\dot{V}O_2$ during the competitive season.

Energy Cost

Figure 7-2 depicts the energy cost of cycling at various speeds (McCole et al., 1990; Pugh, 1974; Swain et al., 1987). The energy expended increases gradually until about 30 km/h, when it begins to increase rapidly due to wind resistance, which is proportional to the square of the air velocity and is nearly proportional to the cyclist's frontal area. For larger body sizes, the frontal area increases at approximately the ⅔ power of body mass (Sjögaard et al., 1982). It has been estimated that the frontal area accounts for up to 20% of the resistive aerodynamic drag forces experienced in racing (Merrill, 1980).

Body size also increases the energy cost of cycling independently of the effect of body size on frontal area. Swain et al. (1987) found that $\dot{V}O_2$ while cycling on a level road increases with body weight for any given speed. The increased oxygen cost was large enough for the authors to conclude that body size is an important factor in competitive long-distance cycling.

A larger body (and muscle) mass increases power production to a greater extent than it increases frontal area and drag. This may be a major reason why 100-km time-trial and pursuit racers tend to be larger cyclists. However, large body size is a distinct disadvantage while cycling up hills because the energy required for the vertical component of ascending a hill is much more dependent on the total weight of the bicycle and rider than

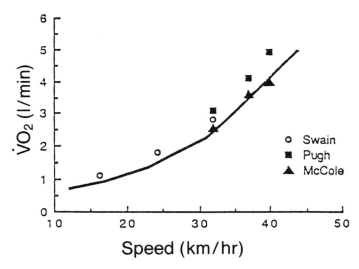

FIGURE 7-2. *Oxygen uptake ($\dot{V}O_2$) at various cycling speeds.* Data shown as open circles are from Swain et al. (1987); closed squares are from Pugh (1974); closed triangles are from McCole et al. (1990). Adapted with permission from J.M. Hagberg and S.D. McCole (1990). Energy expenditure during bicycling. *Cycling Sci.* 2:17.

it is on frontal area (Di Prampero et al., 1979). As the cyclist's speed is reduced during an ascent, the energy required to overcome air resistance is decreased markedly. Smaller cyclists should excel at hill climbing due to a greater ratio of $\dot{V}O_2$max to body mass (Swain et al., 1988).

McCole et al. (1990) also studied the relationship between cycling speed and $\dot{V}O_2$ and demonstrated an 8% lower $\dot{V}O_2$ at 32 km/h than did Swain et al. (1987). This difference may be explained by the fact that the subjects in the study of McCole et al. (1990) were more experienced cyclists and may have been more efficient in pedaling and positioning on the bicycle than were the subjects in the study of Swain et al. (1987). On the other end of the spectrum, $\dot{V}O_2$ values for cyclists in an investigation by Pugh (1974) were about 7% higher than those for the subjects of Swain et al. (1987). Kyle (1991) suggested Pugh's subjects were required to expend more energy cycling on the hillier course used in his study.

Based on data from nearly 100 trials conducted under the same conditions, McCole et al. (1990) derived the following equation to predict the $\dot{V}O_2$ required for different riding speeds.

$$\dot{V}O_2 = -4.50 + 0.17\ \dot{V}_R + 0.052\ \dot{V}_W + 0.22\ W_R,$$

where $\dot{V}O_2$ is expressed in L/min, $\dot{V}_R$ is the cycling speed in km/h, $\dot{V}_W$ is the headwind speed in km/h, and W_R is the rider mass in kg. This equation accounted for more than 70% of the differences in $\dot{V}O_2$ observed among the different trials in the study. While this equation will not give a rider an absolutely precise value for $\dot{V}O_2$ under all conditions, it will provide a general estimate of a cyclist's energy expenditure, at least across the 32–40 km/h range of speeds utilized in the study (Hagberg & McCole, 1995).

Power Output

Several years ago, it was reported that Eddy Merckx produced 450 W for 1 h while on a cycle ergometer (Kyle & Caiozzo, 1986). Recreational cyclists can only hold this power output for about 1 min (Whitt & Wilson, 1982a). At the other end of the scale, an Italian sprinter has produced 1644 W for 5 s (Dal Monte & Faina, 1989). Healthy untrained subjects can produce more than 700 W for a few seconds, and about 180 W for 1 h (Kyle & Caiozzo, 1986; Whitt & Wilson, 1982a). The speed at which a bicycle will travel with a fixed power output is dependent upon the resistance forces against the bicycle (Kyle, 1991).

FACTORS THAT MAY LIMIT CYCLING PERFORMANCE

Disturbances in Acid-Base Balance

Craig et al. (1989) showed that peak lactate concentrations in the blood reached 17 mM in elite track cyclists after a 1-km race that lasted approximately 70 s. Mean postrace blood lactate concentrations have been reported to be 12.1 mM for the team pursuit events, 13.7 mM for the match sprints, 15.2 mM for the individual pursuit, and 19.9 in the 1-km event (Burke et al., 1981). The high blood lactates seen after match sprinting show that anaerobic glycolysis occurs in cycling events that are as brief as 10 s.

Changes in lactate concentrations in the active muscles are consistent with the high blood lactate values. Lactate concentrations in muscle biopsies that were obtained from both men and women immediately after maximal cycle ergometer exercise lasting 10 s or 30 s averaged 36 and 61 mmol/kg dry weight, respectively (Jacobs et al., 1983). Directionally similar results were reported by Jones et al. (1985), who reported that muscle lactate concentrations for two subjects who cycled on an isokinetic ergometer for 10 s increased to 15–17 mmol/kg dry weight at 140 rpm and to 14 mmol/kg at 60 rpm. In this latter study, glycogenolysis was activated very rapidly at both pedal speeds.

Insufficiently Aerodynamic Body Position and Equipment

At speeds greater than 40 km/h, wind resistance is responsible for 90% of the total resistance on the bicycle and cyclist. Unfortunately, the human body and most of the parts of the bicycle resemble cylinders and thus have a relatively high aerodynamic drag. The wind resistance of the human body in both track and road cycling is responsible for about ⅔ of the wind drag losses, whereas the bicycle causes approximately ⅓ of the drag (Kyle & Burke, 1984). The greatest reduction in wind resistance comes from changing the position of the human body on the bicycle. This has been accomplished in recent years by using so-called aerodynamic handlebars that cause the rider to assume a more aerodynamic body posture. Clip-on handlebars and other models of aerodynamic handlebars can trim 0.45 pounds from a rider's total drag at 48 km/h compared with using normal dropped bars (Kyle, 1989). Thus, riding in an aerodynamic position can decrease drag by about 10–15% and can shorten race time by about 2.7 s/km.

Faria et al. (1978) found that riding a standard cycle ergometer while grasping the lowest part of the standard dropped handle bars increased oxygen uptake, power output, and pulmonary ventilation without affecting heart rate, compared to grasping the upper portion of the bars. In contrast, Johnson and Shultz (1990), whose subjects rode ergometers set up to resemble their road bikes, detected no additional energy cost using standard dropped bars when aerodynamic clip-on handlebars were used. Finally, Origenes et al. (1993) reported that moderately trained cyclists exhibited similar absolute power outputs, ventilatory responses, and oxygen uptakes when upright posture and aerodynamic cycling posture were compared. These latter two studies suggest that the reduction in wind drag afforded by aerodynamic handlebars is obtained with little or no apparent increase in physiologic costs. Still, it remains unclear if riding for long periods in an aerodynamic position alters muscle fiber recruitment and accelerates fatigue processes. The rider's kinetics and kinematics on the bike, especially at the hip joint, are altered significantly while riding in this position.

Spacing between riders is also critical for minimizing drag. The closer one cyclist follows another, the greater the drag reduction. For the team pursuit, a reduction of clearance from 30 cm to 15 cm between the leader's back wheel and the following rider's front wheel will reduce wind resistance for the following rider by 2%. This can result in a 1.5–2.0 s advantage in a 4000-m race (Faria, 1992).

In addition to maintaining an aerodynamic body position with the aid of specialized handlebars and allowing appropriate spacing between bicycles, the use of aerodynamic wheels, helmets, clothing, and bicycle components can further reduce aerodynamic drag in all cycling events (Kyle, 1991).

Disturbances in Thermoregulation and Inadequate Fluid Replacement

During strenuous cycling in a laboratory setting with little or no air flow past the rider, body core temperature can rise dangerously within 30 min; during cycling at the same intensity on the road or track, air flow over the skin surfaces speeds heat loss by convection and evaporation so that cycling can be continued for many hours with little increase in core temperature (Whitt & Wilson, 1982b).

The effects of various types of skintight clothing on heat load from solar radiation were studied in resting subjects seated in racing position on bicycles in a laboratory where temperature was maintained at 27° C, the humidity was held constant, and the air was still (Berglund et al., 1987). The bicycles were placed on a sensitive balance so that weight loss caused by the evaporation of sweat could be carefully monitored while the riders were exposed intermittently to four intensities of simulated solar radiation: 0, 190, 360, and 480 W. An aluminized fabric was best for reducing radiative heat gain—even better than bare skin—followed by white and light-colored fabrics. Dark, tightly woven fabrics were projected to increase sweat loss by 692 mL. Thus, the nature of the fabric covering the skin of a road cyclist can be an important factor in determining the extent of potential dehydration during endurance cycling races.

It is widely known that consuming fluids during prolonged exercise decreases hyperthermia and the risk of heat illness, but until recently, the precise relationship between the volume of fluid ingested during cycling and its affect on thermoregulation was unknown. Montain and Coyle (1992b) documented the effects of different degrees of dehydration on thermoregulation, heart rate, and stroke volume during prolonged cycling. On four separate occasions, trained endurance cyclists rode for 2 h in a warm environment (33° C dry bulb, 50% relative humidity) at 62–67% of $\dot{V}O_2$max. During the rides, the cyclists randomly drank no fluid (NF) small volumes (SF, 300 mL/h), moderate volumes (MF, 700 mL/h), or large volumes (LF, 1,200 mL/h) of a sports drink containing 6% carbohydrate and small amounts of electrolytes. These fluid volumes replaced 0%, 20%, 50%, and 80%, respectively, of the sweat produced during the rides, which translated into body weight losses of 4%, 3%, 2%, and 1% during the NF, SF, MF, and LF trials, respectively. Several cyclists had great difficulty completing the 2-h rides during the NF trial, and the increases in core temperature, heart rate, and ratings of perceived exertion were inversely related to the amounts of fluid consumed, i.e., the greatest increases in temperature, heart rate, and perceived exertion occurred in the NF condition and the least in the LF trial. Each liter of dehydration was associated with a 0.3° C rise in core temperature and an 8 beats/min elevation in heart rate. The mechanism underlying the beneficial effects of fluid replenishment apparently involves an increased blood flow to the skin that helps dissipate body heat (Montain & Coyle, 1992a).

Montain and Coyle (1992b) reported that none of their cyclists experienced gastrointestinal distress, even during the 1,200 mL/h trial. In contrast, Mitchell and Voss (1991) found that some cyclists ingesting 1,200 mL/h fluid and all subjects ingesting 1,600 mL/h were "visibly uncomfortable." Interestingly, 25% of their subjects developed diarrhea when ingesting 1.6 L/h, indicating that the rate of fluid ingestion exceeded the combined maximal rate of absorption of both the large and small intestines (Mitchell & Voss, 1991).

Insufficient Carbohydrate Supply

Many studies have clearly demonstrated that carbohydrate feedings during prolonged cycling can delay fatigue. One of these investigations was conducted on experienced cyclists who intermittently consumed either a placebo or a carbohydrate solution while they rode to fatigue at 74% $\dot{V}O_2$max in a laboratory environment (Coyle et al., 1983). In the carbohydrate trial, the cyclists maintained at least 90% of their assigned power output for 157 min, whereas they cycled at that intensity for only 134 min in the placebo trial.

Coyle et al. (1986) then tested the hypothesis that carbohydrate feedings improved performance by slowing down the depletion of glycogen in the vastus lateralis muscle; he found that cyclists could cycle at 70% $\dot{V}O_2$max for 3 h when drinking a placebo at 20-min intervals throughout the ride and 4 h at the same intensity when provided with about 27 g of carbohydrate every 20 min. The carbohydrate feedings appeared to improve performance by better maintaining blood glucose levels, not by reducing the extent of muscle glycogen depletion.

In a further investigation of the hypothesis that the maintenance of blood glucose concentrations was the explanation for the beneficial effects of carbohydrate feedings during endurance cycling, Coggan and Coyle (1987) had cyclists ride to exhaustion at 70% $\dot{V}O_2$max while drinking only water. Next, the subjects rested for 20 min before beginning a second ride to exhaustion. During the rest period, they drank either a placebo beverage or a 50% solution of maltodextrins (3 g/kg). A third treatment included the placebo beverage ingestion during the rest period plus an intravenous infusion of glucose just prior to and during the second ride. On average, exhaustion occurred after 170 min during the water feeding trial, during which there were gradual decreases in blood glucose concentrations and carbohydrate oxidation. Fatigue was reversed by the carbohydrate feeding and by the glucose infusion, which was the only treatment that maintained stable blood glucose concentrations; during the second ride, the cyclists rode for 10 min after ingesting the placebo drink, 26 min after the carbohydrate feeding, or 43 min during glucose infusion. An intravenous supply of glucose at a rate of about 1 g/min was needed to maintain blood glucose levels, indicating that skeletal muscle was utilizing glucose at a similar rate and that carbohydrate feedings at the rate of about 60 g/h may be appropriate for carbohydrate replenishment during prolonged exercise.

FLUID AND CARBOHYDRATE RECOMMENDATIONS DURING CYCLING

Both runners (Costill et al., 1970) and cyclists (Mitchell & Voss, 1991) develop symptoms of "fullness" when ingesting fluid at a rate of 800 mL/h or greater. Also, Brouns et al. (1991) showed that the rate of fluid ingestion for subjects encouraged to drink as much as possible during a simulated triathlon was two to three times higher in the cycling leg (600–800 mL/h) than during running (100–300 mL/h). Furthermore, as discussed earlier, some cyclists can tolerate up to 1,200 mL/h before gastrointestinal distress occurs (Montain & Coyle, 1992a, 1992b). Thus, the evidence suggests that it is easier to consume large amounts of fluids during cycling than during running (Brouns et al., 1987), and peak rates of fluid ingestion under ideal conditions for cycling are seldom greater than 800–1,200 mL/h. Finally, it is advisable for cyclists to practice drinking large volumes of fluids in training before doing it during competition (Maughan, 1991).

A practical nutritional problem for cyclists in long events such as the Tour de France is the difficulty they experience eating enough ordinary food to obtain the amount of carbohydrate needed for optimum performance (Brouns et al., 1989a). There are several explanations for this phenomenon: intense, prolonged exercise can decrease appetite; eating a large volume of food can cause gastrointestinal distress during cycling; and the cyclists are spending so much time on the bicycles that there is little time available for eating in relaxed conditions. To determine if adequate carbohydrate intake could be achieved with a high-energy drink, Brouns et al. (1989b) had a group of cyclists consume a high-carbohydrate drink throughout a simulated Tour de France. The drink was a 20% solution of carbohydrates, 85% of which consisted of maltodextrins and 15% of which was fructose. Subjects who drank this beverage were able to consume enough energy and carbohydrate to match their needs, whereas those who relied on conventional foods or a high-fructose beverage (a 20% carbohydrate solution containing 50% fructose and 50% maltodextrins) failed to ingest enough energy and exhibited impairments in their cycling performances. The high-fructose drink was deemed too sweet, and it caused gastrointestinal distress.

Research on the formulation of sport drinks and on the drinking schedule that will optimally supply both fluids and carbohydrate suggests that drinking 200–300 mL of a 6–20% solution of carbohydrate every 15–20 min is effective in delaying fatigue and is generally well-tolerated by cyclists (Coyle & Montain, 1992). For optimal absorption of both carbohydrate and fluids under most conditions, drinks containing 5–10% carbohydrate should be used during competitive cycling (Maugh n, 1991). Glucose, sucrose, or maltodextrins, but not fructose, are equally effective as carbohydrate sources to improve performance during prolonged cycling (Maughan, 1991).

Rough terrain or a particularly fast speed can make drinking awkward, so cyclists in competition often do not drink fluids until late in the race. By then, blood glucose and muscle glycogen stores may be severely depleted. Still, if carbohydrate and fluid consumption begins late in the race but before exhaustion, it can be effective in extending performance. Coggan and Coyle (1989) required cyclists to drink 400 mL of a 50% solution of maltodextrins after 135 min of cycling at 70% $\dot{V}O_2$max, i.e., about 35 min before exhaustion occurred in a placebo trial. In the carbohydrate trial, the cyclists boosted their blood glucose concentrations, increased the use of carbohydrate as fuel, and improved their endurance by 35 min or 21% (Coggan & Coyle, 1989). Anecdotal evidence suggests that many cyclists cannot tolerate drinking 400 mL of a 50% solution of carbohydrate. Therefore, it is more practical for the cyclists to drink throughout the ride rather than to wait until late in exercise.

In summary, carbohydrate should be ingested during cycling at the rate of about 1 g/min, particularly during the later stages of training rides or competitive races. This can be accomplished in a 3 h race by ingesting approximately 45–75 g/h throughout exercise or about 200 g late in exercise. When ingested at 600–1000 mL/h during cycling, carbohydrate solutions of 5–10 g carbohydrate/100 mL can supply both fuel and fluid needed to enhance cycling performance (Coggan, 1992; Coyle & Montain, 1992).

NUTRITION WHILE RECOVERING FROM ENDURANCE CYCLING

To restore diminished carbohydrate reserves, cyclists should ingest carbohydrate following strenuous prolonged training or competition. Muscle glycogen replenishment appears to predominate over liver glycogen replenishment during such postexercise carbohydrate feedings (Sherman, 1991). If a diet of at least moderate carbohydrate content (5 g·kg^{-1}·d^{-1}) is consumed following exhaustive exercise, liver glycogen will be normalized within 24 h. To optimize muscle glycogen stores, carbohydrate must be consumed immediately after exercise and at frequent intervals thereafter (Sherman, 1991, 1992). Approximately 1.5 g carbohydrate/kg body weight should be consumed at 2-h intervals for up to 6 h after exercise. Total carbohydrate intake in the first 24 h after exercise should be 8–11 g·kg^{-1}·d^{-1} (Sherman, 1992).

Zawadzki et al. (1992) showed that a drink containing both carbohydrate and protein increased the rate of muscle glycogen storage after cycling by 38% when compared to a drink containing only carbohydrate. It was suggested that the protein had a positive effect on insulin secretion, which enhanced glycogen resynthesis. These results remain to be confirmed.

MEDICAL CONCERNS

In cycling, injuries can be avoided not only by anticipating dangerous circumstances and by skillful riding but also by assuming a proper position on the bicycle, ensuring that the bicycle is in first-class working order, and wearing protective equipment, including an approved helmet, gloves, and clothing. Fitness is also important because some injuries result from inadequate training for the event. The main causes of injury on the bicycle are overuse injuries and accidents.

Overuse Injuries

Acute and chronic pain in muscles and joints, especially the knees and the vertebral column, are the most common symptoms of overuse injury in cycling (Holmes & Pruitt, 1991; Leadbetter & Schneider, 1982). Neck and back pain are extremely common, occurring in up to 60% of competitive cyclists (Mellion, 1991). Ulnar neuropathy, characterized by tingling, numbness, and weakness in the hands, is common in serious cyclists after a few days of riding. Improper fit of the bicycle and use of large gears may also lead to problems such as trochanteric bursitis, iliopsoas tendinitis, and patellofemoral pain syndrome (Mellion, 1991). Other factors, including genetic variation in joint anatomy and inadequate fitness (Mellion, 1991), may also predispose a cyclist to overuse injuries.

Over a 5-y period, Holmes and Pruitt (1991) studied 99 professional and amateur elite cyclists who complained of cycling-related knee problems. In addition to a standard orthopedic exam, each athlete was evaluated on his bicycle to check for possible biomechanical imbalances. Problems of the anterior knee, especially chondromalacia and patellar tendinitis, were the most common diagnoses and were found in 64% of these athletes. Surprisingly, medial knee injuries, diagnosed in 21.2% of the cyclists, accounted for the second largest category of overuse injuries. Other injuries reported were medial plica, iliotibial band syndrome, and other soft tissue problems.

Overuse injuries usually result from improper biomechanics combined with the highly repetitive motion of pedaling. During steady-state cycling, the forces applied to the pedal are often equal to body weight (Davis & Hull, 1981; Gregor et al., 1991; Soden & Adeyefa, 1979). In addition, forces equivalent to three times body weight are applied to the bicycle pedals during periods of intense hill climbing and sprinting (Soden & Adeyefa, 1979). Extremely rapid extension and flexion of the knees produces these great forces when cycling at 70–110 rpm and makes the knees particularly susceptible to overuse injuries.

Proper fit of the rider to the bicycle is critical for the prevention of overuse injuries. One of the best ways to ensure proper and accurate fit on the bicycle is to use the Fitkit®, which can be found at any good bicycle shop. It is a system of measuring devices and tables used to provide a customized fit on the bicycle for the cyclist. An optional rotational adjustment device can be used to provide accurate cleat adjustments for cyclists with traditional cleated shoes or clip-in pedals. Proper frame selection and adjustment can be made by following simple guidelines for frame size, seat height, fore and aft saddle adjustment, saddle angle, and handlebar reach and height. To help prevent cycling injuries, it is important to remember that the bicycle is somewhat adjustable and the athlete is somewhat adaptable. The ultimate riding position for speed and performance is secondary to a higher priority—a fit that minimizes vulnerability to pain and injury. For a more detailed discussion of proper fit on the bicycle the reader is directed to excellent reviews of the subject by Mellion (1991) and by Phinney and Carpenter (1992).

Management of overuse injuries in cycling generally involves mechanical adjustment of the bicycle as well as medical treatment of the cyclist. Overall, conservative therapies, i.e., application of ice, use of nonsteroid anti-inflammatory drugs, prescription of exercises, and correction of bicycle position, are the most effective forms of treatment of knee injuries (Holmes & Pruitt, 1991). However, cyclists who fail to respond to such conservative treatment may require surgery (Holmes & Pruitt, 1991).

Cycling Accidents

Over half of all cycling accidents involve motor vehicles, but poor road surfaces and mechanical bicycle problems are also common causes of accidents. Cycling accidents account for 500,000 visits per year to emergency rooms in U.S. hospitals (Sacks, 1991). From 1984–1988, bicycling accounted for 2,985 deaths due to head injuries (62% of all bicycling deaths) and 905,752 head injuries (32% of bicycling injuries treated in an emergency department) (Sacks, 1991). Forty-one percent of cycling-related head injury deaths and 76% of head injuries occurred among children less than 15 y of age (Sacks, 1991).

Sacks (1991) calculated that universal use of helmets by all bicyclists could have prevented as many as 2,500 deaths and 757,000 head injuries in his 5-y study, i.e., more than one death every day and one head injury every 4 min. Many cyclists risk injury by not wearing helmets during training and competition because they believe that the increased heat load caused by wearing the helmet will detract from their performances; there is no evidence to substantiate this belief. For example, Gisolfi et al. (1988) asked six competitive cyclists, each of whom had ridden over 800 km in the previous month, to ride for 2 h at 70% $\dot{V}O_2$max with and without a helmet. The laboratory environment was maintained at 33° C (92° F) and 20–30% relative humidity; a fan blew air on the cyclists' faces to simulate outdoor conditions. Wearing the helmets did not significantly affect rectal temperatures, skin temperatures, heart rates, perceived exertion, or $\dot{V}O_2$.

In another study that addressed the issue of thermoregulation while wearing cycling helmets, Wood (1986) compared seven commercially available helmets during rides in the heat in laboratory experiments and concluded that the better ventilated helmets were almost as comfortable as riding helmetless. The results of the work of Wood (1986) and Gisolfi et al. (1988) are consistent with the absence of any published reports attributing heat illness during cycling to helmet use in events such as U.S. Cycling Federation races, the Iron Man Triathlon, and the Race Across America. In each of these events, athletes ride in hot, humid conditions for many hours, often over hilly terrain. It seems abundantly clear that cyclists can wear helmets to minimize their chances of serious head injury or death without detracting from their competitive performances.

FUTURE RESEARCH

Future research in cycling should include more cycling-specific experimental designs, equipment, subject selection, and protocols to address questions unique to the competitive and recreational aspects of the sport.

Both laboratory and field studies should use experienced competitive or recreational cyclists performing on their own bicycles.

- Studies should be conducted to evaluate interactive effects on energy expenditure and wind drag when alternative positions of the body are employed while cycling in events such as pursuits. Such studies should also track adaptations in energy expenditure that may occur as cyclists become habituated to new body positions.
- Instrumentation needs to be developed to continually inform cyclists about their cycling mechanics and force application while riding their own bicycles. This will allow for better application of force to the pedals during the cycling stroke. A compact computerized analyzer carried on the bicycle could be developed for monitoring and storing data on the physiological and mechanical responses of cyclists during outdoor training sessions and competition.
- The physiological responses of women cyclists during long-distance competitions should be comprehensively documented. The growth of women's cycling is being restrained at the international level because of the dearth of this type of information.
- With the advent of new shoe and pedal systems, more research needs to be done on the effects of these systems on pedaling mechanics, force applications, and overuse injuries. It is important to evaluate these effects after several hours of cycling on the road, especially because most of the available biomechanical information has been obtained during brief periods of ergometer cycling in a laboratory.
- Bicycle helmet and clothing design can be improved. What is the ideal design to maximize convective cooling in protective bicycle helmets? What tests can accurately simulate human head cooling? How can clothing improve the cooling of endurance cyclists? What are the effects of various types of clothing on thermal balance in a rider cycling in the sunshine?
- We need to know how various pedaling motions, e.g., oval, linear, variable angular velocity, etc., affect efficiency, fatigue, maximum speed, and other performance variables. What other alternative drive systems appear promising? Considering only event performance, what crank length is best for each leg length or riding style? For example, is the optimal crank length for sprinting different from that for racing in time trials?
- More research on optimal nutrition for cyclists is important. A more comprehensive examination of the effects of solid feedings upon cycling performance during events lasting 4–8 h or more on the bicycle is needed. It is obvious that athletes want some solid food while competing for such extended periods of time. What are

the best feeding patterns during events lasting over 4 h? What effects do protein and amino acid feedings and/or supplements have upon long-term cycling endurance and recovery between stages of a race or between training sessions? Do antioxidants aid in recovery and performance in endurance cycling? How does the administration of medium chain triglycerides (MCT) affect energy provisions during endurance cycling?

SUMMARY

Competitive cycling includes a variety of individual and team events that are as brief as 10 s or as long as 3 wk. Accordingly, the physiological requirements for cycling range from the ability to produce exceptionally high power anaerobically to the ability to sustain moderately high power aerobically for many consecutive hours. Thus, sprint cyclists generally have a greater proportion of larger Type II muscle fibers in their thigh muscles, whereas endurance cyclists have more Type I fibers. Endurance cyclists are also able to produce greater power before accumulating excessive amounts of lactic acid in their blood than are sprint cyclists.

Because of the tremendous effect of air resistance on the performance of high-speed cycling, every cyclist must attempt to achieve the maximal aerodynamic body position on the bicycle that is consistent with optimal energy expenditure and power production. In addition, the various parts of the bicycle must be aerodynamically designed if performance is to be maximized. Other factors that can limit cycling performance include acid-base disturbances, impairments in thermoregulation (including those associated with dehydration), and insufficient carbohydrate supply.

To optimize both fluid and carbohydrate replenishment, endurance cyclists are advised to consume large volumes of 5–10% carbohydrate solutions every 15–20 min during both training and competition. Carbohydrate foods should also be consumed in large amounts during recovery from a hard training session or from exhaustive competition to hasten the replenishment of glycogen stores in the muscles and the liver.

The major medical concerns associated with cycling are overuse injuries and cycling accidents. Improper body position and other biomechanical factors are often the causes of overuse injuries, whereas interactions with motor vehicles and failure to wear cycling helmets contribute to many cycling accidents.

ACKNOWLEDGEMENT

The author expresses his gratitude and appreciation to those fellow researchers, coaches, and athletes whose works are cited and discussed in this chapter.

BIBLIOGRAPHY

Ahlquist, L.E., D.R. Bassett, R. Sufit, F.J. Nagle, and D.P. Thomas (1992). The effect of pedaling frequency on glycogen depletion rates in type I and type II quadriceps muscle fibers during submaximal cycling exercise. *Eur. J. Appl. Physiol.* 65:360-364.

Berglund, L., D. Fashena, and X. Su (1987). Evaporative weight loss as a measure of absorbed thermal radiation in the human. *8th Conference on Biometeorology and Aerobiology.* Boston, MA: American Meteorological Society, pp. 338-340.

Brouns, F., E. Beckers, B. Knopfli, B. Villiger, and W. Saris (1991). Rehydration during exercise: effect of electrolyte supplementation on selective blood parameters. *Med. Sci. Sports Exerc.* 23:S84.

Brouns, F., W.H.M. Saris, and N.J. Rehrer (1987). Abdominal complaints and gastrointestinal function during long-lasting exercise. *Int. J. Sports Med.* 8:175-189.

Brouns, F., W.H.M. Saris, J. Stroecken, E. Beckers, R. Thijssen, N.J. Rehrer, and F. Hoorten (1989a). Eating, drinking, and cycling, a controlled Tour de France simulation study. Part 1. *Int. J. Sports Med.* 10:S32-S40.

Brouns, F., W.H.M. Saris, J. Stroecken, E. Beckers, R. Thijssen, N.J. Rehrer, and F. Hoorten (1989b). Eating, drinking, and cycling, a controlled Tour de France simulation study. Part 2. *Int. J. Sports Med.* 10:S41-S48.

Burke, E.R. (1980). The physiological characteristics of competitive cyclists. *Physician Sportsmed.* 8:78-84.

Burke, E.R., F. Cerny, D. Costill, and W. Fink (1977). Characteristics of skeletal muscle in competitive cyclists. *Med. Sci. Sports* 9:109-112.

Burke, E.R., S. Fleck, and T. Dickson (1981). Post-competition blood lactate concentrations in competitive track cyclists. *Brit. J. Sports Med.* 15:242-245.

Capelli, C., and P.E. Di Prampero (1991). Maximal explosive power and aerobic exercise in humans. *Schweiz. Z. Sportmed.* 39:103-111.

Carter, J.E.L. (1982). Physical Structure of Olympic Athletes Part 1. The Montreal Olympic Games Anthropological Project. *Medicine and Sport*, Vol. 16. Basel: S. Karger, pp. 38-39.

Coggan, A.R. (1992). Nutritional manipulations before and during endurance exercise: effects on performance. *Med. Sci. Sports Exerc.* 24:9:S331-S335.

Coggan, A.R., and E.F. Coyle (1987). Reversal of fatigue during prolonged exercise by carbohydrate infusion or ingestion. *J. Appl. Physiol.* 62:2388-2395.

Coggan, A.R., and E.F. Coyle (1988). Effect of carbohydrate feedings during high-intensity exercise. *J. Appl. Physiol.* 65:1703-1709.

Coggan, A.R., and E.F. Coyle (1989). Metabolism and performance following carbohydrate ingestion late in exercise. *Med. Sci. Sports Exerc.* 21:59-65.

Costill, D.L., W.F. Krammer, and A. Fisher (1970). Fluid ingestion during distance running. *Arch. Environ. Health* 21:520-525.

Coyle, E.F. (1991). Cycling techniques of elite 40 kilometer time trialists. *Cycling Sci.* 3:8-12.

Coyle, E.F., A.R. Coggan, M.K. Hemmert, and J.L. Ivy (1986). Muscle glycogen utilization during prolonged strenuous exercise when fed carbohydrates. *J. Appl. Physiol.* 61:165-172.

Coyle, E.F., A.R. Coggan, M.K. Hopper, and T.J. Walters (1988). Determinants of endurance in well-trained cyclists. *J. Appl. Physiol.* 64:6:2622-2630.

Coyle, E.F., M.E. Feltner, S.A. Kautz, M.T. Hamilton, S.J. Montain, A.M. Baylor, L.D. Abraham, and G.W. Petrek (1991). Physiological and biomechanical factors associated with elite endurance cycling performance. *Med. Sci. Sports Exerc.* 23:93-107.

Coyle, E.F., J.M. Hagberg, B.F. Hurley, W.H. Martin, A.A. Ehsani, and J.O. Holloszy (1983). Carbohydrate feedings during prolonged strenuous exercise can delay fatigue. *J. Appl. Physiol.* 55:230-235.

Coyle, E.F., and S.J. Montain (1992). Carbohydrate and fluid ingestion during exercise: are there trade-offs? *Med. Sci. Sports Exerc.* 24:671-678.

Coyle, E.F., L.S. Sidossis, J.F. Horowitz, and J.D. Beltz (1992). Cycling efficiency is related to the percentage of Type I muscle fibers. *Med. Sci. Sport Exerc.* 24:7:782-788.

Craig, N.P., F.S. Pyke, and K.I. Norton (1989). Specificity of test duration when assessing the anaerobic lactic acid capacity of high-performance track cyclists. *Int. J. Sports Med.* 10:237-242.

Dal Monte, A., and M. Faina (1989). Human anaerobic power output. *Cycling Sci.* 1:13.

Davies, C.T.M. (1992). The physiology of cycling, with reference to power output and muscularity. *Ann. Physiol. Anthrop.* 11:309-312.

Davis, R., and M. Hull (1981). Measurement of pedal loading in bicycling II: analysis and results. *J. Biomech.* 14:857-872.

de Caray, A.L., L. Kevine, and J.L. Carter (1974). *Genetic and Anthropological Studies of Olympic Athletes.* New York: Academic Press.

Desipres, M. (1974). An electromyographic study of competitive road cycling conditions simulated on a treadmill. In: R.C. Nelson and C. Morehouse (eds.) *Biomechanics IV.* Baltimore: University Park Press, pp. 349-355.

Di Prampero, P.E., G. Cortili, P. Mognoni, and F. Saibene (1979). Equation of motion of a cyclist. *J. Appl. Physiol.* 47:201–206.

Fagard, R., A. Aubert, R. Lysens, J. Staessen, L. Vanhees, and A. Amery (1983). Noninvasive assessment of seasonal variations in cardiac structure and function in cyclists. *Circulation* 67:896–901.

Fananapazir, L., B. Ryan-Woolley, C. Ward, and J.A. White (1982). Echocardiographic left ventricular dimensions in two groups of road race cyclists during a training season. *Br. J. Sports Med.* 16:113–114.

Faria, I.E. (1992). Energy expenditure, aerodynamics and medical problems in cycling. *Sports Med.* 14:43–63.

Faria, I., C. Dix, and C. Frazer (1978). Effect of body position during cycling on heart rate, pulmonary ventilation, oxygen uptake and work output. *J. Sports Med. Phys. Fit.* 18:49–56.

Foley, J.P., S.R. Bird, and J.A. White (1989). Anthropometric comparison of cyclists from different events. *Br. J. Sports Med.* 23:30–33.

Foster, C., A.C. Snyder, N.N. Thompson, M.A. Green, M. Foley, and M. Schrager (1993a). Effect of pacing strategy on cycle time trial performance. *Med. Sci. Sports Exerc.* 25:383–388.

Foster, C., M.A. Green, A.C. Snyder, and N.N. Thompson (1993b). Physiological responses during simulated competition. *Med. Sci. Sports Exerc.* 25:877–882.

Gisolfi, C.V., D.P. Rohlf, S.N. Navarude, C.L. Hayes, and S.A. Sayeed (1988). Effects of wearing a helmet on thermal balance while cycling in the heat. *Physician Sportsmed.* 16:139–146.

Gregor, R.J., J.P. Broker, and M.M. Ryan (1991). The biomechanics of cycling. In: J.O. Holloszy (ed.) *Exercise and Sport Science Reviews: Vol 19.* Baltimore: Williams & Wilkins, pp. 127–169.

Gregor, R.J., and S.G. Rugg (1986). Effects of saddle height and pedaling cadence on power output and efficiency. In: E.R. Burke (ed.) *Science of Cycling.* Champaign, IL: Human Kinetics Publishers, pp. 69–90.

Hagberg, J., and S. McCole (1995). Energy expenditure during cycling. In: E.R. Burke (ed.) *High Tech Cycling.* Champaign, IL: Human Kinetics Publishers. (In press.)

Holmes, J.C., and A.L. Pruitt (1991). Cycling knee injuries. *Cycling Sci.* 3:11–14.

Horowitz, J.F., L.S. Sidossis, and E.F. Coyle (1994). High efficiency of type I muscle fibers improves performance. *Med Sci. Sport Exerc.* (In press.)

Jacobs, R., P.A. Tesch, O. Bar-Or, J. Karlsson, and R. Dotan (1983). Lactate in human skeletal muscle after 10 and 30 s of supramaximal exercise. *J. Appl. Physiol.* 55:365–367.

Johnson, S., and B. Shultz (1990). The physiological effects of aerodynamic handlebars. *Cycling Sci.* 2:9–12.

Jones, N.L., N. McCartney, T. Graham, L.L. Spriet, J.M. Kowalchuk, G.J.F. Heigenhauser, and J.R. Sutton (1985). Muscle performance and metabolism in maximal isokinetic cycling at slow and fast speeds. *J. Appl. Physiol.* 59:132–136.

Kautz, S.A., M.E. Felter, E.F. Coyle, and A.M. Baylor (1991). The pedaling technique of elite endurance cyclists: changes with increasing workload at constant cadence. *Int. J. Sport Biomech.* 7:29–53.

Krebs, P., S. Zinkgraf, and S. Virgilio (1983). The effects of training variables, maximal aerobic capacities, and body composition upon cycling performance time. *Med. Sci. Sports Exerc.* 15:133.

Kyle, C.R (1989). The aerodynamics of handlebars and helmets. *Cycling Sci.* 1:23–25.

Kyle, C.R. (1991). Ergogenics for bicycling. In: D.R. Lamb and M.H. Williams (eds.) *Perspectives in Exercise Science and Sports Medicine, Vol. 4: Ergogenics—Enhancement of Performance in Exercise and Sport.* Indianapolis, IN: Brown and Benchmark, pp. 373–413.

Kyle, C.R., and E.R. Burke (1984). Improving the racing bicycle. *Mech. Engineer.* 109:35–45.

Kyle, C.R., and V.J. Caiozzo (1986). Experiments in human ergometry as applied to the design of human powered vehicles. *Int. J. Sport Biomech.* 2:6–19.

Leadbetter W.B., and M.J. Schneider (1982). Orthopedics. In: J. Krausz (ed.) *The Bicycle Book.* New York: Dial Press, pp. 195–214.

Mackova, E., J. Melichna, Z. Placheta, D. Blahova, and B. Semiginovsky (1986). Skeletal muscle characteristics of sprint cyclists and nonathletes. *Int. J. Sports Med.* 7:295–297.

Maughan, R. (1991). Carbohydrate-electrolyte solutions during prolonged exercise. In: D.R. Lamb and M.H. Williams (eds.) *Perspectives in Exercise Science and Sports Medicine, Vol. 4: Ergogenics—Enhancement of Performance in Exercise and Sport.* Indianapolis, IN: Brown and Benchmark, pp. 35–86.

McCole, S.D., K. Claney, J.C. Conte, R. Anderson, and J.M. Hagberg (1990). Energy expenditure during bicycling. *J. Appl. Physiol.* 68:748–853.

Mellion, M.B. (1991). Common cycling injuries: management and prevention. *Sports Med.* 11:52–70.

Merrill, E.G. (1980). The B.C.C.S. physiological test program. British Cycling Coaching Scheme. *Coaching News,* Summer, 13–25.

Mitchell, J.B., and K.W. Voss (1991). The influence of volume on gastric emptying and fluid balance during prolonged exercise. *Med. Sci. Sports Exerc.* 23:314–319.

Montain, S.J., and E.F. Coyle (1992a). Fluid ingestion during exercise increases skin blood flow independent of increases in blood volume. *J. Appl. Physiol.* 73:903–910.

Montain, S.J., and E.F. Coyle (1992b). The influence of graded dehydration on hyperthermia and cardiovascular drift during exercise. *J. Appl. Pysiol.* 73:1340–1350.

Origenes, M.M., S.E. Blank, and R.B. Schoene (1993). Exercise ventilatory response to upright and aero-position cycling. *Med. Sci. Sports Exerc.* 25:608–612.

Phinney, D., and C. Carpenter (1992). *Training for Cycling.* New York: Perigee Books, pp. 65–88.

Pugh, L.G.C.E. (1974). The relation of oxygen intake and speed in competition cycling and comparative observations on the bicycle ergometer. *J. Physiol.* (London) 241:795–808.

Sacks, J.J., P. Holmgren, S.M. Smith, and D.M. Sosin (1991). Bicycle-associated head injuries and deaths in the United States from 1984 to 1988. *J. Am. Med. Assoc.* 266:3016–3018.

Saris, W.H.M., A.M.J. van Erp-Baart, K.R. Westerterp, and F. ten Hoor (1989). Study on the food intake during extreme sustained exercise: The Tour de France. *Int. J. Sports Med.* 10:S26–S31.

Sherman, W.M. (1991). Carbohydrate feedings before and after exercise. In: D.R. Lamb and M.H. Williams (eds.) *Perspectives in Exercise Science and Sports Medicine, Vol. 4: Ergogenics—Enhancement of Performance in Exercise and Sport.* Indianapolis, IN: Brown and Benchmark, pp. 1–34.

Sherman, W. M. (1992). Recovery from endurance exercise. *Med. Sci. Sports Exerc.* 24:S336–S339.

Sjögaard, G., B. Nielsen, F. Mikkelsen, B. Saltin, and E.R. Burke (1982). *Physiology of Cycling.* Ithaca, NY: Movement Publications, pp. 33–37.

Soden, P.D., and B.A. Adeyefa (1979). Forces applied to a bicycle during normal cycling. *J. Biomech.* 12:527–541.

Swain, D.P., J.R. Coast, P.S. Clifford, M.C. Milliken, and J. Stray-Gundersen (1987). Influence of body size on oxygen consumption during cycling. *J. Appl. Physiol.* 62:668–672.

Swain, D.P., J.R. Coast, M.C. Milliken, P.S. Clifford, R. Vaughan, and J. Stray-Gundersen (1988). Is there an optimum body size for competitive cycling? In: E.R. Burke and M.M. Newsom (eds.) *Medical and Scientific Aspects of Cycling.* Champaign, IL: Human Kinetics, pp. 39–46.

van Ingen Schenau, G.J., J.J. de Koning, and G. de Groot (1992). The distribution of anaerobic energy in 1000 and 4000 meter cycling bouts. *Int. J. Sports Med.* 13:447–451.

White, J.A., G. Quinn, M. Al-Dawalibi, and J. Mulhall (1982a). Seasonal changes in cyclists' performance—part 1. The British Olympic road race squad. *Br. J. Sports Med.* 16:4–12.

White, J.A., G. Quinn, M. Al-Dawalibi, and J. Nulhall (1982b). Seasonal changes in cyclists' performance—part 2. The British Olympic track squad. *Br. J. Sports Med.* 16:13–21.

Whitt, F.R., and D.G. Wilson (1982a). *Bicycling Science.* Cambridge: MIT Press, pp. 29–67.

Whitt, F.R., and D.G. Wilson (1982b). *Bicycling Science.* Cambridge: MIT Press, pp. 71–80.

Wood, J. G. (1986). An investigation of the relative thermal comfort of bicycle helmets. (Unpublished B.Sc. dissertation, Faculty of Engineering, University of Southampton, England.)

Zawadzki, K.M., B.B. Yaspelkis, and J.L. Ivy (1992). Carbohydrate-protein complex increases the rate of muscle glycogen storage after exercise. *J. Appl. Physiol.* 72:1854–1859.

DISCUSSION

COYLE: The conventional training programs of cyclists are obviously not specifically designed for particular events. The physiological demands of track cycling events, e.g., the 1-km sprint of 1 min duration and the 4-km race of about 5 min, are similar to those of track running and swimming events of equivalent duration. But cyclists do little anaerobic, high-intensity training. Cyclists could improve a great deal by following the simple principle of specificity. Ordinary athletes who have not followed the conventional "road distance" program but have trained specifically for the short-duration events have been placing very well in national championships. Of course, we hear the old claims that "elite performers wouldn't respond the same way to that kind of training" and "those non-elite cyclists still haven't won any gold medals," but I just don't buy that sort of rationalization.

KNUTTGEN: Is this failure to follow the principle of specificity in cycling training a national or an international phenomenon? Is there any evidence from the training programs of cyclists from the former Soviet Union, East Germany, France, Spain, Denmark, etc., that cyclists and coaches from other countries are similarly unenlightened?

BURKE: Some countries seem to be on target. Given the level of talent available, the Australian national team has been very successful in cycling in 1993, perhaps because their coach, Charlie Walsh, trains his cyclists more according to the specificity principle. Likewise, the coaches of the former East German team were more advanced in their training techniques.

COYLE: There are some rather strange findings in cycling research. For example, you have noted that some of the best sprint cyclists in the world do not have high proportions of fast twitch fibers in their knee extensors; in fact, they have mostly slow twitch fibers. Furthermore, it is often assumed that more fast twitch muscle fibers are used at faster pedal revolutions, but the glycogen depletion data of Ahlquist et al. indicate that fast twitch fibers are recruited less frequently at 100 rpm than at slower rates; i.e., more glycogen is used in fast twitch fibers at slower pedaling rates. It turns out that, at lower rpm, more fast twitch fibers must be recruited to produce more force per revolution.

TERJUNG: Is there evidence of a fiber type difference between competitors who are "spinners" (high rpm during a climb) versus those who are "grunters" (relatively low rpm during a climb)?

BURKE: Not to my knowledge. It is interesting that some of the spinners think they are using higher pedaling rates than they actually are while climbing. They might tell you that they are spinning at 80–90 rpm when they are really down around 60 rpm.

COYLE: We sometimes go overboard in suggesting that the aerodynamic properties of the cycling equipment are the most important factors in determining aerodynamics. In fact, two-thirds of the resistance is offered by the cyclist's body. If you can use the bikes to make the cyclist's body more aerodynamic, that is by far the most important factor. As I understand it, that is the reason that the Chris Boardman bicycle was superior. It positioned him in such a way that he was flatter and the air was able to flow more easily between his legs.

BURKE: I agree with you.

HAGERMAN: Boardman finished eighth in the world's championships after failing to qualify for the finals the year before. Are there any factors other than his equipment to help explain his improvement?

BURKE: I think his training did improve, and they did do more fine tuning of his position on the bike. Psychological changes associated with the new bike may also have played a role. When the USA National Team cyclists showed up with their new bikes, new wheels, etc., at the 1984 Olympic Games, they felt they could not be beat. I am sure Chris Boardman experienced similar feelings; he suddenly felt at least the equal of if not superior to the other athletes because he knew he had the fastest bike on the track.

KRAEMER: I am impressed by the amount of hypertrophy in the thigh muscles of sprint cyclists. How much supplementary resistance training is done to help produce it?

BURKE: I have no solid evidence on that issue. As in most sports, the highly mesomorphic athlete tends to migrate toward the sprint and power events.

HORSWILL: Do some of the sprinters use anabolic steroids to increase muscle mass and power?

BURKE: Yes, they do, along with growth hormone and other drugs. It has been said that, if there is anything new in ergogenic aids, it is being used by cyclists.

HAGERMAN: Are all fruits easily digestible? In training for marathon running, I can not eat apples because they seem to produce intestinal gas and cause a lot of esophageal reflux. Should all fruits be described as easily digestible?

BURKE: Relative to the ham and cheese sandwiches most road cyclists eat, I think all fruits are easily digestible. Also, remember that the exercise intensity while riding in a large pack is probably less than 50% $\dot{V}O_2$max; this might give fewer problems with digestion than marathon running.

COYLE: Road cyclists who do not ingest carbohydrate throughout exercise and need energy to delay fatigue must consume highly concentrated carbohydrate solutions in order to deliver sufficient carbohydrate to the intestines. The more concentrated it is, the greater the rate of delivery of carbohydrate (not fluid) from the stomach to the intestines. We used 400 mL of a 50% carbohydrate solution in our initial studies to make sure we had enough carbohydrate. That is a large volume of concentrated carbohydrate, and cyclists can more easily tolerate 200 mL of a 50% solution without having adverse effects. A 100 g dose is certainly tolerable. By the way, the 50% solution should be a solution of maltodextrins, starch, or some homogenized solid carbohydrate, not simple sugars, which would be disgustingly sweet.

KANTER: One hundred g of carbohydrate may be tolerable, but is it optimal? Would not it be better to ingest small doses of carbohydrate at the rate of 15 g every 15 min or so? Then you wouldn't be in a position of having to take a bolus dose of 100 g of carbohydrate in the latter stages of a race.

COYLE: Yes, it is better to ingest carbohydrate throughout exercise at 30–60 g/h, but if you can not do that in the early stages of the race, we recommend more concentrated solutions to provide a lot of energy late in the race.

BURKE: You are pointing out some of the dilemmas that I have raised as to how tolerable the concentrated carbohydrate solutions can be when compared to apples and bananas for each of 10 individual riders in a race. One person may tolerate a 10% solution, another a 6% solution, and another loves apples, etc. I can guarantee that I have cyclists taking in 200–400 g of carbohydrate over a 2-h period and somehow emptying it. I wonder whether it is the intermittent intensity of road cycling that allows rapid emptying at certain times during the race.

COYLE: There is tremendous interindividual variability, e.g., two-to three-fold differences, in rates of gastric emptying and delivery to the intestine. Subjects have to experiment with various carbohydrate solutions to see what works for them.

NADEL: Why would people want to take in more than 2 g of glucose per minute or 120 g/h? Maximal glucose oxidation rate is probably not more than 1.5 to 2 g/min during strenuous steady-state exercise.

BURKE: I do not know the scientific explanation, but talk to good stage riders and they will tell you that they are eating during that stage in preparation for tomorrow's stage. When they get off the bikes, they are exhausted; they can't sit down and eat big meals. A cyclist who consumes 6,000 kcal/d must eat a lot of that during the 8-h ride.

MAUGHAN: A large part of the carbohydrate that is ingested can not be accounted for, at least over the time scale in which we are interested. It is not oxidized. Some of it sits in the gut, but much of it seems to disappear. Therefore, if the goal is to oxidize 1 g/min, the cyclist probably must consume carbohydrate at a much greater rate than that.

EKBLOM: Why don't road cyclists eat fat during long races so they can spare glycogen and get ready for the race on the following day?

BURKE: Actually, cyclists traditionally do eat plenty of fat in their race food.

COYLE: There may be a role for fat during cycling races. During intense exercise, i.e., 85% of $\dot{V}O_2$max, fatty acid entry into the plasma from fat depots is slow, resulting in suboptimal fatty acid concentrations in the blood. It is possible that medium chain triglycerides, which are easily digested and absorbed and do not require transport across the mitochondrial membrane, might be readily oxidized so that glycogen can be spared. On the other hand, ingesting long-chain triglycerides probably would not help much.

SPRIET: It is not the fat store that is critical, but getting free fatty acids into the blood stream. It has been suggested that athletes might use small doses of heparin, which will mobilize the lipoprotein lipase from the various tissues and hydrolyze the triglycerides that are already circulating in the blood stream. This is another way to increase free fatty acids in the plasma, but this is a dangerous procedure and should not be advocated.

Ed, you gave me the impression that cycling sprints lasting about 10 s require energy primarily from the ATP and phosphocreatine system. The glycolytic system is also activated maximally or near-maximally during the initial 6–10 s of a sprint bout and makes a major contribution to the energy requirements of match sprinting.

BURKE: I have realized that recently, because the blood lactates we recorded after maximal 10–12 s sprints reached almost 14 mM.

GISOLFI: Many years ago we noticed a high incidence of hypertension is some cyclists we were studying. Is there any systematic evidence that cyclists tend to become hypertensive?

BURKE: I know of nothing in the literature.

NADEL: Carl, we have observed that subjects who are dehydrated tend to be hypertensive during exercise, relative to euhydrated controls. Perhaps a decreased preload on the heart in these dehydrated subjects causes reflexes to protect against a fall in arterial blood pressure during exercise, and they overcompensate. Could dehydration have played any part in your observations on cyclists?

GISOLFI: No. Our subjects were not dehydrated. Good try, though, Ethan!

8

Physiology and Nutrition for Middle Distance and Long Distance Running

Ron Maughan, Ph.D.

INTRODUCTION

For the purposes of this review, running events at all distances from 1,500 m upwards will be considered. Among runners, events from 1500–5000 m are usually classified as middle distance and events at 10,000 m or longer as distance races. Races at distances longer that the marathon (42.2 km, or 26.2 miles) are commonly termed ultra-distance. In recent years, participation in marathon races has declined, and the popular city marathons have been largely replaced by events at distances of 10,000 m or at the half marathon distance. Among serious athletes, there has been a growing interest in ultra-distance races, especially over 100 km or 24 hours; although these are still very much minority events, they do raise some interesting physiological problems. Based on the physiological demands of the events, the runners' distinction between middle distance and long distance is realistic, although the classification is based solely on the experiences of coaches and athletes. The requirements for successful performance at the marathon distance are quite different from those at 1500 m, and these differences will emerge in the discussions which follow.

CHARACTERISTICS OF ELITE COMPETITORS

Physical Characteristics

Age. It is a matter of common experience that athletic performance deteriorates with age, but the age at which optimum performance can be expected to occur in different events is not clear. Most elite performers in distance running events record their best performances between the ages of 20 and 30 years, and a study of the ages of medal winners at major championships and of world record holders tends to confirm this. There is a general trend for sprinters to be younger than distance runners, and most runners find that their preferred racing distances increase as they grow older. This was demonstrated by Moore (1975), who plotted world age bests at different distances; the updated records suggest that performance deteriorates in both sprint and long distance events, but that the rate of decrease in sprinting ability is greater than that in endurance capacity. Some confirmation of this trend was provided from a comparison of the results of a 30-km running event with those from a 90-km cross-country ski race: the best performances in the 30-km race were achieved by runners in the 26–30 age group, whereas the fastest times in the ski race were recorded by individuals aged 31–36 years (Böttiger, 1973).

In the past, marathon runners were generally athletes who turned to distance running after racing careers over shorter distances on the track. Although it is now more common for younger runners to attempt the marathon distance without experience over shorter distances, the data referred to above show that it is still the case that most successful competitors in long distance races are older than those in shorter distance events. Schulz and Curnow (1988) studied the records of competitors in the Olympic Games since the first Games in 1896; these results again confirm the suggestion that success occurs at a greater age in the longer distance events. As with all generalizations, however, there are many exceptions, e.g., several of the top male sprinters at the Barcelona Olympics, including the 100-m gold medalist, were considerably older than all of the medalists in the marathon. In spite of regulations that prevent young athletes from running marathons in some countries, outstanding performances can be achieved by some young competitors, e.g., the sixth fastest time ever for the marathon by a woman (2:24:07 by Wang Junxia) was recently set by an 18-year-old.

Body Composition. Although it is immediately apparent that there are substantial differences in physical characteristics between sprinters and long distance runners, elite distance runners come in a variety of shapes and sizes, and there are perhaps too many exceptions to make all but the broadest generalizations. The one outstanding anthropometric characteristic of successful competitors in all distance running events is a low body fat content (Carter, 1982). In a study of a population of runners who were rather heterogeneous with respect to training status and athletic ability, Housh et al. (1986) observed a significant relationship between body composition and the best time that could be achieved over a distance of 2 miles. This relationship may at least in part be explained by an association between the amount of training carried out and the body composition: body fat content tends to decrease as the volume of training increases (Figure 8-1).

There are problems in applying the standard methods for assessing body composition to athletic populations, and it is not clear that any of the commonly used methods is entirely reliable. Pollock et al. (1977) demonstrated that predictive equations based on indirect methods are unreliable, i.e., equations generated from normal populations are not applicable to elite athletes. However, such methods have been widely used, and in the absence of any method of body composition analysis that can be accepted as free from error, these results will be referred to here.

Skinfold thickness estimates of body composition in 114 male runners at the 1968 U.S. Olympic Trial race gave an average fat content of 7.5% of body weight, less than half that of a physically active but not highly trained group (Costill et al., 1970). The low body fat content of female distance runners is particularly striking: values of less than 10–15% are commonly reported among elite performers (Wilmore & Brown, 1974; Graves et al., 1987). These observations will be discussed below in relation to the nutritional habits of these individuals. The occasional exceptions to the generalization that a low body fat content is a prerequisite for success are most likely to occur in women's ultra-distance running, and

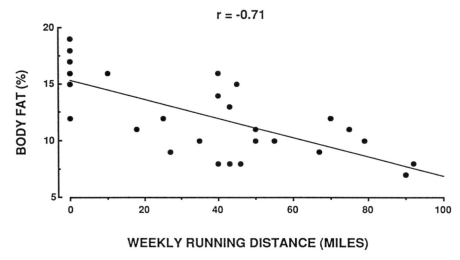

FIGURE 8-1. *Body fat content was estimated in a group of male runners who were in a steady state with respect to training load and body composition, and in a group of six weight-stable sedentary control subjects (shown at 0 miles training). The runners had all been training for at least 2 y and had completed the same weekly training distance without any change in body weight for at least 10 wk prior to the time of measurement. One of the effects of a high training load is to maintain a low body fat content.*

even world record holders at some distances have a high (in excess of 30%) body fat content. This probably reflects the under-developed state of women's long distance running; as more women take part, the level of performance can be expected to rise rapidly, and the elite performers are likely to conform to the model of their male counterparts and of successful women competitors at shorter distances.

Excess body fat serves no useful function (although a certain minimum amount of fat is necessary) but adds to the weight that has to be carried and thus increases the energy cost of running. Even in an event as long as the marathon, the total amount of fat oxidized does not exceed about 200 g. A 60-kg runner with 5% body fat will have 3 kg of fat, and a typical 55-kg female runner with 15% body fat will have more than 8 kg of body fat. Non-elite runners will commonly have at least twice this amount. Although not all of this is available for use as a metabolic fuel, the amount of stored fat is greatly in excess of that which is necessary for immediate energy production.

Anaerobic Power and Capacity

Muscular exercise is possible only if the ATP resynthesis rate is equal to the rate of ATP hydrolysis. Anaerobic ATP formation is necessary to supplement oxidative metabolism in the first few minutes of exercise until oxygen delivery increases to meet the demand and in circumstances where the power output demands a rate of energy utilization greater than that which can be met by oxidative metabolism alone. The proportion of the total energy cost met by anaerobic metabolism is clearly higher in events of shorter duration. In middle distance running, the rate of energy expenditure is much greater than the rate at which oxidative metabolism can supply energy, and a high capacity for anaerobic metabolism is essential for successful performance. Åstrand and Rodahl (1986) estimated the relative contribution of anaerobic metabolism to the total energy demand to be about 30% in a maximum effort of 4 min duration, decreasing to 5% over 30 min, and to 1% in exercise lasting for 2 h.

Snell (1990) estimated the oxygen cost of running at 4 min per mile to be about 84 mL·kg^{-1}·min^{-1} and calculated that the oxygen deficit incurred in running one mile (1604 m) at this speed is about 4.9 L for a 70-kg runner with a $\dot{V}O_2$max of 70 mL·kg^{-1}·min^{-1}. Medbø et al. (1988) estimated the anaerobic capacity, measured as the maximum oxygen deficit that could be accumulated, to be equivalent to about 52–90 mL·kg^{-1}; values in male middle-distance runners were about 70–80 mL·kg^{-1}, and the lowest values were recorded by untrained subjects. Although peak power output can be attained within a few seconds of the onset of exercise, Medbø et al. (1988) showed that at least 2 min of exercise were necessary to maximally tax the anaerobic capacity; in exercise lasting about 9 min or longer, there was no further change in the total contribution of anaerobic metabolism.

In events of longer duration, the overall contribution of anaerobic metabolism to energy production declines, and the requirement for a high anaerobic capacity is of correspondingly less importance. Exercise at an intensity corresponding to $\dot{V}O_2$max typically cannot be sustained for longer than a few minutes; however, elite performers can run 5000 m-races at an intensity at or close to $\dot{V}O_2$max, and the substantial oxygen deficit incurred in the first few minutes will persist or even increase as the race progresses. Even at longer distances, anaerobic energy production will occur at intermediate points in a race if the pace is increased or if the course includes uphill phases. Some anaerobic effort is also normally involved in the closing stages during a sprint finish. Most of the outstanding performers at distances of 10,000 m or less are capable of running 1 mile in less than 4 min.

The anaerobic power that can be produced by endurance runners in standardized laboratory tests is, as might be expected, rather low compared with that of trained sprint athletes (Lorentzon et al., 1988). Marathon runners demonstrate low isometric strength of the quadriceps muscles relative to sprinters and tend to have less strength than healthy but untrained individuals (Maughan et al., 1983a). These observations are perhaps unsurprising in view of the smaller mass of the muscles of distance runners and in view of the high proportion of Type I fibers present in their muscles, but they may also reflect the training patterns of these athletes.

Aerobic Power

As the duration of running events increases, so does the proportion of the total energy demand that must be met by oxidative metabolism; thus, a high maximal oxygen uptake ($\dot{V}O_2$max) is a prerequisite for success in distance running. Running speed declines as the distance increases; based on current world records, it is apparent that the decrease in speed, and hence in oxygen demand, is rather gradual with increasing duration of effort (Figure 8-2). Few successful male runners have failed to record values of $\dot{V}O_2$max of less than 70 mL·kg^{-1}·min^{-1}, compared with typical values of 40–50 mL·kg^{-1}·min^{-1} for sedentary individuals. There have been several reports of individual values of 80–85 mL·kg^{-1}·min^{-1}, and it is notable that such exceptionally high values are more common in middle distance than in long distance athletes (see Noakes [1991] for references to individual values). Average $\dot{V}O_2$max values for elite women runners are only slightly less than the those for their male counterparts, but the highest reported values for female runners are generally substantially lower

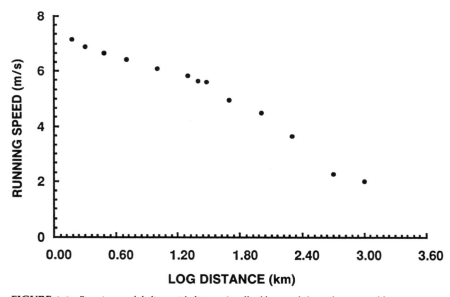

FIGURE 8-2. *Running speed declines with distance for all athletes, and this is demonstrated by an examination of the current world records at different distances. The shape of the curve, however, is not the same for an individual as it is for these composite data; the decline in the maximum sustainable speed with increasing distance will be more pronounced for the middle distance runner than for the ultra-marathoner.*

than the greatest values reported for males. The highest individual value ($73.3 \ mL \cdot kg^{-1} \cdot min^{-1}$) recorded for women appears to be that of Grete Waitz, who established a best marathon time of 2:25:29 (Noakes, 1991). In a group of elite female distance runners, including specialists at both middle and long distance events, Pate et al. (1987) found $\dot{V}O_2max$ values ranging from 61–73 $mL \cdot kg^{-1} \cdot min^{-1}$, with a mean value of 68.0 for the middle distance (5 km or less) runners and 66.4 for the long distance (10 km or more) specialists. A large part, but not all, of the difference between male and female runners can be accounted for by differences in body fat content. When values are expressed relative to lean body mass, the values obtained by women are closer to, but still less than, those of the best men.

When comparisons are made within groups of runners of widely different levels of performance, a good relationship between performance and $\dot{V}O_2max$ values is apparent. This is true for middle distance events (Foster et al., 1978; Ramsbottom et al., 1992; Camus, 1992) as well as for long distance events (Costill et al, 1973; Foster et al., 1977; Maughan & Leiper, 1983). The relationship between finishing time in a marathon race and $\dot{V}O_2max$ measured within a few weeks of the race is shown in Figure 8-3. Within groups of individuals of comparable levels of performance, however, there is no good relationship between $\dot{V}O_2max$ and performance (Conley & Krahenbuhl, 1980; Costill, 1972; Noakes, 1991), suggesting that, although a high capacity for oxidative metabolism is necessary for

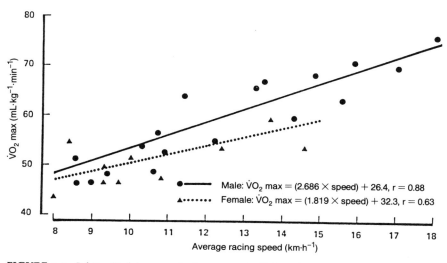

FIGURE 8-3. *Relationship between maximal oxygen uptake ($\dot{V}O_2max$) achieved in a laboratory treadmill running test and performance in male and female competitors in a marathon (42.2 km) race. Performance is expressed as the average running speed for the complete distance. All subjects took part in the same race, and all measurements were made within 2 wk of completion of the race. Reproduced with permission from Maughan and Leiper (1983).*

success in distance running, it does not, in itself, distinguish the elite performer. It is not unusual to find club athletes who can achieve $\dot{V}O_2$max values of 70–75 mL·kg^{-1}·min^{-1} in spite of their relatively modest performances. Similarly, much has been made of the fact that some exceptional athletes have failed to produce outstanding results in the laboratory. An athlete holding the current world's best marathon performance (2:08:33) was found to have a $\dot{V}O_2$max of 70 mL·kg^{-1}·min^{-1} (Costill et al., 1971), and a 2:10 marathon runner was more recently reported to have reached only 67 mL·kg^{-1}·min^{-1} (Sjödin & Svedenhag, 1985). Similarly modest values have been recorded for some elite middle distance runners. As an example, a value of 72 mL·kg^{-1}·min^{-1} was reported for Peter Snell, whose best mile time was 03:54.5, compared with 84.4 mL·kg^{-1}·min^{-1} for Steve Prefontaine, whose best mile performance was almost identical (03:54.6) (see Noakes [1991] for references). Although there have been dramatic improvements in world records over the years, measurements made on Don Lash, whose best mile time of 04:07.2s in 1937 was achieved with an oxygen uptake of 81.5 mL·kg^{-1}·min^{-1} (Dill et al., 1967), suggest that improvements in records cannot be attributed simply to greater aerobic power.

Before looking for a physiological explanation for these seemingly anomalous results, however, it should be remembered that in many of these studies measurements were made at times when the athletes who were tested were not at their peak fitness levels. The information is not usually given, but it is apparent that in some cases the laboratory tests were separated by a period of months or even years from the times when their best performances (to which the laboratory tests are related) were achieved. In addition, the exercise protocol in some cases involved horizontal running at increasing velocities, which is likely to result in termination of the test before $\dot{V}O_2$max is reached.

Fractional Utilization of Aerobic Capacity

In middle distance events, runners are exercising at intensities close to or above $\dot{V}O_2$max. Åstrand and Rodahl (1986) have estimated that trained athletes can sustain 100% of $\dot{V}O_2$max for 10 min, 95% for 30 min, 85% for 60 min, and 80% for 120 min. In the longer events, where the demand is met almost entirely by aerobic metabolism, runners with a high $\dot{V}O_2$max can meet the oxygen requirement by employing a relatively low fraction of their $\dot{V}O_2$max; runners who have a lower $\dot{V}O_2$max have to exercise at a relatively higher intensity to run at the same speed. Part of the apparent lack of a close association between $\dot{V}O_2$max and performance in long distance races may be accounted for by differences between individuals in the fraction of $\dot{V}O_2$max that can be sustained for the duration of a race. Although a good relationship between marathon running performance and the fraction of $\dot{V}O_2$max that can be sustained for the duration of the race is seen when runners of widely different levels of ability are compared (Figure 8-4), there is generally no such relationship seen when homogeneous groups are compared. The general trend does suggest that the fastest runners are characterized by an ability to run at a high fraction of $\dot{V}O_2$max over any given distance. This is hardly surprising, as the fraction of $\dot{V}O_2$max that can be maintained is more closely related to time than to distance, and the faster runners take less time to cover any given distance (Maughan, 1990). For any individual, however, the fraction of $\dot{V}O_2$max that can be sustained decreases with the distance. Davies and Thompson (1979) found that a group of highly trained marathon runners employed 94% of $\dot{V}O_2$max over 5 km (0:15:49), 82% over 42.2 km (2:31:00), and 67% over 84.4 km (5:58:00). One of the major effects of endurance training is to increase the ability to utilize a large fraction of $\dot{V}O_2$max for prolonged periods, and substantial improvements in racing performance can be achieved without any measurable change in $\dot{V}O_2$max.

Biomechanics and Running Economy

It requires no sophisticated laboratory analysis to distinguish between the elite runner and the jogger. Even the untrained eye can see the difference between the fluent running action of the best distance runners and the movement of the more modest performer. There are some prominent exceptions to this generalization, but they are rather few in number. An effective running style is partly an innate characteristic, but is also the result of a modification of this style by training. There is some evidence

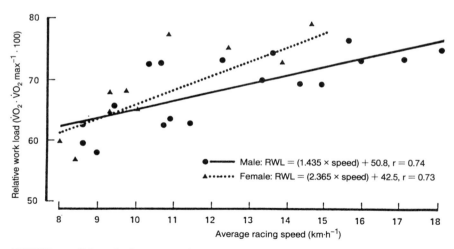

FIGURE 8-4. *Relationship between marathon performance and fractional utilization of maximal oxygen up-take ($\dot{V}O_2$max) in the same group of marathon runners as presented in Figure 8-3. Reproduced with permission from Maughan and Leiper (1983).*

that training status is an important determinant of running economy, which is a measure of the energy cost of running at a given speed. For example, Scrimgeour et al. (1986) showed that runners covering more than 100 km per week in training could run at a variety of speeds with a lower oxygen consumption than runners who did less training. As might be expected, running economy is a more important determinant of success at long rather than at short distances. Based on a review of the literature, Costill (1972) concluded that marathon runners use 5–10% less oxygen than middle distance runners to run at the same speed. Pollock (1977) later confirmed this observation. At a running speed of 16 km/h (10 mph), Cavanagh et al. (1977) found that the oxygen consumption of elite runners was about 6% less than that of well-trained non-elite competitors. Similar results were reported by Pate et al. (1987) for elite and non-elite female runners.

Even among elite runners, however, there may be large differences in the oxygen cost of running. In a group of world-class runners, Pollock et al. (1980) found the oxygen cost of treadmill running at a speed of 20 $km \cdot h^{-1}$ (12 mph) to range from 60.5 to 70.0 $mL \cdot kg^{-1} \cdot min^{-1}$. Rather surprisingly, Karlsson et al. (1972) reported that the oxygen cost of treadmill running at the same speed of 20 $km \cdot h^{-1}$ was remarkably constant: in a group of 20 elite runners, oxygen consumption varied from 67 to 71 $mL \cdot kg^{-1} \cdot min^{-1}$. In highly trained 10 km runners, the oxygen cost of running at a range of different speeds has been shown to be closely related to the best time that can be achieved (Conley & Krahenbuhl, 1980). Farrell et al. (1979) observed a significant relationship between the oxygen cost of running at a fixed speed and marathon running performance, but Costill et al. (1973), Foster et al. (1977), and Davies and Thompson (1979) all failed to find evidence for such a relationship. In spite of this conflict, a review of published data shows that the lowest oxygen uptake values at fixed running speeds have been recorded by the world's best distance runners (Sjödin & Svedenhag, 1985), suggesting that running economy is a factor in successful performance.

There have been several attempts to identify the factors that might account for the differences in running economy existing among runners. Cavanagh et al. (1977) compared elite and non-elite runners and found a slightly shorter stride length (and correspondingly higher stride frequency) in the elite runners when running at the same speed; these differences, however, were not statistically significant. The extent of vertical oscillation of the center of gravity was not different between the groups, and yet the energy cost of running was less for the better runners. In contrast, Matsuo et al. (1985) studied a group of non-elite female 3000-m runners, and found a good relationship between performance time and the displacement of the center of gravity during running. Williams and Cavanagh (1987) were unable to identify any single variable that could account for differences in running economy in a group of 31 trained runners; they concluded that many different factors each made a small contribution to the differences they observed among individuals.

In summary, these studies imply that differences in running economy exist when heterogeneous groups are studied and that large differences may exist even between runners of similar ability.

Muscle Fiber Composition and Metabolic Profile

It has been clearly established that Type I fibers predominate in the muscles of elite endurance athletes and that elite sprinters have muscles that consist mostly of Type II fibers (Saltin et al., 1977). Although early investigations commonly reported muscle fiber composition simply as the proportions of the different fiber types present, it is more meaningful, because of differences in the size of the major fiber types, to express composition as the proportion of total muscle cross-sectional area occupied by Type I or Type II fibers. For example, Sjöstrom et al. (1988) observed that the cross-sectional area of the Type IIA fibers of sprinters was almost twice as great as that of their Type I fibers, but that no such size differences between fiber types were apparent in marathon runners. They also reported structural abnormalities in the muscles of the distance runners that were not apparent in the muscles of the sprinters.

The muscles of endurance-trained individuals, or at least those muscles which have been trained, also have a high capacity for oxidative metabolism, i.e., the mitochondrial density is high, and activity of the enzymes involved in substrate oxidation is correspondingly high. These muscles also have a well-developed capillary network, allowing an increased perfusion of the muscle and an increased capillary transit time. The time course of adaptation of the muscles to training and detraining is, however, different from that of the observed changes in $\dot{V}O_2$max, and the magnitude of the responses is quite different. Enzyme activity changes rapidly in response to changes in the training load, and the changes are rather large relative to the changes in $\dot{V}O_2$max (Henriksson & Hickner, 1992).

Exercise intensity is a major factor influencing the adaptive response of muscle and of the different muscle fiber types (Dudley et al., 1982). Training volume is generally proportional to racing distance, and intensity is inversely related to volume; therefore, the higher training intensities of runners competing at distances of 1500-5000 m will result in greater adaptations of the Type II fibers. High-speed running that elicits more than 80% of $\dot{V}O_2$max appears to be necessary to produce a training response in Type IIB fibers. Marathon runners whose training consists primarily of long slow runs will seldom reach this intensity in training, and it is perhaps unsurprising that, even among long distance runners, there has been a trend towards a reduction in training volume and an increase in intensity in recent years.

The high oxidative capacity of the muscles of the elite endurance athlete is in part a reflection of the high proportion of Type I fibers present, reflecting a genetically determined predisposition to success in these events (Costill et al., 1976; Saltin et al., 1977). The muscles of these individuals also contain few Type IIB fibers, most of the fast twitch fibers being high oxidative Type IIA fibers. The activity of enzymes involved in oxidative metabolism is, however, generally high in both of the major fiber types in these individuals, reflecting an adaptation to the training program. Such is the capacity for adaptation that the oxidative capacity of the Type II fibers of the highly trained endurance athlete may exceed that of the Type I fibers of the sedentary individual. There are still, however, distinct fiber types present in the trained muscle, and the oxidative capacity of Type II fibers does not exceed that of Type I fibers from the same individual.

The major significance of the local adaptations within the muscle may be an increased capacity for the use of fat as a fuel, leading to a slower rate of depletion of the limited muscle glycogen stores. At the same exercise intensity, the trained individual has a greater rate of fat oxidation, reflecting an increased delivery of blood-borne free fatty acids secondary to the increased capillary supply of the muscle as well as the enhanced capacity of the muscle to oxidize fat.

Gender

In 1960, the best time ever recorded by a male marathon runner was 2:15:16. The best performance by a woman was 3:40:22, a record dating back to 1926. In 1970, the men's record was 2:08:33, and the women's record 2:52:53—the gap had narrowed to 54:19. A decade later, the men's record had not improved, but the women's record had been lowered to 2:25:24, so that the gap between the sexes was 17:08. At the time of writing this chapter, the men's record was 2:06:50, and the women's record 2:21:06. The rapid improvement in women's distance running performances has led to speculation that women's records will soon be superior to those of men (Whipp & Ward, 1992). The evidence does not, however, support this interpretation. Performances are generally improving in all women's events at a faster rate simply because relatively few women have participated in sport in the past—we are now seeing a catching-up phase. Men's performances will remain generally superior to those of women; exceptions to this rule will tend to occur in events or at distances that are contested only rarely.

Current world record performances for men and women at a variety of distances are compared in Table 8-1. The ratio of these performances is relatively constant across a wide range of distances; the relatively poorer performances of women at the long distances reflects the comparatively short history of women's participation in these events. Factors that may account for performance differences between men and women are identified in Table 8-2. Peak power output of women is generally lower than that of men, reflecting in part the lower muscle mass; muscle strength per unit of muscle mass is generally similar in men and women (Ikai & Fukunaga, 1968; Maughan et al., 1983b). Female athletes generally achieve lower $\dot{V}O_2$max values than those of men competing in the same events. Part of this difference is a consequence of the higher body fat content of women, but the differences persist even after correction for body mass and body fat content. A number of factors contribute to the lower $\dot{V}O_2$max of women. These include a lower maximum cardiac output that, because maximal heart rates are similar, reflects a smaller stroke volume. Blood hemoglobin concentration is generally lower in women than in men, and this may have some significance for oxygen transport (Woodson, 1984). Hard endurance training tends to lower the circulating hemoglobin concentration, and anemia may be a problem for some female athletes. The low hemoglobin concentration of highly trained endurance athletes,

TABLE 8-1. *World record performances for men and women at distances from 1500 m to 100 km. All performances are track records, except for the marathon distance (42.2 km). In the right-hand column, the women's record is expressed as % of the men's best time. This ratio is remarkably consistent, except for the ultra-distance events, where the relatively poor women's record reflects the limited participation of women at these distances. The greatest distance run by a woman in 24 h (240 km) is 84% that of men (286 km).*

Distance (km)	Time Men	Women	%
1.5	3:28.9	3:52.7	90
1.6 (1 mile)	3:46.3	4:15.6	89
2	4:50.8	5:28.7	88
3	7:29.5	8:22.6	89
5	12:58.3	14:37.3	89
10	26:58*	30:13.7	89
42.2	2:06:50	2:21:06	90
50	2:48:06	3:36:58	77
100	6:10:20	8:01:01	77

*This performance, recorded in Oslo on July 10, 1993, has been included, although it was not yet ratified at the time of writing.

TABLE 8-2. *Factors that may account for performance differences between male and female runners*

Factor	Factor Potentially Affects:
Muscle mass	force production
	peak power output
Body composition	oxygen cost of running
Heart size	maximum oxygen uptake
Hemoglobin concentration	maximum oxygen uptake
Muscle enzyme activity	relative use of fat and carbohydrate as fuels
Biomechanical differences	running economy

whether male or female, is, however, most commonly a pseudo-anemia resulting from a disproportionate expansion of the plasma volume. The potentially adverse effects of a low hemoglobin concentration may be offset, at least in part, by the raised 2,3-DPG content of red blood cells seen in endurance-trained women (Pate et al., 1985).

Muscle fiber types are normally distributed in both sexes, with no sex difference in the relative proportions of the major fiber types present (Nygaard, 1981). There have been suggestions of an increased reliance on fat as a metabolic fuel during exercise in women, leading to a sparing of glycogen, but there are conflicting reports in the literature (Maughan, 1990).

POTENTIAL LIMITATIONS TO PERFORMANCE

Although the existence of a single factor that limits the performance of all individuals in all situations is unlikely, several clues as to the possible limitations to performance in distance running are readily apparent from the study of the characteristics of elite performers. Other information comes from measurements made during competition or in the laboratory, but the evidence is inevitably circumstantial at best.

Cardiovascular and Pulmonary Function

The primary requirement in middle distance running is the ability to sustain a high power output for short periods of time, whereas the challenge facing the long distance runner is that of maintaining a submaximal effort over prolonged periods. For the middle distance runner, a high $\dot{V}O_2$max is, therefore, a prerequisite, whereas the long distance runner can compensate to some degree for a lower $\dot{V}O_2$max by the ability to sustain a high fraction of aerobic power for prolonged periods. The significance of $\dot{V}O_2$max, of the fraction of $\dot{V}O_2$max that can be sustained, and of running economy is discussed elsewhere in this chapter.

The limitations to $\dot{V}O_2$max have recently been reviewed (Maughan, 1992). There has been considerable debate as to where the limitation to $\dot{V}O_2$max resides. Endurance-trained individuals have a highly developed cardiovascular system, and their muscles also have a high capacity for oxidative metabolism. The balance of the available evidence suggests that in circumstances in which a large muscle mass is involved, as in running, oxygen utilization is limited by the rate at which it can be delivered to the working muscles rather than by the capacity of those muscles to utilize oxygen. There remain, however, several potential limitations to oxygen delivery.

Until recently, it was generally considered that there was no limitation on oxygen uptake imposed by the lungs, but a number of recent reports demonstrate arterial desaturation during intense exercise in endurance-trained subjects. The implication of these observations is that there may be a pulmonary limitation to oxygen transport (Powers et al., 1993). In as many as 50% of elite distance runners, the arterial oxygen saturation may fall during sea-level exercise at intensities close to $\dot{V}O_2$max; these runners will be particularly liable to suffer decrements in performance during events held at altitude. The oxygen content of the blood may fall in exercise at intensities close to maximum because of a mismatch between perfusion of the vascular bed and local diffusion capacity (Dempsey, 1986; Wagner et al., 1986). When the cardiac output is very high, pulmonary capillary transit time may be too short to allow complete equilibration to occur. The fact that desaturation occurs in athletes rather than in sedentary individuals may be a consequence of the relative insensitivity of the lungs to training (Dempsey, 1986). Elite distance runners can achieve cardiac outputs 2–3 times greater than those of sedentary individuals, but the differences in maximum ventilatory function and pulmonary diffusion capacity are small. Perhaps distance runners should give some thought to efforts to improve functional lung capacity.

An individual's $\dot{V}O_2$max is closely related to the maximum cardiac output that can be achieved. Because maximal heart rate is little influenced by training status and tends, if anything, to decrease, it is clear that stroke volume is a major determinant of $\dot{V}O_2$max (Savard et al., 1986, 1987) and, hence, of distance running performance. Blood volume and the circulating hemoglobin concentration also have an influence on $\dot{V}O_2$max (Kanstrup & Ekblom, 1984), and the practice of removal and subsequent re-infusion of whole blood or red blood cells has been employed by athletes to improve performance, with apparent success. Coyle et al. (1990) have shown that the use of plasma volume expanders to increase the circulating volume by about 4% can increase $\dot{V}O_2$max; larger increases are not effective, presumably because of the hemodilution that results. In view of these observations and of the importance of the oxygen-carrying capacity of the blood for oxygen transport, the decrease in circulating hemoglobin concentration that commonly occurs in trained athletes seems surprising. Often referred to as sports anemia, this condition is not a true anemia; the total red cell mass is unchanged or even increased. It is the result of a disproportionate increase in the plasma volume in response to the training stimulus.

Energy Metabolism

The relative contributions of anaerobic and aerobic metabolism to energy production in events over different distances have been referred to above. The primary factor influencing the metabolic response to exercise is the intensity; the higher the intensity, the greater the energy demand and the greater the proportion of the total energy turnover that is met by carbohydrate metabolism. When the exercise intensity exceeds about 95% of $\dot{V}O_2$max, the contribution of fat oxidation to energy metabolism is negligible. Using Snell's estimate of 5.6 L/min as the oxygen cost of running at a 4-min-mile pace for a 70-kg runner, and assuming that the entire energy demand could be met by oxidation of muscle glycogen, it can be calculated that the rate of carbohydrate oxidation necessary to meet this rate of energy expenditure would be 7.5 g/min. Assuming, however, that the energy supply was met entirely by anaerobic glycolysis, the rate of carbohydrate degradation would be approximately 100 g/min. For a runner with a $\dot{V}O_2$max of 70 mL·kg^{-1}·min^{-1}, who can use 75% of that value in the first minute and 100% thereafter, and ignoring the contribution of creatine phosphate hydrolysis, the total carbohydrate degradation during the 1-mile race would be about 110 g. Of this amount, some 85 g would be converted to lactate, which, if distributed equally throughout 85% of the body water space, would reach a concentration of just over 26 mmol/L. Osnes and Hermansen (1972) reported a post-race blood lactate concentration of approximately 24 mmol/L in an athlete who ran 1500 m at a slightly slower pace in 03:48, which is equivalent to about 04:06 for 1 mile; they also found a similar value in a runner who completed 5000 m in a time of 13:46.

These rough calculations show that the amount of muscle glycogen used is small relative to the whole body glycogen store and that substrate availability should not be limiting in events over this distance. There are, however, suggestions that the availability of muscle glycogen may limit the performance of events of this duration (Maughan & Greenhaff, 1991), perhaps because of depletion in specific muscle fiber pools. The implications of lactate accumulation for acid-base status and fatigue are discussed below.

At submaximal exercise intensities, the contribution of fat oxidation to energy production increases with time, but the contribution of fat to energy metabolism is likely to be insignificant at distances of less than 10 km run at race pace. Even at the marathon distance, where the energy demand can be met almost entirely by aerobic metabolism, the total amount of fat oxidized is small; if fat was the only fuel used, the total amount oxidized in a race would be no more than about 300 g. In contrast, if carbohydrate was the only fuel used, the total would be about 700 g, and this amount is considerably in excess of the amount that is normally stored. Carbohydrate availability is widely recognized as a potential limitation to long distance running performance, and carbohydrate ingestion during running is effective in improving performance (Wilber & Moffatt, 1992; Williams, 1989).

Disturbances in Acid-base Status

From the study of the energy metabolism in distance running, it is apparent that anaerobic glycolysis is a major factor in middle distance races, but is relatively unimportant in long distance events. When the rate of carbohydrate breakdown by the glycolytic enzymes in the cytoplasm exceeds the rate at which the pyruvate produced can be converted to carbon dioxide and water in the mitochondria, regeneration of cytoplasmic NAD is achieved by conversion of some of the pyruvate to lactate. At physiological pH, both pyruvate and lactate are essentially completely dissociated, and hydrogen ions also accumulate. Some of these hydrogen ions are buffered by the intracellular buffers (primarily proteins) and some diffuse into the extracellular space, where further buffering occurs (primarily by bicarbonate). The buffering, however, is incomplete, and pH of the intracellular and extracellular spaces will fall when there is significant lactate accumulation. There is some debate at present as to how far the pH in exercising muscle falls during exercise, partly as a result of methodological differences between biopsy data and data from nuclear magnetic resonance techniques, and there appear to be no reliable measurements on middle distance running.

There are several possible mechanisms by which a fall in pH may result in fatigue (Maughan & Greenhaff, 1991). It must be emphasized, however, that anaerobic glycolysis does allow a high rate of ATP production to be maintained. Reductions in the glycolytic rate, if not compensated for by other sources of energy production, would therefore have the effect of reducing exercise capacity. Increasing buffering capacity, on the other hand, might be expected to improve performance if the fall in pH is indeed limiting. There is evidence that performance in simulated competition over a distance of 800 m is significantly improved by ingestion of sodium bicarbonate in the pre-race period; Wilkes et al. (1983) observed a mean improvement of 2.9 s in a group of trained runners who achieved a time of 02:05.8 in the control trial. Several other studies involving high-intensity exercise of short duration have produced similar findings (Maughan & Greenhaff, 1991), and these results provide circumstantial evidence to support the idea that the fall in pH that occurs in this type of exercise can limit performance.

Fluid Balance and Thermoregulation

Most (about 75–80%) of the chemical energy liberated during substrate oxidation appears as heat. In an activity such as running on the level, the rate of heat production is a function of speed and body mass. If the rate of heat production exceeds that rate of heat loss from the body, as is normally the case during running, body temperature will rise. The direction of heat exchange between the body and the environment depends on skin temperature and climatic conditions, but heat is gained by radiation and convection in hot conditions. Evaporation of sweat is then the only available avenue of heat loss.

The rate of heat production during distance races obviously declines as the distance increases. In middle distance races, the rate of heat production is high, but the duration is short; only small changes in core temperature occur, although there is a substantial increase in muscle temperature. In longer races, hyperthermia and dehydration consequent upon sweat loss are potentially major problems, even to the extent of fatality. Heat exhaustion and collapse occur most often on hot days, but even at moderate (23°C) environmental temperatures, rectal temperatures may be elevated above 40°C in marathon runners (Pugh et al., 1967). Many of the highest values of rectal temperatures in distance runners have been seen after races at intermediate distances: among competitors in a 14-km road race, Sutton (1990) reported more than 30 cases over a period of years where rectal temperatures exceeded 42°C. In a single 10-km road race, England et al. (1982) reported 29 cases of heat illness, but their diagnostic criteria are unclear, and only 13 of these individuals recorded rectal temperatures of 39.7°C or greater. These data do, however, suggest that hyperthermia may be more common when the rate of heat production is very high. At very high exercise intensities, skin blood flow is likely to be reduced, with a larger fraction of the cardiac output being directed to the working muscles, so heat loss will be reduced. Among athletes, it is well recognized that performance is impaired in conditions of high temperature and humidity. This recognition is usually translated into a more cautious pace, helping to reduce the incidence of heat illness.

Although severe hyperthermia is associated with a reduction in the ability to continue running, the secondary problem of dehydration resulting from prolonged sweating may be more significant. Even in conditions of high temperature and humidity, sweat losses are small when the exercise duration is short. In the shorter middle distance events, sweat loss is negligible, but performance is reduced by prior dehydration (Armstrong et al., 1985), and athletes competing in these events may be dehydrated prior to exercise if proper attention is not paid to replacement of losses. In more prolonged exercise, sweat losses may be large, resulting in significant losses of body water and electrolytes, especially sodium. The rate of loss during distance running is generally in excess of the rate at which fluid is consumed, so some degree of hypohydration normally occurs. Even in the same race and with the same fluid intake, however, there is a large variation between runners in the extent of sweat loss; this may vary from 1–6% of body weight in a marathon run in moderate environmental conditions (Whiting et al., 1984). According to Sawka and Pandolf (1990), dehydration results in a greater impairment of performance in endurance events that rely primarily on aerobic metabolism than in those events where there is a significant contribution from anaerobic metabolism. This is supported by the results of Armstrong et al. (1985), who found that dehydration resulted in a 3.1% reduction in performance in a 1500-m race compared with a 6.3% reduction in a 10-km race. The factors influencing fluid and electrolyte homeostasis during exercise and the effects of disturbances in fluid balance on exercise performance have been the subject of extensive reviews (Gisolfi & Lamb, 1990; Maughan, 1991).

Current and recommended fluid intake practices of distance runners are described below.

Nutritional Limitations to Performance

The fuels used for energy production in distance running are fat and carbohydrate, with the contribution of carbohydrate increasing as the intensity of effort increases. In middle distance races, the contribution of fat is negligible. Because the demand for carbohydrate is high and the body's carbohydrate store is meager, its availability may limit performance. Many laboratory studies using bicycle exercise have shown a close association between the point at which the glycogen content of the exercising muscles falls close to zero and the subjective feeling of exhaustion. Studies using running exercise also show a fall in the muscle glycogen content, but significant amounts remain even at the point of exhaustion. Sherman et al. (1981) measured the glycogen content of the gastrocnemius muscle after a 20.9-km time trial (mean running time 83 min) and found postexercise muscle glycogen values of about 100 mmol/kg wet weight; this was about 50–65% of the pre-exercise value. Karlsson and Saltin (1971) found that the muscle glycogen content had fallen to about 30% of the preexercise value after a 30-km race. However, if a high carbohydrate diet was fed in the few days prior to exercise, the pre-exercise value was increased by 100%, and the post-exercise glycogen content was actually greater than the pre-exercise value observed after the normal diet. These results suggest that muscle glycogen depletion may be a less likely candidate for the limitation of exercise performance in running than in cycling. Again, however, the possibility of a limitation imposed by glycogen depletion in a specific fiber type cannot be ignored.

In middle distance running, the rate of glycogen breakdown is high, but the duration is short. Although it might be possible to use more than 100 g of muscle glycogen during a race over a distance of 1 mile, the total muscle glycogen content is likely to be at least 350 g, so glycogen availability should not be limited (Åstrand & Rodahl, 1986).

In cycling, there is an obvious relationship between the pre-exercise muscle glycogen content and the time for which exercise at a fixed intensity can be sustained (Sherman, 1991). Using similar models, it has also been clearly established that carbohydrate feeding during exercise can improve performance in prolonged exercise (Coyle, 1991; Maughan, 1991). There is also evidence to suggest that performance in exercise of only a few minutes duration is also influenced by the availability of carbohydrate as a metabolic fuel (Maughan & Greenhaff, 1991).

Although it is common for marathon runners to consume a high-carbohydrate diet in the days prior to exercise, there have been relatively few studies where the effects of carbohydrate feeding, either before or during exercise, have been investigated using running rather than cycling exercise. In the study of Karlsson and Saltin (1971) referred to above, it appeared that runners in a 30-km race slowed down less in the later stages of the race if they had consumed a high-carbohydrate diet in the days prior to the race; there was no difference between the trials in running speed at the beginning of the race, but the overall performance time was better after the high-carbohydrate diet.

Ingestion of carbohydrate during treadmill running can extend the running time at a fixed speed (Wilber & Moffatt, 1992) and can allow runners to maintain higher speeds in the later stages of a long run (Williams, 1989). These results suggest that an insufficient supply of carbohydrate as a metabolic fuel may limit performance during prolonged running.

HISTORY OF TRAINING AND NUTRITIONAL PRACTICES

Training

Distance running had its origins in England in the middle of the eighteenth century, when the sport was almost entirely professional, with rather few serious participants. Although the early pedestrians seem to have done little serious training, some of the performances were remarkable. For example, in 1753, the record for 10 miles was set at 54:30. After a race, it was common for no training to be done, and athletes then began preparations some weeks before the next race. Captain Barclay Allardice was an outstanding long distance pedestrian who, in 1810, walked 1000 miles in 1000 hours, covering 1 mile in each successive hour. His regimen of training, purging, sweating, and diet would have eliminated the weak and the poorly motivated. His approach to training was to develop stamina by large amounts of low-intensity exercise, and his recommendations to the athlete, which he appears to have followed himself, are as follows (Downer, 1902):

> He must rise at five in the morning, run half a mile at the top of his speed up hill, and then walk six miles at a moderate pace, coming in about seven to breakfast, which should consist of beef-steak or mutton chop, under-done, with stale bread and old beer. After breakfast, he must again walk six miles at a moderate pace, and at twelve lie down in bed without his clothes for half an hour. On getting up, he must walk four miles, and return by four to dinner, which should also be beef-steaks or mutton chops, with bread and beer as at breakfast. Immediately after dinner, he must resume his exercise by running half a mile at the top of his

speed, and walking six miles at a moderate pace. He takes no more exercise for that day, but retires to bed about eight, and next morning proceeds in the same manner.

It was another 100 y before the amateurs offered a serious challenge to the top professionals; a systematic approach to training and accurate record keeping date from this time. The history of training methods for distance running since that time is largely a history of the outstanding athletes who have progressively advanced the world records, and it is common for athletes to slavishly follow the training program of a success-ful competitor. There must be a suspicion, however, that most elite ath-letes would have succeeded whatever type of training they had followed.

An example of the training of elite middle distance runners of the late nineteenth century is that of W. G. George. Shortly after taking up athlet-ics, and at a time when the world record for 1 mile was 04:24.5, George announced publicly that he had prepared a schedule for a mile to be run in 04:12; this consisted of successive laps of 59, 63, 66 and 64 s. His training and racing were based on this schedule. Although the total amount of training was small by today's standards, he followed a regular schedule. He also introduced a novel form of indoor exercise, which he termed his "hundred up" and which he claimed to have performed throughout his career. This consisted of an alternate knee-raising and springing exercise. He set records at distances from 1 mile to 10 miles, but his times were generally inferior to the professional records of his contemporary William Cummings.

Because of financial difficulties, however, George turned professional and issued a challenge to Cummings. In 1885, Cummings beat George at 10 miles in a time of 51:06.6; this time would have won the AAA Cham-pionships every year up to 1958. In the summer of 1886, in preparation for a challenge at 1 mile, George regularly ran time trials over distances of ¾ mile and 1¼ miles, but rarely exceeded 2 miles per day in training. Cummings' preparation for the race consisted mostly of walking; he walked distances of 2-4 miles four times per day. Only once or twice per week did he run. On the day they met, George ran almost exactly to the schedule prepared 8 y earlier, to remove almost 4 s from the world record by finishing in a time of 04:12.75. This time was not beaten until 1915. These performances show that outstanding times could be achieved with little hard training.

An excellent account of the training of athletes of the late nineteenth century is contained in Downer (1902). This shows that walking remained a significant part of the training program of both middle distance and long distance runners, but that repeated sprints were beginning to be featured. These tended to be relatively few in number and to be run at speeds close to maximum effort, with long recovery periods. Time trials over various distances were a prominent part of the race preparation.

Since the beginning of the present century, the amount and intensity of training undertaken has progressively increased. Outstanding middle distance athletes, such as Nurmi, Zatopek, Elliot, and Snell, were renowned for the severity of their training schedules. One thing common to the training programs of all these athletes is the inclusion of a variable amount of high-intensity interval training. Nurmi appears to have relied heavily on long, slow walking in the early stages of his career, but later included some repeated sprints over distances of 80–120 m. Zatopek relied almost exclusively on interval training at some stages in his career, and would run up to 30 km per day, consisting of relatively fast intervals of 200–400 m separated by 200 m of slower running. Zatopek was of the opinion that better results were obtained with a greater volume of training, even if the intensity had to be reduced. Kuts followed the principles established by Zatopek, but increased the intensity and reduced the quantity of the intervals; he also ran more long intervals over distances of up to 3000 m— the total training volume remained high. The training program of Chataway, who achieved performances at 5000 m that were very similar to those of Kuts, was, however, totally different. Chataway relied on rather few high-intensity efforts, and the total volume of training was small.

Much emphasis was placed on the training programs of the most successful athletes, and these have been extensively copied by aspiring champions. The dramatic differences in the training programs of different athletes, suggests, however, that Roger Bannister was correct when he expressed the opinion that "training methods, being dependent on more factors than it is possible at present to analyze, are likely to remain empirical" (Bannister, 1955). The situation has changed little since then.

Nutrition

The training programs of the early years of distance running were light, but bore recognizable similarities to the schedules of modern athletes. The same cannot be said of their dietary habits. Some examples of the recommendations of Barclay Allardice at the beginning of the nineteenth century are as follows:

Animal diet is alone prescribed, and beef and mutton are preferred. Biscuit and stale bread are the only preparations of vegetable matter which are permitted. Vegetables are never given as they are watery and of difficult digestion. Fish must be avoided. Salt, spices, and all kind of seasonings, with the exception of vinegar, are prohibited. Liquors must always be taken cold, and home brewed beer, old but not bottled, is best. Water is never given alone. It is an established rule to avoid liquids as much as possible. (Downer, 1902)

It was a strong man who could survive this regimen, to which was added emetics, purgatives, and "sweating liquors." To be able to run after submitting to this treatment is nothing short of remarkable.

It will be noted that the diet emphasized a high protein intake, a limited amount of carbohydrate, very little in the way of fruit or vegetables, and a restricted fluid intake. The belief in the need for high protein consumption and restricted fluids remained fashionable at least until the end of the century (Downer, 1902), and these ideas persist to some degree at the present time.

CONTEMPORARY TRAINING AND NUTRITION PRACTICES

Talent Selection and Laboratory Assessment

The ultimate test of an athlete's ability is performance on the road or running track, and most athletes inevitably gravitate to the events to which they are genetically and constitutionally best suited. Laboratory tests are no substitute for this evaluation process, but they may have some uses in identification of the individual strengths and weaknesses of the athlete, and in monitoring progress in response to training.

There is an enormous body of literature providing descriptive information on the physical and physiological characteristics of athletes of all standards. Although some general patterns emerge, as described above for the elite performer, the predictive power of laboratory tests is generally not high because of the multiplicity of factors that contribute to athletic success. In many, perhaps even most, cases, the results of physiological assessments of elite athletes are of more value to the scientist who wishes to understand the limitations to human performance than to the athlete or coach.

Identification of predisposition to success in specific events has been attempted based on measurement of variables that are largely genetically determined; these include muscle fiber composition, cardiovascular dimensions, and anthropometric characteristics (MacDougall et al., 1982). Such measurements, however, ignore several important characteristics, of which the most significant might be the responsiveness to training, the resistance to injury, and the psychological component.

Measurement of $\dot{V}O_2$max has traditionally been the laboratory procedure of choice for the evaluation of endurance fitness. The realization that both a high $\dot{V}O_2$max and the ability to run at a high fraction of this value for prolonged periods are important has led to a re-assessment of testing procedures for endurance athletes. Many different laboratory tests that take both of these factors into account have been introduced in recent years. Most of these rely on some measurement of the running speed at which a contribution to total energy production from anaerobic metabolism becomes apparent. This can be established by measurement of the blood lactate accumulation, or of changes in ventilation consequent to the resulting metabolic acidosis, and is commonly referred to as the "anaerobic threshold." An alternative to the establishment of a threshold value, which is associated with some methodological difficulties, is the estimation of running speed at which a fixed blood lactate concentration (most commonly 2 or 4 mmol/L) is achieved. This latter value is referred to at the onset of blood lactate accumulation (OBLA). In reviewing the available information on the physiological variables associated with marathon running performance, Sjödin and Svedenhag (1985) concluded that some measure of the onset of anaerobic metabolism is the single variable that shows the closest relationship with race performance.

Training

As in the past, training practices of the elite performers show little consistency among individuals, and it seems possible to achieve success at the highest level with very different methods of preparation. This appears, at least to the author, to indicate that genetic endowment is of greater significance than the precise details of the training schedule. There appear to be differences among individuals in the trainability of the cardiovascular system and of the muscles, and this may be an important part of the genetic endowment. It is undoubtedly true that many mediocre athletes train more intensively than most elite performers, although they remain unable to achieve comparable levels of performance.

There have always been debates among athletes and coaches as to whether the training emphasis should be on quantity or on quality, and there are certainly some indications that the intensity of the effort in training may be of greater significance than the total volume of training (Wenger & Bell, 1986). Because of the difficulties involved in the quantification of the intensity at which training is carried out, it is not possible to verify whether or not this is reflected in the training programs of elite runners. Every serious runner, however, keeps a record of the distance covered in training, and training volume is thus easy to measure.

Several studies have related training indices to running performance, mostly at the marathon distance. In a group of runners of diverse ability (n = 50, 2:19:00–4:58:00), Hagan et al. (1981) showed that the mean weekly running distance in the two months immediately preceding a race showed the highest correlation with racing performance. Even in a more heterogeneous group (n = 12, best performance <2:30) Sjödin and Svedenhag (1985) observed a statistically significant relationship between weekly training distance and performance. The association between training volume and performance, although statistically significant, should not be taken to imply a cause-and-effect relationship; more is not necessarily better, and in many cases, increasing training volume is associated with an increased risk of injury, infectious illness, and psychological problems.

High training volumes may have some effects on the economy of running and may also play a role in keeping the body fat content low. There seems, however, to be a need for the inclusion of some high-intensity effort in the training program. This seems reasonable because low-intensity efforts will not recruit the Type II muscle fibers, and the local adaptations that result in an increased oxidative capacity of the muscle will not occur unless fibers are active. If the exercise duration is sufficiently long to result in fatigue of the Type I fibers, recruitment of the Type II fibers will occur, even when the intensity is low. Training exclusively by running long distances at slow speeds has been proposed, and long slow distance (LSD) training was popular in North America in the 1970s. Although one or two successful marathon runners claimed to employ this training strategy, it quickly fell into disuse, suggesting a lack of effectiveness. Most distance runners include some such training runs in their schedule, but the emphasis at present is more on fast runs over shorter distances.

Nutrition

It is now widely recognized that nutrition plays an important role in supporting an intensive training load and in allowing optimum performance in competition. Although runners, relative to athletes in other sports, are generally well-informed on nutritional issues, they are often more concerned with nutritional preparation for competition, whereas nutrition may have its biggest impact on performance by supporting the routine training load.

Diet for Training. Hard training increases the body's energy requirement, and the energy intake must be increased to meet extra expenditure. Much of the training will inevitably be at a relatively high intensity and will place heavy demands on the limited carbohydrate stores that are available in the liver and muscle glycogen depots. For runners in steady state with respect to training load and body weight, both total energy intake (Figure 8-5) and carbohydrate intake (Figure 8-6) are closely related to the distance covered in training each week (Maughan et al., 1989).

It is recommended that all athletes consume a high-carbohydrate diet in training, with carbohydrate contributing 60% or more of total energy intake (Williams & Devlin, 1992). This is substantially higher than the amount of carbohydrate supplied by the typical Western diet, where carbohydrate supplies no more than about 40–45% of energy intake (Gregory et al., 1990), and has led to repeated calls for athletes to increase their intake of sugars and starches. Although the idea that a high-carbohydrate diet is

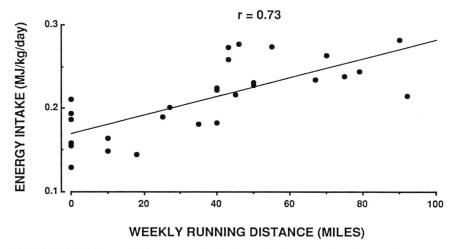

FIGURE 8-5. *Total energy intake increases with the volume of training carried out. A statistically significant relationship is observed between these two variables even without correction for body weight. Expression of energy intake relative to body weight increases the closeness of the relationship. These data were obtained from the subjects described in Figure 8-1.*

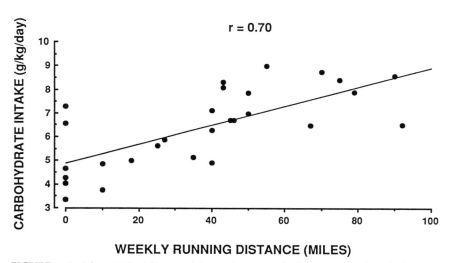

FIGURE 8-6. *A large intake of dietary carbohydrate is often stated to be necessary to allow a high training load to be sustained. These data, obtained from the same group of subjects as described in Figure 8-1, show that there is a significant relationship between the self-selected carbohydrate intake and the training load, but also show a wide variability among individuals.*

essential to sustain high-intensity training on a daily basis is intuitively attractive, there is little experimental support (Sherman et al., 1993; Sherman & Wimer, 1991). A large number of experimental studies have manipulated the diets of runners and other endurance athletes for short periods during which intensive training is continued. These studies have generally shown that a diet which provides 5 g of carbohydrate per kg body weight per day to athletes training hard over 7 d is insufficient to prevent a progressive fall in the muscle glycogen content, whereas 10 $g \cdot kg^{-1} \cdot d^{-1}$ will maintain the muscle glycogen content. However, provided that the energy intake is adequate, there is no evidence that exercise capacity is different between these two experimental conditions. Whether these results can be applied to the athlete who trains hard on a long-term basis is not presently known, but it is clear that a low-carbohydrate intake will impair the capacity for hard exercise (Costill, 1988). It remains sensible to recommend that runners consume a diet that is low in fat and relatively high in carbohydrate.

The requirement for dietary protein is increased by hard training, and it is possible that there may also be small increases in the requirement for some of the vitamins, minerals, and trace elements (Williams & Devlin, 1992). The available evidence suggests, however, that athletes who eat a varied diet that is adequate to meet their energy demands are unlikely, because of the increased total nutrient intake, to be deficient in any of these dietary components. In spite of this, it must be recognized that not all athletes eat diets that contain sufficient variety to meet their requirements; in this respect they are not different from the general population.

The dietary habits of female distance runners have been the focus of much attention in recent years. In common with female competitors in other sports where a low body fat content is an important factor in performance, many elite performers have a surprisingly low energy intake. There must be some concern that the energy intake of these women is not sufficient to support consistent hard training, and also that micronutrient intake (especially that of iron and calcium) may be inadequate.

Diet for Competition. It has been known since the 1930s that the capacity for endurance exercise is increased by a high-carbohydrate diet during the days preceding the exercise and is reduced by a diet low in carbohydrate (Christensen & Hansen, 1939). Only with the application of the percutaneous needle biopsy technique in the 1960s did the reasons for this effect become apparent as the relationships among diet, glycogen storage, and endurance capacity were elucidated. These studies using bicycle exercise as a model made it clear that endurance capacity was directly related to the magnitude of the pre-exercise muscle glycogen stores, which were in turn dependent on the pattern of exercise and dietary carbohydrate intake in the preceding few days. Being aware of these results, and assuming that they would apply also to running, Ron Hill used a glycogen depletion/supercompensation regimen prior to the European Championship marathon in 1969. His pre-race program consisted of a hard run 6 d before the race, followed by two further days of training with a low-carbohydrate diet; he consumed a high-carbohydrate diet and did no hard running for the last three days. In the race, Hill ran strongly in the later stages, moving from third to first, to win in a time of 2:16:48. Since then the carbohydrate-loading diet in one form or another (Costill, 1988) has been a feature of marathon racing, even though few runners now follow such a strict regimen as that employed by Hill.

Runners competing in races at distances shorter than the marathon have been slow to recognize that an adequate muscle glycogen store is essential for optimum performance. This is perhaps because the early studies, carried out on a cycle ergometer, indicated that glycogen depletion was a possible cause of fatigue only when the exercise intensity was about 75% of $\dot{V}O_2$max and the exercise duration was about 1.5–3 h (Saltin & Karlsson, 1971). At higher exercise intensities, exhaustion occurred when there were still substantial amounts of glycogen in the muscles. Two points need to be borne in mind, however, when attempts are made to apply these results to runners. The first is that there is no good evidence for complete depletion of muscle glycogen in any muscle group during running, as opposed to cycling, at any distance. Secondly, glycogen depletion in a specific sub-group of muscle fibers cannot be eliminated as a possible cause of fatigue, even when glycogen is present within other fibers in the same muscle.

Fluid Intake. Athletes are often confused as to the optimum fluid replacement regimen for enhancement of performance. The current recommendation of the American College of Sports Medicine, in a position statement on the prevention of heat injuries in distance running, is that cool water is the optimum fluid for distance runners (ACSM, 1984). However, examination of the extensive literature published in this area in recent years can leave no doubt that suitably-formulated carbohydrate-electrolyte drinks are more effective in improving performance in prolonged exercise than is plain water. Several extensive reviews of the subject have recommended the use of solutions containing about 5–10% carbohydrate and 20–30 mmol/L sodium; this has been the consensus view at three major conferences that have debated this topic (Committee on Military Nutrition Research, 1992; Gisolfi & Lamb, 1990; Williams & Devlin, 1992).

The precise composition of fluids to be ingested, and the volumes and frequency at which drinks should be taken, cannot be stated with any certainty. It is clear, however, that distance runners generally consume only small amounts of fluid during races, and very few runners habitually drink during training. Surveys of the drinking habits of marathon runners suggest that they ingest only small amounts of fluid during races (Noakes, 1991). There are undoubtedly practical problems associated with drinking while running, but these can be minimized with regular practice. When runners have been required, for experimental purposes, to ingest much larger volumes of fluid than they would normally consume during a race, they appeared to tolerate the changes very well (Whiting et al., 1984).

The aims of fluid ingestion during distance running are as follows:

1. To provide a substrate for energy production. This fuel should be primarily in the form of carbohydrate, but there is no good evidence that different types of carbohydrate confer particular benefits. Glucose, sucrose, and maltodextrin appear to be equally effective. Fructose in low concentrations, especially when mixed with other sugars, is acceptable, but high concentrations of fructose are best avoided because of the risk of gastrointestinal distress.
2. To provide water to offset the risk of dehydration. Optimal rates of water replacement are achieved by the addition of low concentrations of carbohydrate and sodium to drinks. These do not substantially delay gastric emptying, but stimulate water absorption in the small intestine.
3. In extreme endurance exercise where sweat losses are large (with a correspondingly large electrolyte loss) replacement with plain water or with solutions containing only low levels of sodium may lead to hyponatremia, and the addition of some sodium may be necessary.

Fluid ingestion during training or racing will only be of benefit when there is sufficient time for absorption to take place, and there is unlikely to be any benefit in events lasting less than 30–40 min. During longer runs, however, fluid intake is essential for optimum performance, and the reviews referred to above give guidelines for the composition and timing of drinks. It must be emphasized, however, that individual requirements and preferences vary greatly, even in a given runner, depending on the environmental conditions.

Pre-existing dehydration will severely impair performance at all distances, even when the exercise duration is too short for significant sweat loss to occur during the race itself (Armstrong et al., 1985). Runners must, therefore, ensure that water losses incurred during training in the days prior to competition are adequately replaced. When runners, especially those resident in temperate climates, compete in events held in hot climates, they must be informed that large water losses occur even at rest and that appropriate steps must be taken to ensure adequate replacement. There are, however, real problems encountered in trying to suddenly increase fluid intake from a level of 2–4 L/d, which might be adequate for training in a cool climate, to the 10–12 L/d that might be necessary when training in the heat.

MEDICAL CONSIDERATIONS

Although occasional problems are associated with distance races, they are rather infrequent. The sudden death of a recreational runner inevitably attracts media attention, but such events are extremely rare. Various medical problems encountered by distance runners are most often the result of the severe training regimens that they undertake. Much attention has been paid to musculoskeletal injuries, and these, especially chronic overuse injuries to the lower limbs, are undoubtedly common in runners (Crandall, 1986). It appears that injuries to the knee are most common, with injury to the Achilles tendon, foot, and shin also being rather frequent. Many of the injuries reported in surveys of runners are, however, trivial and result in little or no disruption of the training and racing program. The ability to tolerate a high training load without succumbing to injury must, nonetheless, be seen as a characteristic of the elite competitor. Other minor or uncommon complaints, such as jogger's nipple and penile frostbite, have received an undue amount of attention.

Hematological Concerns

A low circulating hemoglobin concentration is a recognized characteristic of distance runners and is commonly referred to as "runners' anemia." In most cases, this is a dilutional anemia due to expansion of the plasma volume, i.e., the total red cell mass is usually normal or even elevated, and other indices of iron status may be normal. The distinction between true anemia and pseudo-anemia is important. In the former intervention and supplementation are warranted; in the latter, they will be ineffective.

The available evidence suggests that there is little difference in the prevalence of iron-deficiency anemia between athletic populations and the normal population, at least in Western countries (Weight, 1993). There is evidence that, in addition to a reduced blood hemoglobin content, a low serum ferritin level may be more common in endurance-trained athletes than in the general population, supporting the concept of a true anemia, but the validity of these measures in athletes has been questioned (Newhouse & Clement, 1988). Some indicators of hemolysis, including serum haptoglobin and bilirubin concentrations, are altered after exercise, and hard exercise may result in blood loss in stools and urine, although the quantitative significance of these losses is questionable.

As with sedentary individuals, athletes may suffer from anemia as a consequence of low iron intakes rather than from high rates of iron loss. Although the high energy intake associated with hard training should ensure a high dietary iron intake, this is by no means certain. Robertson et al. (1992) showed that the iron intakes of male runners with high weekly training distances (80–147 km/week) were not different from those of sedentary subjects. Female distance runners are more susceptible to anemia because of their greater obligatory monthly blood losses in combination with inadequate dietary intakes (Weight et al., 1992).

Although the significance of the traditional markers of hematological status can be ambiguous when applied to runners, anemia remains a potential problem. Monitoring of iron status may be justified, and supplementation is warranted when a deficiency is apparent.

Bone Mineral Content

At a time when osteoporosis is becoming widely recognized as a problem for both men and women, an increase in bone mineral content is one of the benefits of participation in exercise programs. Regular exercise results in an increased mineralization of those bones subjected to stress (Bailey & McCulloch, 1990), and an increased peak bone mass may delay the onset of osteoporotic fractures; exercise may also delay the rate of bone loss. The specificity of this effect is demonstrated by the unilateral increase in bone density that occurs in the dominant arm of tennis players (Pirnay et al., 1987).

In athletes training hard on a regular basis, the circulating levels of sex steroids are likely to decrease. Estrogen plays an important role in the maintenance of bone mass in women, and low estrogen levels cause bone loss (Drinkwater et al., 1984). Many of these women also have low body fat and, because of their low body mass, also have low energy (and calcium) intakes in spite of their high activity levels. All of these factors are a threat to bone health. The loss of bone in these women may result in an increased predisposition to stress fractures and other skeletal injury and must also raise concerns about bone health in later life (Martin & Bailey, 1987). It should be emphasized, however, that this condition appears to affect only relatively few athletes. Hard sustained training is a relatively new phenomenon, particularly among female athletes, and it remains to be seen whether the long-term effects are clinically significant.

Immune Function, Infection, and Overtraining

One of the acute effects of a hard bout of exercise is suppression of immune function. Much attention has recently been focused on the overtraining syndrome that is occasionally apparent in elite athletes. Although this often manifests itself as a sudden and unexplained decrease in performance, it is often accompanied by an increased susceptibility to minor infective illnesses, particularly those affecting the upper respiratory tract. The mechanisms underlying this effect and the implications for health and performance have been the subject of a number of extensive reviews (Sharp, 1992; Shephard et al., 1991; Sparling et al., 1993).

Parry-Billings et al. (1992) have proposed that the impaired immunity of the highly trained runner is a consequence of a reduced plasma concentration of glutamine, which is the major fuel of both lymphocytes and macrophages. Since exercise reduces glutamine release from skeletal muscle, their theory proposes that excessive levels of exercise reduce the circulating glutamine concentration to the point that the activation of cells of the immune system may be compromised.

Peters et al. (1993) have confirmed that there is a higher than expected incidence of upper respiratory tract infections in the days after an ultra-marathon (90-km) race. They also reported that supplementation with vitamin C (600 mg/d for 21 d prior to the race) reduced the incidence of symptoms in runners and in sedentary control subjects. The authors related this finding to the antioxidant properties of vitamin C, since it is known that exercise is associated with increased formation of free radicals that may inhibit leukocyte function (Duthie et al., 1990).

DIRECTIONS FOR FUTURE RESEARCH

Many of the outstanding questions that can be raised in relation to training and competition in distance running are fundamental questions in exercise physiology. The causes of fatigue are not clearly understood, and it seems certain that many factors are involved. The fatigue experienced by the 1500-m runner is probably related in some way to the high rate of anaerobic metabolism, which results in a metabolic acidosis. Fatigue in marathon running is related to depletion of the available carbohydrate reserves, but dehydration and thermoregulatory problems also play a role. If the mechanisms underlying these effects can be clarified, then appropriate training and nutritional strategies to delay the onset of fatigue can be devised.

Training studies to investigate the effectiveness of different training programs for elite runners will never be possible. Elite runners are not prepared to make long-term changes to their schedules to accommodate experiments that may not produce direct benefits, and non-elite runners cannot sustain the training loads of the top competitors.

Overtraining and associated declines in performance have recently been the focus of much attention. There appear to be links between overtraining and impairment of immune function, possibly leading to an increased susceptibility to infection. Changes in mood and in the perception of effort may also occur. There is also a suggestion that excessive training loads may be linked to reduced antioxidant status, which may in turn result in free radical damage to skeletal muscle and perhaps also to other tissues. Evidence for these effects is, however, mostly indirect; systematic investigation is needed. Once again there are formidable obstacles to the conduct of such studies.

Nutritional studies are both necessary and possible. The effectiveness of different nutritional strategies in improving the ability to tolerate training and enhance performance should be investigated for events at different distances. At the present time, a high-carbohydrate diet is generally recommended for all athletes, but there is little evidence that this improves training and racing performances over short distances. Recent evidence has even cast doubt on the need for a high-carbohydrate intake to sustain high training loads.

BIBLIOGRAPHY

Armstrong, L.E., D.L. Costill, and W.J. Fink (1985). Influence of diuretic-induced dehydration on competitive running performance. *Med. Sci. Sports Exerc.* 17:456–461.
Åstrand, P-O., and K. Rodahl (1986). *Textbook of Work Physiology*. 3rd ed. New York: McGraw-Hill.
Bailey, D.A., and R.G. McCulloch (1990). Bone tissue and physical activity. *Can. J. Sport Sci.* 15:229–239.
Bannister, R.G. (1955) *The first four minutes*. London: Putnam.
Böttiger, L.E. (1973). Regular decline in physical working capacity with age. *Br. Med. J.* 2:270–271.
Camus, G. (1992). Relationship between record time and maximal oxygen consumption in middle-distance running. *Eur. J. Appl. Physiol.* 64:534–537.
Carter, J.E.L. (Ed) (1982). *Physical Structure of Olympic Athletes*. New York: Karger.
Cavanagh, P.R., M.L. Pollock, and J. Landa (1977). Biomechanical comparison of elite and good distance runners. In: P. Milvy (ed.) *Marathon: Physiological, Medical, Epidemiological, and Psychological Studies*. New York: New York Academy of Sciences, Part 4, pp. 328–345.
Christensen, E.H., and O. Hansen (1939). Arbeitsfähigkeit und Ernährung. *Skand. Arch. Physiol.* 81:160–171.
Committee on Military Nutrition Research. (1992). *Nutritional Needs in Hot Environments: Applications for Military Personnel in Field Operations*. B.M. Marriott (Ed.). Washington, D.C.: National Academy Press.
Conley, D.L., and G.S. Krahenbuhl (1980). Running economy and distance running performance of highly trained athletes. *Med. Sci. Sports. Exerc.* 12:357–360.
Costill, D.L. (1972). Physiology of marathon running. *JAMA* 221:1024–1029.
Costill, D.L. (1988). Carbohydrates for exercise: dietary demands for optimal performance. *Int. J. Sports Med.* 9:1–18.
Costill, D.L., R. Bowers, and W.F. Kammer (1970). Skinfold estimates of body fat among marathon runners. *Med. Sci. Sports* 2:93–95.
Costill, D.L., G. Branam, D. Eddy, and K. Sparks (1971). Determinants of marathon running success. *Int. Z. Angew. Physiol.* 29:249–254.
Costill, D.L., W.J. Fink, and M.L. Pollock (1976). Muscle fiber composition and enzyme activities of elite distance runners. *Med. Sci. Sports* 8:96–100.
Costill, D.L., H. Thomason, and E. Roberts (1973). Fractional utilization of the aerobic capacity during distance running. *Med. Sci. Sports* 5:248–252.
Coyle, E.F. (1991). Timing and method of increased carbohydrate intake to cope with heavy training, competition and recovery. *J. Sports Sci.* 9(Special Issue):29–52.
Coyle, E.F., M.K. Hopper, and A.R. Coggan. (1990). Maximal oxygen uptake relative to plasma volume expansion. *Int. J. Sports Med.* 11:116–119.
Crandall, R.C. (1986). *Running: The Consequences*. Jefferson: McFarland.
Davies, C.T.M., and M.W. Thompson (1979). Aerobic performance of female marathon and male ultramarathon athletes. *Eur. J. Appl. Physiol.* 41:233–245.
Dempsey, J.A. (1986). Is the lung built for exercise? *Med. Sci. Sports Exerc.* 18:143–155.
Dill, D.B., S. Robinson, and J.C. Ross (1967). Longitudinal study of 16 champion runners. *J. Sports Med. Phys. Fit.* 7:4–27.
Downer, A.R. (1902) *Running Recollections and How to Train*. London: Gale & Polden.
Drinkwater, B.L., K. Nilson, C.H. Chesnut, W.J. Bremner, S. Shainholtz, and M.B. Southworth (1984). Bone mineral content of amenorrheic and eumenorrheic athletes. *New Engl. J. Med.* 311:277–281.
Dudley, G.A., W.M. Abraham, and R.L. Terjung (1982). Influence of exercise intensity and duration on biochemical adaptations in skeletal muscle. *J. Appl. Physiol.* 53:844–850.
Duthie, G.G., J.D. Robertson, R.J. Maughan, and P.C. Morrice (1990). Blood antioxidant status and erythrocyte lipid peroxidation following distance running. *Arch. Biochem. Biophys.* 282:78–83.
England, A.C., D.W. Fraser, A.W. Hightower, R. Tirrinazi, D.J. Greenberg, K.E. Powell, C.M. Slovis, and R.A. Varsha (1982). Preventing severe heat injury in runners: suggestions from the 1979 Peachtree road race experience. *Ann. Int. Med.* 97:196–201.
Farrell, P.A., J.H. Wilmore, E.F. Coyle, J.E. Billing, and D.L. Costill (1979). Plasma lactate accumulation and distance running performance. *Med. Sci. Sports* 11:338–344.
Foster, C., J.T. Daniels, and R.A. Yarbrough (1977). Physiological and training correlates of marathon running performance. *Aust. J. Sports Med.* 9:58–61.

Foster, C., D.L. Costill, J.T. Daniels, and W.J. Fink (1978). Skeletal muscle enzyme activity, fiber composition and V̇O₂max in relation to distance running performance. *Eur. J. Appl. Physiol.* 39:73–80.

Gisolfi, C.V., and D.R. Lamb (Eds.) (1990). *Perspectives in Exercise Science and Sports Medicine. Vol 3. Fluid Homeostasis During Exercise.* Indianapolis: Benchmark Press.

Graves, J.E., M.L. Pollock, and P.B. Sparling (1987). Body composition of elite female distance runners. *Int. J. Sports Med.* 8:96–102.

Gregory, G., K. Foster, H. Tyler, and M. Wiseman (1990). *The Dietary and Nutritional Survey of British Adults.* London: HMSO.

Hagan, R.D., M.G. Smith, and L.R. Gettman. (1981). Marathon performance in relation to maximal aerobic power and training indices. *Med. Sci. Sports Exerc.* 13:185–189.

Henriksson, J., and R.C. Hickner (1992). Skeletal muscle adaptations to endurance training. In: D.A.D. Macleod et al. (Eds.) *Intermittent High Intensity Exercise.* London: Spon, pp. 5–25.

Housh, T.J., W.G. Thorland, G.O. Johnson, R.A. Hughes, and C.J. Cisra (1986). Body composition and body build variables as predictors of middle distance running performance. *J. Sports Med.* 26:258–262.

Ikai, M., and T. Fukunaga. (1968). Calculation of muscle strength per unit of cross sectional area of a human muscle by means of ultrasonic measurements. *Int. Z. angew. Physiol.* 26:26–31.

Kanstrup, I.L., and B. Ekblom (1984). Blood volume and hemoglobin concentration as determinants of maximal aerobic power. *Med. Sci. Sports Exerc.* 16:256–262.

Karlsson, J., L. Hermansen, G. Agnevik, and B. Saltin (1972). Löping. Idrottsfysiologi, rapport no. 4. Stockholm: Trygg-Hansa.

Karlsson, J., and B. Saltin (1971). Diet, muscle glycogen and endurance performance. *J. Appl. Physiol.* 31:203–206.

Lorentzon, R., C. Johansson, M. Sjöstrom, M. Fagerlind, and A.R. Fugl-Meyer (1988). Fatigue during dynamic muscle contractions in male sprinters and marathon runners. *Acta Physiol. Scand.* 132:531–536.

MacDougall, J.D., H.A. Wenger, and H.J. Green. (1982). *Physiological Testing of the High-Performance Athlete.* Champaign, IL: Human Kinetics Books.

Martin, A.D., and D.A. Bailey (1987). Skeletal integrity in amenorrheic athletes. *Aust. J. Sci. Med. Sport* 19:3–7.

Matsuo, A., T. Fukunaga, and T. Asami (1985). Relation between external work and running performance in athletes. In: D.A. Winter, R.W. Norman, R.P. Wells, K.C. Hayes, and A.E. Patla (eds.) *Biomechanics IX-B.* Champaign, IL: Human Kinetics Publishers, pp. 319–324.

Maughan, R.J. (1990). Marathon running. In: T. Reilly et al. (Eds.) *Physiology of Sports.* London: Spon, pp. 121–152.

Maughan, R.J. (1991). Carbohydrate-electrolyte solutions during prolonged exercise. In: D.R. Lamb and M.H. Williams (Eds.) *Perspectives in Exercise Science and Sports Medicine, Vol. 4. Ergogenics—Enhancement of Performance in Exercise and Sport.* Indianapolis: Benchmark Press, pp. 35–89.

Maughan, R.J. (1992). Aerobic function. In: R.J. Shephard (Ed.) *Sport Science Review.* Champaign: Human Kinetics, pp. 28–42.

Maughan, R.J., and P.L. Greenhaff (1991). High intensity exercise and acid-base balance: the influence of diet and induced metabolic alkalosis on performance. In: F. Brouns (Ed.) *Advances in Nutrition and Top Sport.* Basel: Karger, pp. 147–165.

Maughan, R.J., and J.B. Leiper (1983). Aerobic capacity and fractional utilization of aerobic capacity in elite and non-elite male and female marathon runners. *Eur. J. Appl. Physiol.* 52:80–87.

Maughan, R.J., J.S. Watson, and J. Weir. (1983a). Relationships between muscle strength and muscle cross-sectional area in male sprinters and distance runners. *Eur. J. Appl. Physiol.* 50:309–319.

Maughan, R.J., J.S. Watson, and J. Weir. (1983b). Strength and cross-sectional area of human skeletal muscles. *J. Physiol.* 338:37–49.

Maughan, R.J., J.D. Robertson, and A.C. Bruce (1989). Dietary energy and carbohydrate intakes of runners in relation to training load. *Proc. Nut. Soc.* 48:170A.

Medbø, J.I., A.C. Mohn, I. Tabata, R. Bahr, O. Vaage, and O.M. Sejersted (1988). Anaerobic capacity determined by maximal accumulated O₂ deficit. *J. Appl. Physiol.* 64:50–60.

Moore, D.H. (1975). A study of age group track and field records to relate age and running speed. *Nature* 153:264–265.

Newhouse, I.J., and D.B. Clement (1988). Iron status in athletes. *Sports Med.* 5:337–352.

Noakes, T.D. (1991). *Lore of Running.* 3rd Ed. Champaign: Leisure Press.

Nygaard, E. (1981). Women and exercise—with special reference to muscle morphology and metabolism. In: J. Poortmans and G. Niset (Eds.) *Biochemistry of Exercise -IVB* Baltimore: University Park Press. pp. 161–175.

Osnes, J-B., and L. Hermansen (1972). Acid-base balance after maximal exercise of short duration. *J. Appl. Physiol.* 32:59–63.

Parry-Billings, M., V.J. Matthews, E.A. Newsholme, R. Budgett, and J. Koutedakis (1992). The overtraining syndrome: some biochemical aspects. In: D.A.D. Macleod et al. (Eds.) *Intermittent High Intensity Exercise.* London: Spon, pp. 215–225.

Pate, R.R., C. Barnes, and W. Miller (1985). A physiological comparison of performance-matched female and male distance runners. *Res. Q.* 56:245–250.

Pate, R.R., P.B. Sparling, G.E. Wilson, K.J. Cureton, and B.J. Miller (1987). Cardiorespiratory and metabolic responses to submaximal and maximal exercise in elite women distance runners. *Int. J. Sports Med.* 8:91–95S.

Peters, E.M., J.M. Goetzsche, B. Grobbelaar, and T.D. Noakes (1993). Vitamin C supplementation reduces the incidence of postrace symptoms of upper-respiratory-track infection in ultramarathon runners. *Am. J. Clin. Nutr.* 57:170–174.

Pirnay, F., M. Bodeux, J.M. Crielaard, and P. Franchimont (1987). Bone mineral content and physical activity. *Int. J. Sports Med.* 8:331–335.

Pollock, M.L. (1977). Submaximal and maximal working capacity of elite distance runners: cardiorespiratory aspect. *Ann. N.Y. Acad. Sci.* 301:310–322.

Pollock, M.L., L.R. Gettman, A. Jackson, J. Ayres, A. Ward, and A.C. Linnerud (1977). Body composition of elite class distance runners. *Ann. N.Y. Acad. Sci.* 301:361–370.

Pollock, M.L., A.S. Jackson, and R.R. Pate (1980). Discriminant analysis of physiological differences between good and elite distance runners. *Res. Quart. Exerc. Sport* 51:521–532.

Powers, S.K., D. Martin, and S. Dodd. (1993). Exercise-induced hypoxaemia in elite endurance athletes. *Sports Med.* 16:14–22.

Pugh, L.G.C.E., J.L. Corbett, and R.H. Johnson (1967). Rectal temperatures, weight losses and sweat rates in marathon running. *J. Appl. Physiol.* 23:247–253.

Ramsbottom, R., C. Williams, D.G. Kerwin, and M.L.G. Nute (1992). Physiological and metabolic responses of men and women to a 5-km treadmill time trial. *J. Sports Sci.* 10:119–129.

Robertson, J.D., R.J. Maughan, A.C. Bruce, and R.J.L. Davidson (1992). Hematological status of male runners in relation to the extent of physical training. *Int. J. Sports Nutr.* 2:366–375.

Saltin, B., J. Henriksson, E. Nygaard, and P. Andersen (1977). Fiber types and metabolic potentials of skeletal muscles in sedentary man and endurance runners. In: P. Milvy (ed.) *Marathon: Physiological, Medical, Epidemiological, and Psychological Studies.* New York: New York Academy of Sciences, Part 1, pp. 3–29.

Saltin, B., and J. Karlsson (1971). Muscle glycogen utilization during work of different intensities. In: B. Pernow and B. Saltin (Eds.) *Muscle Metabolism During Exercise.* London: Plenum, pp. 289–299.

Savard, G., B. Kiens, and B. Saltin. (1986). Central cardiovascular factors as limits to endurance. In: D. Macleod et al. (Eds.) *Exercise: Benefits, Limits and Adaptations.* London: Spon, pp. 162–180.

Savard. G., B. Kiens, and B. Saltin. (1987). Limb blood flow in prolonged exercise: magnitude and implications for cardiovascular control during muscle work in man. *Can. J. Sport Sci.* 12 (Suppl. 1):89S–101S.

Sawka, M.N., and K.B. Pandolf (1990). Effects of body water loss on physiological function and exercise performance. In: C.V. Gisolfi and D.R. Lamb (Eds.) *Perspectives in Exercise Science and Sports Medicine, Vol 3. Fluid Homeostasis During Exercise.* Indianapolis: Benchmark Press, pp. 1–38.

Schulz, R., and C. Curnow (1988). Peak performance and age among superathletes: Track and field, swimming, baseball, tennis, and golf. *J. Gerontol.* 43:P113–P120.

Scrimgeour, A.G., T.D. Noakes, B. Adams, and K. Myburgh (1986). The influence of weekly training distance on fractional utilization of maximum aerobic capacity in marathon and ultramarathon runners. *Eur. J. Appl. Physiol.* 55:202–209.

Sharp, N.C.C. (1992). Immunological aspects of exercise, fitness and competition sport. In: D.A.D. Macleod et al. (Eds.) *Intermittent High Intensity Exercise.* London: Spon, pp. 201–213.

Shephard, R.J., T.J. Verde, S.G. Thomas, and P. Shek (1991). Physical activity and the immune system. *Can. J. Sport Sci.* 16:163–185.

Sherman, W.M. (1991). Carbohydrate feedings before and after exercise. In: D.R. Lamb and M.H. Williams (eds.) *Perspectives in Exercise Science and Sports Medicine, Vol. 4: Ergogenics—Enhancement of Performance in Exercise and Sport* Indianapolis, IN: W.C. Brown and Benchmark Publishers, pp. 1–34.

Sherman, W.M., and G.S. Wimer (1991). Insufficient dietary carbohydrate during training: does it impair athletic performance? *Int. J. Sport Nutr.* 1:28–44.

Sherman, W.M., D.L. Costill, W.J. Fink, and J.M. Miller (1981). Effect of exercise-diet manipulation on muscle glycogen and its subsequent utilization during performance. *Int. J. Sports Med.* 2:114–118.

Sherman, W.M., J.A. Doyle, D.R. Lamb, and R.H. Strauss (1993). Dietary carbohydrate, muscle glycogen, and exercise performance during 7 d of training. *Am. J. Clin. Nutr.* 57:27–31.

Sjödin, B., and J. Svedenhag (1985). Applied physiology of marathon running. *Sports Med.* 2:83–99.

Sjöstrom, M., C. Johansson, and R. Lorentzon. (1988). Muscle pathomorphology in m. quadriceps of marathon runners. Early signs of strain disease or functional adaptation? *Acta Physiol. Scand.* 132:537–542.

Snell, P. (1990). Middle distance running. In: T. Reilly et al. (Eds.) *Physiology of Sports.* London: Spon, pp. 101–120.

Sparling, P.B., D.C. Nieman, and P.J. O'Connor (1993). Selected scientific aspects of marathon racing. *Sports Med.* 15:116–132.

Sutton, J.R. (1990). Clinical implications of fluid imbalance. In: C.V. Gisolfi and D.R. Lamb (Eds.) *Perspectives in Exercise Science and Sports Medicine, Vol 3. Fluid Homeostasis During Exercise.* Indianapolis: Benchmark Press, pp. 425–448.

Wagner, P.D., G.E. Gale, R.E. Moon, J.R. Torre-Bueno, J.W. Stolp, and H.A. Saltzman. (1986). Pulmonary gas exchange in humans exercising at sea level and simulated altitude. *J. Appl. Physiol.* 60:260–270.

Weight, L.M. (1993). 'Sports anaemia': does it exist? *Sports Med.* 16:1–4.

Weight, L.M., T.D. Noakes, and P. Jacobs. (1992). Dietary iron intake and 'sports anaemia.' *Br. J. Nutr.* 68:253–260.

Wenger, H.A., and G.J. Bell (1986). The interactions of intensity, frequency and duration of exercise training in altering cardiorespiratory fitness. *Sports Med.* 3:346–356.

Whiting, P.H., R.J. Maughan, and J.D.B. Miller (1984). Dehydration and serum biochemical changes in marathon runners. *Eur. J. Appl. Physiol.* 52:183–187.

Whipp, B.J., and S.A. Ward (1992). Will women soon outrun men? *Nature* 355:25.

Wilber, R.L., and R.J. Moffatt (1992). Influence of carbohydrate ingestion on blood glucose and performance in runners. *Int. J. Sports Nutr.* 2:317–327.

Wilkes, D., N. Gledhill, and R. Smyth (1983). Effect of acute induced metabolic alkalosis on 800-m racing time. *Med. Sci. Sports Exerc.* 15:277–280.

Williams, C. (1989). Diet and endurance fitness. *Am. J. Clin. Nutr.* 49:1077–1083.

Williams, C., and J.T. Devlin (1992). *Foods, Nutrition and Sports Performance.* London: Spon.

Williams, K.R., and P.R. Cavanagh (1987). Relationship between distance running mechanics, running economy, and performance. *J. Appl. Physiol.* 63:1236–1245.

Wilmore J.H., and C.H. Brown (1974). Physiological profiles of women distance runners. *Med. Sci. Sports* 6:178–181.

Woodson, R.D. (1984). Hemoglobin concentration and exercise capacity. *Am. Rev. Resp. Dis.* 129(Suppl): 572–575.

DISCUSSION

KRAEMER: Is more muscle damage caused by running than by other endurance sports such as cycling? Also, is there any physiological basis for the contention of some marathon runners that they have the potential for only a small number of high quality marathon performances?

MAUGHAN: The conventional wisdom is that any activity that involves a large component of eccentric muscle actions will cause muscle damage, i.e., running downhill will cause a large amount of damage, whereas running on the flat will not. If we look at delayed-onset muscle soreness and at activities of creatine kinase and lactate dehydrogenase in the serum after exhausting exercise, those values are higher in runners than they are in cyclists. They are also higher after running a hilly course than after a flat course. How physiologically important that muscle damage is I am not certain. Good runners can repeat their performances week after week in spite of evidence of muscle damage, so that it appears that the muscles can recover between the competitive runs. Otherwise, there would be a progressive loss of muscle tissue over time, and there is no evidence for such a phenomenon; runners can continue to participate for many years. There is, of course, less delayed-onset muscle soreness after training with downhill running than before such training. I suspect this is a true adaptation to eccentric exercise, but it is possible that sensitive fibers are simply destroyed during the training. After an exhausting bout of swimming or cycling, there are some signs of muscle damage. For example, serum creatine kinase is slightly elevated to 100–200 U/L. This effect can be explained partly by hemoconcentration and, I suspect, partly by transport of enzymes from the interstitial space into the blood.

With regard to the suggestion of a limited potential for performing well in a finite number of marathons, this is obviously true in a general sense. However, many ultra-distance runners will run a 100-km race every week if they get the chance. Is there something unique about the marathon races so they cannot be run that frequently? Certainly the top-class middle distance runners in Europe can run 2–3 times per week during the competitive season in different cities across Europe. They have all the problems of traveling and time changes, and they can still race well. Obviously it is psychologically very difficult to participate in more than a few marathons in any given season, but I am not certain there is any special physiological limitation for the marathon.

HAGERMAN: There is evidence from biopsy studies of selective necrosis of fast twitch fibers during recovery from the marathon. Intuitively, this seems to favor the runner for subsequent races because he would then have a greater proportion of slow twitch fibers. Do you think that slow recovery of energy stores or slow regeneration of damaged fibers might limit one's ability to recover from a marathon?

MAUGHAN: Both are important. There are persistent signs of muscle damage for 10–12 days following a marathon, and recovery of muscle glycogen stores can also be delayed for several days. It seems likely that it would be difficult to compete successfully until the energy stores have been replenished and until there is some regeneration of damaged or destroyed muscle fibers.

It is not clear what the best way to recover after a marathon race is. The marathon runners I used to train with would go running the day after a marathon, no matter how sore they felt. These athletes would even try and run a mile or two immediately following the marathon. Actually, it was not so much running as it was limping around the track, but the idea was to get out the next day and limp a few miles, no matter what. One of these runners I trained with went running the day after setting a 100-km world record. Many of these runners were convinced that taking a day off would slow their recovery. Today there are more runners who take a few days off following a big race, but I am not sure there is much evidence favoring one approach versus the other. My guess is that low-intensity recovery exercise is important to speed the recovery process.

HAGERMAN: In the U.S., the Olympic trials occur shortly before the actual Olympic Games. Do you think this short interval for recovery is harmful for the U.S. marathon runners' chances in the Olympics?

MAUGHAN: Yes. This is a big problem in events like the marathon. Many of the best marathon runners have to achieve their best performances to qualify and they then do not perform as well as they should at the time of the Olympics. In the United Kingdom, they have tried pre-selection procedures to avoid the problem you describe, but that hasn't always been successful, either. You have to pre-select 6–12 months in advance, and it is difficult to predict how somebody is going to perform that far in advance.

GISOLFI: You suggest that pre-race muscle glycogen stores may be important for an event such as the 1500-m run; this is contrary to the notion that this event is too brief to deplete muscle glycogen substantially, even when considering the effect of training for several days before the competition. To be adequately prepared to compete in the 1500-m run, how would you advise a runner from a nutritional standpoint?

MAUGHAN: Our results on cycling demonstrate that a moderate depletion of muscle glycogen before an event lasting 3–4 minutes can impair performance; if the athlete practices glycogen supercompensation, there is a suggestion of a slight improvement in performance. Certainly, if glycogen is depleted, performance is worse. My recommendation would be to err on the side of caution and make sure the muscle glycogen level is high before the start of the competition. The tendency has been for middle distance runners to say that glycogen loading is not important. However, the total amount of glycogen used may be misleading. There may be a limitation caused by glycogen depletion in specific fiber types.

SPRIET: I find it difficult to accept the suggestion that glycogen depletion could occur in either fiber type in a 1500-m race. It is not possible to deplete glycogen aerobically in something like a 1500-m race. If that is the case, what you are suggesting is that glycogen depletion in a specific fiber would be due to anaerobic glycolysis. The evidence suggests that this is impossible to achieve because of the associated acid load. Even when you do maximal sprints that activate all the fibers, you only break down about a quarter of the normal glycogen store. Therefore, I don't think it is likely that glycogen depletion could occur in Type I or IIa fibers in a 1500-m race. The single fiber techniques that Paul Greenhhaff and Eric Hultman are using will soon settle this issue. They could certainly simulate a 1500-m run on the treadmill and take the pre- and post- exercise biopsies, separate the fibers, and examine the glycogen depletion. Then we will have our answer.

MAUGHAN: I agree that we will have the answer fairly soon. The issue, though, is not so much whether glycogen can be depleted during a 1500-m race, but rather whether a low pre-race glycogen concentration will allow the runner to finish in his or her best time. One of the reasons for making the dietary suggestions was based on treadmill sprinting data showing a 25% depletion of muscle glycogen after a 30-second sprint. It seems likely to me that glycogen may be substantially reduced in the muscles of a middle-distance runner who trains fairly hard during mid-week by doing repeated 200-400-m sprints. If he then competes on the weekend, I think his performance is likely to suffer. This is certainly somewhat speculative, but a high glycogen level at the start of the race certainly will not hurt, and it might help. If I were advising someone for the Olympic

1500-m final, there is no doubt that I would recommend a high-carbohydrate diet to insure a high level of glycogen before the race.

COYLE: Milers have often run two of their best races separated by only a few hours. They apparently can run very close to their top performances without much glycogen resynthesis between races.

MAUGHAN: Those cases, such as the winner of the 1500-m and the 5000-m races in the 1924 Olympics in Paris, have been exceptions. It is very difficult to produce that sort of performance more than once or twice in a season. Generally speaking, when preliminary heats and finals are run in the same day, performance times are relatively slow.

EKBLOM: We should consider not only total glycogen content in a muscle and glycogen content in specific fibers, but also the location of glycogen in those fibers. I believe one can load the glycogen in different compartments of the fiber in different ways. This means that measuring only the content of glycogen in the entire fiber may not show the complete story.

MAUGHAN: I am sure that in the next few years that evidence will emerge. Right now we can only speculate.

KANTER: Is there any evidence that exercising while glycogen stores are low might make a runner more susceptible to exercise-induced muscle damage?

MAUGHAN: Fred Brouns reported that there are more injuries in endurance athletes who compete with low glycogen concentrations in their muscles. There are also laboratory studies showing more muscle damage in people who exercise with low muscle glycogen stores. It makes sense that coordination might be impaired if the glycogen stores are low, and this could result in unaccustomed forces in the muscle that could produce damage.

EKBLOM: With electron microscopy we have found that glycogen is always present in the fibers, even after prolonged competitions. This glycogen is not detected with the traditional histochemical methods.

MAUGHAN: It is true that the histochemical technique for identifying glycogen in single muscle fibers is not very sensitive, but the biochemical technique is; it also detects residual glycogen in the muscles of exhausted runners. But some of the biochemical studies on cyclists show quadriceps muscle fibers with essentially no glycogen remaining. There seems to be a difference between cycling and running.

SPRIET: Are there really enough biopsy studies on runners that allow us to conclude that glycogen is not fully depleted in their muscle fibers at fatigue?

MAUGHAN: It is true that there aren't nearly as many studies on runners as on cyclists, for very practical reasons. But the few studies that have been done seem to be consistent in failing to demonstrate total glycogen depletion in runners' muscles at exhaustion.

HORSWILL: Is there a point where carbohydrate loading and supercompensation of glycogen is a disadvantage, particularly for the 1500-m runner, because he ends up carrying the weight of extra water bound to glycogen?

MAUGHAN: I do not think anybody has looked at that. The extra weight is quite small. If there is a problem with carboloading, it is likely to be the large amount of glycogen stored. Eric Hultman has some striking electron micrographs in his 1967 thesis showing muscles that have undergone glycogen supercompensation. The micrographs show so much glycogen that there is hardly room for the contractile machinery, but the muscle seems to function well.

GISOLFI: You pointed out that studies from Cavanagh's group indicated there are no significant differences in stride frequency and stride length that can explain differences in running economy. What other factors might be involved in running economy?

MAUGHAN: I do not know what those other factors are. The fact that Peter Cavanagh's group apparently couldn't detect any critical factors makes me feel a little less ignorant. I am obviously not a biomechanist.

EKBLOM: When estimating running economy, it is important to divide the oxygen uptake by body weight to the $2/3$ power; if you use simple body weight, you cannot correct adequately for different statures. Differences in economy of running among trained runners are quite small if one uses body weight to the $2/3$ power. Another point of interest here is that economy changes among various velocities for different types of runners. Thus, long distance runners have a very good economy in the range of speeds at which they compete, but not at higher speeds. Likewise, middle distance runners are quite economical at their faster racing speeds but not as economical at slower, marathon racing speeds.

MAUGHAN: That is a problem with the literature. Runners are compared at an arbitrary fixed speed. Obviously, a running speed should be chosen that is relevant to the competitive event. Also, we should look at a range of running speeds rather than at a single speed.

BAR-OR: The synchronization of action between muscle agonists and antagonists during the running cycles is another important issue in running economy. In an unsynchronized pattern the agonists and antagonists act simultaneously, which increases the energy cost. We think this may happen relatively frequently in younger children. We are now recording electomyographic (EMG) patterns during running in pre-pubescent children, early pubescent children, and late pubescent children to help explain why children are less economical than adolescents in their running styles. The EMG data are being recorded simultaneously with kinematic, kinetic, and metabolic data. In general, this idea of muscle synchronization has not been studied enough in the analysis of running economy.

MAUGHAN: My guess is that this age effect on running economy is primarily a function of differences in volume of training. This age-related phenomenon is also seen in swimming, cycling, and all the locomotor sports. Younger children apparently simply have not accomplished a large enough volume of training to adequately develop their running style.

BAR-OR: What will this volume prove?

MAUGHAN: I can not tell you the precise mechanism, but it seems to be the case that a large volume of training is critical to improving running style and economy.

EICHNER: You indicate that, in some athletes, iron deficiency is probably caused by insufficient iron in the diet. I think this is true for some women runners, as pointed out in a study by Ann Snyder published in 1989 in *Med. Sci. Sports Exerc.*, but I don't think the case can be made that insufficient iron in the diet is a cause of iron deficiency anemia in men.

MAUGHAN: I agree that iron intake is more of a problem for women than it is for men. At one time, the conventional wisdom was that most runners suffered from anemia. More recently, many have claimed that low hemoglobin concentrations are simply a dilutional effect of an expanded plasma volume and that iron status is of no concern. I think the truth of the matter lies somewhere in between those two views. Just because someone is a runner does not mean he or she is immune to problems such as anemia that other people experience. Generally speaking, the iron intake is higher in the athlete because the total energy intake is higher. But some individuals do not follow normal food consumption patterns; surely there are some males and even more females who have inadequate iron intake.

EICHNER: But the focus in men should be to look for abnormal loss of blood or iron, not for low iron intake.

MAUGHAN: I agree that this is usually the case but, occasionally, we will find an inadequate iron intake in men.

EICHNER: How much of a factor is bicarbonate loading in middle distance and long distance running?

MAUGHAN: It is possibly a factor in middle distance running but is not in long distance running, as far as we can see. Bicarbonate loading has certainly been used by some middle distance runners as a performance enhancer. It has been noticeable in the last 10 y that some athletes who have qualified for finals in the afternoon have not showed up, even though they were seen out on the warm-up track an hour or so beforehand. I suspect that some of those people were experiencing gastrointestinal problems secondary to large bicarbonate intakes. But I do not think bicarbonate loading is a major factor for most elite runners.

HORSWILL: Is it possible that, in ultra-distance events, altered acid-base balance could contribute to fatigue? My rationale for this question is that, as more fat is metabolized, ketone bodies accumulate and this may decrease blood pH. Has this ever been studied?

MAUGHAN: The increase in ketone bodies is quite small and acid-base imbalance is not a major factor in long distance events. To my knowledge, there is no suggestion that manipulating acid-base status will affect long distance running performance. There is some fat metabolism in shorter events, but the overwhelming contribution to energy metabolism in middle distance running is made by carbohydrate. Eddie Coyle might have some more information on the importance of fat in an event lasting 15–30 min.

COYLE: There is some fat oxidation during exercise at 85% $\dot{V}O_2$max, which is the intensity at which a typical 10,000-m runner competes. However, I agree that the contribution of fat as a fuel in such an event is relatively minor. Whether fat supplementation is advantageous, I am not sure. I am not convinced that exercise training improves one's ability to mobilize fatty acids and deliver them to the muscle. Hurley et al. demonstrated that the source of the increased fat oxidation as a result of endurance training was intramuscular fat and not plasma free fatty acids. Furthermore, in our studies we have not seen that trained subjects have a particularly great ability to mobilize fats. Plasma fatty acids might be somewhat limiting, especially in trained subjects during high-intensity exercise.

DAVIS: I do not think that extra plasma free fatty acids will benefit performance at all. We infused lipids and heparin to elevate free-fatty acids to very high levels and saw absolutely no beneficial effect on time to fatigue in cycling exercise at approximately 78% $\dot{V}O_2$max for the first hour and 65% for the next two hours. We also saw no changes in RER, blood glucose, or in other related variables. Endurance performance was simply not effected by raising plasma free fatty acid concentrations to high values.

COYLE: At 65–70 % $\dot{V}O_2$max the concentration of plasma fatty acids is in excess of 1 mM and is not limiting. However, at higher exercise intensities, e.g., 85% $\dot{V}O_2$max, the concentration of fatty acids declines to 0.1–0.2 mM, presumably because the fatty acids being produced are trapped in adipose tissue. When the subjects stop exercise, the plasma fatty acids go from 0.2 mM to 1.2 mM in 5 min. This huge overshoot appears to follow the same time course as the post-exercise hyperemia to skin and possibly to adipose tissue. So it appears that, at an exercise intensity of 85% $\dot{V}O_2$max, an increase in the concentration of plasma fatty acids can spare muscle glycogen and perhaps enhance performance.

SPRIET: There are two studies from Dave Costill's lab, one in 1977 and another in 1992, that point out that you have to be exercising at an intensity of 70% $\dot{V}O_2$max or higher to see a carbohydrate-sparing effect of enhanced fatty acid availability. I believe their subjects exercised at 70% $\dot{V}O_2$max for 1 h. The 1992 experiment studied the effects of both a high-fat meal and a lipid and heparin infusion and reported quite a substantial glycogen sparing after 1 h of exercise. Our own study demonstrated a

40% glycogen sparing during 15 min of exercise at 85% $\dot{V}O_2$max following a lipid and heparin infusion. The problem of reduced fat availability appears at a certain intensity of exercise and that intensity may vary depending on the training status of the population being examined.

COYLE: Costill's subjects were not well-trained and their blood lactates were relatively high; it was quite high-intensity exercise for the subjects.

DAVIS: The intensity of exercise during the first hour of our study was above 75% $\dot{V}O_2$max before we dropped to 65% and continued until fatigue. Time to fatigue wasn't affected at all; if glycogen had been spared during that first hour, it should have affected performance, but it did not.

COYLE: If the plasma free fatty acids were already high during the control trial, there was no reason to think the fatty-acid concentration was suboptimal.

SPRIET: I think Mark's point is well taken. If the glycogen had been spared, there should have been an enhanced performance.

EKBLOM: Endurance training reduces the respiratory exchange ratio at 70–80% $\dot{V}O_2$max, which is telling us that we are metabolizing more fat, wherever it comes from, than before training.

SPRIET: That's a good point. We did not use particularly well-trained people in our studies, whereas Ed Coyle has used well-trained cyclists. The training effect on fat metabolism should be kept in mind as we try to interpret these findings.

MAUGHAN: Perhaps one important reason that distance runners engage in prolonged warm-up runs at low intensity is that this helps them mobilize fatty acids so they start the race with elevated concentrations of fatty acids in their blood. The intensity of the warmup may be low enough that it does not draw down on their glycogen stores but gives them an edge on fatty acid mobilization, which might later help spare muscle glycogen until the end of the race.

NADEL: George Sheehan, a man of considerable wisdom, advised middle distance runners to run for time on a cool day, but to run for place on a hot day. On a race day, it is probably critical to be well-hydrated. How should middle distance runners maintain a state of optimal hydration on hot days so they can suffer the heat-induced decrements in performance to a lesser extent than do their competitors?

MAUGHAN: Most of the recent major championships for the middle distance runners have been held in hot environments. A runner coming from a temperate zone will surely be dehydrated for a few days after exposure to a hot climate. Many of these athletes are not aware that dehydration is a problem. It should not be difficult to encourage them to increase their fluid intake if they can be made aware of the potential for dehydration. Electrolytes need to be replaced as well as water, and there is probably also a need for a carbohydrate source to provide fuel.

9

Physiology and Nutrition for Cross-Country Skiing

Björn Ekblom, M.D., Ph.D.

Ulf Bergh, Ph.D.

INTRODUCTION

Cross-country skiing has been practiced for about 4000 y, mostly for hunting and basic transportation. Today, recreational touring, endurance training, and racing are more common objectives. Skiing equipment has also changed considerably and has become much more specialized. For example, in the beginning of this century racing skies were about 3 m long, 10 cm wide, and 2-3 kg in weight. Nowadays, the corresponding values are 2 m, 4 cm, and about 0.5 kg. An example of the specialization is that skis and boots for classic cross-country skiing are different from those for freestyle ski racing.

The courses have changed as well. In the beginning of this century, the ski tracks usually followed trails used for other purposes. There was rarely any additional preparation of these trails before competition. Since the 1960s, grooming machines have been used, at least for the more advanced levels of competition. These machines make the tracks very hard and durable, rendering the conditions more or less constant for the competitors. However, considerable variations may still occur due to weather changes and differences in snow characteristics.

Skiing competitions are classified into two different styles: classic and freestyle. Three main techniques are used in classic skiing: double pole, kick double pole, and diagonal. In freestyle events, skating techniques dominate. These are characterized by leg movements similar to those used in ice skating combined with various forms of double poling.

Elite skiing competitions are performed over distances ranging from 5-90 km. In the Olympic Games and the World Championships, the distances range from 5-30 km for women and from 10-50 km for men. Relay races require four women to ski 5 km each or four men to ski 10 km each. At present, individual races last from 15-100 min for women and 25-150 min for men.

Racing speed in international championships has increased dramatically since the 1920s. This change is partly due to the greater number and improved physical capacity of the skiers but also to better equipment and faster courses.

Modern rules stipulate that the length of courses for international races must be equally divided into segments requiring uphill, downhill, and level skiing. Because the racing speeds differ among these three parts of the course, the time spent in uphill skiing is more than half of the total racing time, whereas downhill skiing time is correspondingly less than 10% of the total (Frost et al., 1984). Even so, downhill skiing ability is important. A fall in a downhill segment causes loss of speed and rhythm in skiing and a resultant increase in overall race time. This is illustrated in Figure 9-1, which shows the average time lost in uphill, level, and downhill segments of the course for each competitor according to the order of finish. Because so much more time was spent on uphill and level segments of the course, the absolute time lost for the skiers depicted in Figure 9-1 was greatest in uphill and level skiing; still, the small amount of time lost in the downhill segments could easily have affected the order of finish.

The exact relationships among times spent skiing different segments of a course are, of course, dependent on many factors, such as gender, level of competition, and type of terrain, but because of the typical emphasis on time during uphill and level skiing, most of the following discussion will be focused on factors important during those two segments. We will especially discuss maximal oxygen uptake ($\dot{V}O_2$max), endurance, and skiing efficiency.

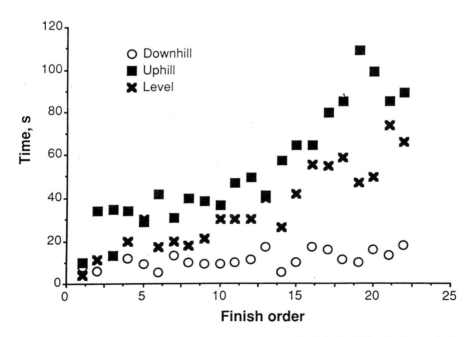

FIGURE 9-1. *Average time lost, relative to the race winner, in several uphill, downhill, and level segments of the course in relation to the finish order of a ski race* (modified from Forsberg, 1988)

CHARACTERISTICS OF ELITE SKIERS

Age

Judging from data on skiers of international caliber, elite competitors may vary considerably in age; average ages were 27 and 29 y for women and men, respectively, with a standard deviation of four years in each case (Bergh & Forsberg, 1992a). Moreover, no junior skier has ever won an individual gold medal in the Olympic Games or World Championships, indicating that it takes years of training to achieve that level of performance.

Body Composition

The elite cross-county competitor does not differ very much in body size and appearance from other non-obese persons. The elite skier usually has relatively little body fat, but not to an extreme (Wilmore, 1983). As a group, elite skiers are heavier than long-distance runners, but considerably lighter than rowers (Bergh, 1987). The average body mass index (mass · height^{-2}) for men who finished among the top 20 in the 1991 World Cup was similar to that for ordinary males, whereas the female skiers had a somewhat lower average body mass index than did non–athletic age-matched women (Bergh & Forsberg, 1992b). The coefficient of variation for this variable was about 6% for both sexes.

Muscle Fiber Types

Type I (slow twitch) fibers predominate in the leg muscles of elite cross-country skiers, but the variability is considerable (Rusko, 1976). A similar distribution of fibers types occurs in the deltoid muscle, where there is an even greater variation. Young elite skiers have lower percentages of Type I fibers than do older skiers (Rusko, 1976), perhaps because of differences in total training exposure or because skiers with fewer Type I fibers tend to abandon the sport earlier in life. Consistent with, but not definitively proving, the former explanation, Rusko (1992) reported that skiers who had increased their training also increased the average percentage of Type I fibers in their muscles from 57% to 68%, whereas skiers who stopped training displayed a slight decrease in their average percentage of Type I fibers.

The predominance of Type I fibers in cross-country skiers is logical because the metabolism in cross-country skiing is predominantly aerobic, and Type I fibers have a high aerobic capacity. Furthermore, the number of capillaries is greater around a Type I than around a Type II (fast twitch) fiber. This enhances the transportation of gases and nutrients between blood and muscle cells, thus enabling an effective metabolism. All these findings are consistent with the hypothesis that physical training for many years increases local aerobic metabolic capacity; i.e., training improves muscle endurance (Rusko, 1992; Saltin & Gollnick, 1983).

Movement Speed

Elite competitors have longer strides (i.e., more distance is covered during each stride), but the stride rates are about the same as those for less successful skiers who use the diagonal technique or the skating technique; during double poling, however, the stride frequency is higher for elite skiers (Smith, 1992). Speed is increased mainly by increasing the stride rate in both elite and non-elite skiers. Elite skiers also are better able to change potential to kinetic energy within body segments than are recreational skiers; this reduces the energy demand for changing the velocity of body segments (Norman et al., 1985).

As mentioned earlier, the speed in cross-country ski racing has increased over the years. The average speed is now usually about 6–7 m·s^{-1}, with a relatively large variation among different races due to variations in snow conditions and topographic profiles of the courses. The type of skiing technique also affects racing time. Faster speeds usually occur over shorter distances, but this phenomenon is not as evident in skiing as it is in running and speed skating (Bergh & Forsberg, 1992a). Males are reported to be approximately 14% faster than females (Bergh & Forsberg, 1992a). This figure, however, is based on data obtained in elite competitions, in which males and females rarely are racing on the same course. One exception is the Vasa Race (90 km) in Sweden, where men and women have raced together on the same course and started at the same time since 1981. In this race, male winners were, on the average, 16% faster than female winners; interestingly, the difference between genders in $\dot{V}O_2$max (when expressed per unit of body mass) is of the same magnitude.

From the view of the spectator, the motions of a cross-country skier do not appear to be very fast. This impression is probably created by the fact that arms and legs do not move at high frequencies because there is a gliding phase within the cycle of motion. There are, however, parts of the skiing cycle that include fairly rapid movements, e.g., during the kicking phase of the diagonal stride technique (Ekström, 1980) and during the extension of the elbow while double poling. These motions must be fast; otherwise, it would not be possible to create accelerating forces because the body already has considerable speed in the forward direction. The skating technique extends the time available for the accelerating forces to act because the pushing ski moves forward. This lowers the stride rate so that the skier does not have to accelerate various body segments as frequently as during classic skiing. Thus, the skating technique reduces mechanical work and the metabolic cost of skiing.

Maximal Oxygen Uptake

The physiological variable that most vividly distinguishes elite cross-country skiers from either the average person or less successful cross-country skiers is the $\dot{V}O_2$max, expressed either as L/min or as mL·min^{-1}·kg^{-1}. Over the decades, reports have confirmed that elite cross-country skiers have, without exception, very high values for $\dot{V}O_2$max (Åstrand, 1955; Bergh, 1987; Hanson, 1973; Saltin & Åstrand, 1967) (Table 9-1). World class skiers have displayed higher $\dot{V}O_2$max values than less successful skiers (Bergh, 1987; Ingjer, 1991). Skiers of junior age display lower values than do adults (Bergh & Forsberg, 1992a; Rusko, 1976). These differences are also reflected in differences in racing speed and success.

The power generated through aerobic energy metabolism is necessary for moving the body mass in skiing, and the generation of greater power increases speed. More power is needed to move a larger body mass at a given speed. Thus, the expression of power should be corrected for differences in body mass; otherwise, it is invalid to compare aerobic power values among different skiers. Traditionally, such corrections have been made by dividing $\dot{V}O_2$max by body mass. However, it has been demonstrated that the power needed to ski at a given speed on level terrain is not directly proportional to body mass (Bergh & Forsberg, 1992b). Therefore, based upon dimensional analysis and empirical findings, it has been suggested that dividing $\dot{V}O_2$max by body mass$^{2/3}$ may be a more valid expression of aerobic power for cross-country skiing (Bergh, 1987). This recommendation is consistent with the results of Ingjer (1991), who demonstrated that the average $\dot{V}O_2$max of world class skiers was significantly greater than that of medium class and less successful skiers only when $\dot{V}O_2$max was divided by body mass$^{2/3}$, not when it was divided by simple body mass. Thus, it seems logical to relate $\dot{V}O_2$max to body mass$^{2/3}$ if the purpose is to predict the capacity for cross-county skiing.

Central Circulation

At present, there is a consensus that the central circulation limits the $\dot{V}O_2$max during exercise in most non-athletes and in athletes with mod-

TABLE 9-1. *Maximal oxygen uptake ($\dot{V}O_2$max) of groups of male cross-country skiers who competed at various levels of elite competition.* Values listed are means ± SD.

$\dot{V}O_2$max (L/min^{-1})	$\dot{V}O_2$max (mL·kg^{-1}·min^{-1})	Reference
5.5 ± 0.2	80.1 ± 1.4	Åstrand, 1955
5.6 ± 0.3	82.5 ± 1.5	Saltin & Åstrand, 1967
5.5 ± 0.2	75.0 ± 2.7	Hanson, 1973
6.5 ± 0.5	83.8 ± 6.4	Bergh, 1987
5.7 ± 0.6	78.0 ± 6.9	Bergh & Forsberg, 1992

erately high maximal aerobic power when large muscle groups are involved (Åstrand, 1992). However, in athletes whose $\dot{V}O_2$max values are at least 5 L/min, it has been argued that other links in the oxygen transport system chain, such as the oxygen diffusion capacity of the lungs, may limit $\dot{V}O_2$max (Dempsey & Johnson, 1992; Wagner, 1991).

The mitochondrial capacity of the leg muscles to utilize oxygen normally exceeds the capacity of the central circulation to provide the muscle mass with oxygen (cardiac output times arterial oxygen content) during high-intensity exercise with large muscle groups. As pointed out by Saltin (1986), the calculated maximal potential for blood flow to human muscle during strenuous exercise is approximately 2–2.5 $L \cdot min^{-1} \cdot kg$ muscle^{-1}, but the observed muscle blood flow during such exercise is only 0.3–0.4 $L \cdot min^{-1} \cdot kg$ muscle^{-1}. Furthermore, if the oxygen content of arterial blood is increased, the $\dot{V}O_2$max is increased, and time to exhaustion during intense exercise is prolonged without changing maximal cardiac output (Celsing et al., 1987; Ekblom & Berglund, 1991; Ekblom et al., 1976; Kanstrup & Ekblom, 1984). Thus, it is obvious that most of the oxygen offered by the central circulation (cardiac output times arterial oxygen concentration) during intense exercise is used in the exercising muscles, and, if the oxygen delivery is increased, $\dot{V}O_2$max and aerobic performance are also increased. Thus, maximal cardiac output is the most important factor for determining $\dot{V}O_2$max, even in highly trained cross-country skiers.

Maximal cardiac outputs in excess of 40 L/min and stroke volumes over 200 mL have been measured in skiers who had $\dot{V}O_2$max values greater than 6 L/min (Ekblom & Hermansen, 1968). The maximal heart rates and the arterio-venous oxygen differences of those skiers were similar to those for less successful athletes and non-athletes and could not account for the observed differences in $\dot{V}O_2$max among the different groups. Blood volumes are also high in elite skiers, whereas hemoglobin concentrations are ordinary (Ekblom & Hermansen, 1968).

The simultaneous arm and leg exertion in both classical and freestyle skiing involves large muscle groups. Studies of the influence of the active muscle mass on $\dot{V}O_2$max have shown that adding maximal arm exercise to maximal leg exercise increases $\dot{V}O_2$max by only a small percentage (Bergh et al., 1976; Hermansen, 1973; Secher et al., 1974, 1977). When arm exercise is added to leg exercise, the blood flow to the legs is reduced due to vasoconstriction in the legs (Secher et al., 1977; Jensen-Urstad, 1992). Also, vigorous uphill skiing requires an oxygen uptake only about 3% greater than that required for fast running (Strömme et al., 1977), and there is no difference in $\dot{V}O_2$max between the classic and freestyle techniques when used for maximal uphill skiing (Bergh & Forsberg, 1992a). Thus, the muscle mass used during maximal skiing has a metabolic potential that exceeds the capacity of the central circulation to transport oxygen, confirming once again that the central circulation and the regulation of its distribution are of primary importance for skiing capacity.

According to the concept that oxygen delivery limits $\dot{V}O_2$max, hypoventilation, anemia, or other causes of decreased oxygen content in arterial blood may reduce the $\dot{V}O_2$max of an elite skier and may explain some of the variation in performance during a racing season.

Pulmonary Ventilation

The pulmonary ventilation during maximal aerobic exercise in elite cross-country skiers can be greater than 200 L/min and is much higher than in the average person, but the ventilatory equivalent (ventilation per liter of oxygen uptake) for elite skiers is in the same range as that for other well-trained athletes (Ekblom & Hermansen, 1968).

Muscle Strength

According to unpublished observations from the authors' laboratories, the maximal force development by the legs of elite skiers is only slightly greater than that for the average person. However, in endurance tests, such as 50 consecutive knee extensions, skiers show superior endurance values compared to most other endurance athletes. The importance of arm muscle strength for poling (and skiing performance) is illustrated in Figure 9-2. The maximal isokinetic torque produced by the triceps brachii at π rad/s was first determined in well-trained male and female skiers; the skiers then performed a maximal poling test on roller-skis over 60 m from a standing start. As depicted in Figure 9-2, the 60-m poling time was lowest in subjects who produced the greatest arm torque.

Anaerobic Power

Little attention has been paid to the anaerobic power of cross-country skiers, probably because it has not been considered to be a limiting factor in this particular sport. Cross-country skiers can attain about the same blood lactate concentrations during exercise as the average non-athlete (Åstrand et al., 1963). Other indicators of anaerobic power, such as oxygen deficit and power output during brief (< 1 min) high-intensity exercise, have not been reported for elite cross-country skiers relative to other groups.

SKI RACING

Energy Expenditure

The skier must produce power in order to move forward. This power is used for:

1. overcoming friction between ski and snow

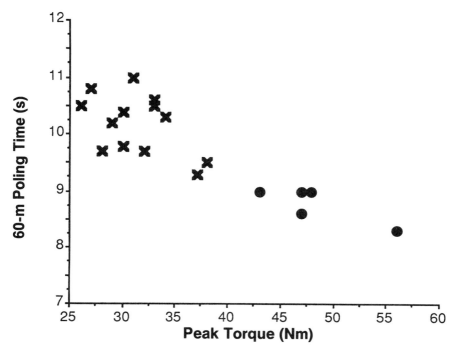

FIGURE 9-2. *Peak isokinetic torque produced at π rad/s by the triceps brachii of well-trained female (X) and male (•) skiers in relation to their times to complete a 60-m double poling test on roller-skis* (unpublished data)

2. elevating the body mass during uphill skiing and during each stride while skiing on level surfaces
3. accelerating the different body segments and the center of mass
4. overcoming air resistance

The relative importance of these energy-consuming processes during skiing is dependent on several factors, such as body composition, type of skiing technique, level of coordination and technique, type of terrain, snow conditions, and racing speed. Hence, quantitative information will only be valid under specific conditions. However, on uphill terrain it is generally true that the cost of elevating the center of the body mass is the dominating factor in determining the energy expenditure. In downhill skiing, the main resistances to forward motion are the friction between the ski and the snow and the air resistance.

To estimate the average metabolic energy cost during a ski race, one can analyze heart rate recordings during the race and blood lactate and core temperature measurements after the race. Core temperatures above

38.8° C after the race indicate an average metabolic energy cost above 75–80% $\dot{V}O_2$max (Saltin & Hermansen, 1966). The average energy expenditure during ski racing 5–30 km is in the range of 90–95% $\dot{V}O_2$max; during the longer ski races, energy cost is some 5–10% lower. There is no reason to believe that genders differ in this respect.

Combining this information with data on maximal oxygen uptake and fractional utilization of oxygen in elite skiers, metabolic rate during racing can be estimated. Such calculations indicate that the metabolic rate of an average male elite skier is about 1.5–2.0 kW during the shorter races. During 50-km or longer races, the metabolic rate is about 10% lower. The total energy cost for a normal 15-km race is about 4–5 MJ; for a 50-km race, the cost is about 13–15 MJ. Corresponding calculations for an average female, who has less body mass to propel, indicates that she uses about 30% less energy than does a typical male for a given distance.

Aerobic Power

Given a constant technical ability, the capacity and effectiveness of the aerobic energy system are the most important determinants of success in ski racing. The relation between $\dot{V}O_2$max and skiing performance during one season is illustrated in Figure 9-3. The skiers with the highest

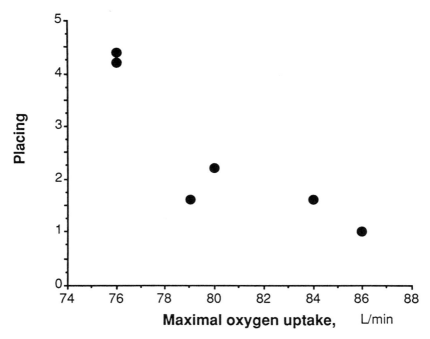

FIGURE 9-3. *Maximal oxygen uptake versus placing (average of the best five results for each skier during January and February, 1972) for six members of the Swedish men's ski team* (modified from Bergh, 1982).

maximal aerobic power have the best ranking over a season, indicating that the probability of winning increases with greater maximal aerobic power. As described later, this does not mean that other factors are of no importance.

Ski racing does not involve large muscle groups all the time. Consequently, the aerobic power attainable during these phases of skiing (e.g., during double poling) will be important. The VO2 max measured during exercise with large muscle groups (e.g., during running) may not mirror $\dot{V}O_2$ max during poling very precisely (Figure 9-4).

The importance of maximal aerobic power in cross-country skiing is illustrated by the heart rates recorded during actual ski races. Figure 9-5 illustrates a profile of the heart rate of a skier who used the classic style during a 21-km ski race. During uphill skiing, the athlete's heart rate was similar to or even exceeded peak heart rate obtained during conventional all-out running on a treadmill. During the downhill segments, heart rate was still only about 20 beats·min^{-1} below maximal, mainly because the strain on the circulation was still high, perhaps because of the requirement to pay back some of the oxygen deficit accumulated during the uphill segment or because, even during downhill racing, poling exercise and some static contractions provide a strain on the circulation.

During level skiing, heart rate averages 10–15 beats/min below maximum; during longer races such as the 50-km, the heart rate is somewhat

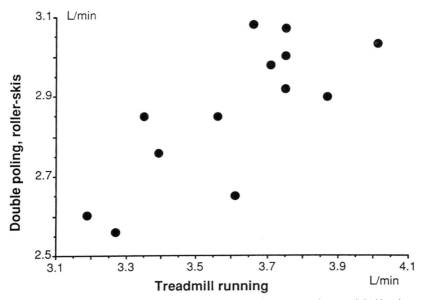

FIGURE 9-4. *Oxygen uptake measured during maximal treadmill running and maximal double poling on roller-skis. The subjects were members of the Swedish junior women's team* (unpublished data)

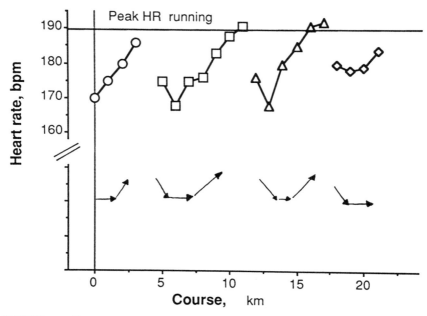

FIGURE 9-5. *Heart rates for the winning skier over various terrains (arrows indicate uphill, downhill, and level terrain) at different stages of a 21-km race in comparison to peak heart rate obtained during a running test (horizontal line at top of graph).* Circles, squares, triangles, and diamonds indicate four different stages of the race (Bergh, 1982).

lower than in the shorter races in the same parts of the track because the intensity of exercise is lower in the longer races.

Endurance

In laboratory tests, endurance is often defined as the time to exhaustion while maintaining a given power output. In contrast, in endurance sports such as cross-country skiing the distance is fixed so that endurance is a function of both maximal aerobic capacity and the ability to utilize a large fraction of that capacity in a sustained manner to cover the required distance in the shortest possible time.

Preparation for a season of skiing competition focuses on improving endurance by increasing maximal aerobic power, especially during exercise that utilizes both the arms and the trunk (Ingjer, 1991), and on increasing the capacity to sustain a high fraction of that aerobic power. As discussed below, training for cross-country skiing is to a large extent focused on long-distance training, often performed on hilly terrain that inevitably varies the load on the muscles and the cardiorespiratory system. A principal aim of such training is to increase capillary density, thereby increasing mean transit time of the blood in the capillaries to enhance the transfer of oxygen, fuels, and metabolites between the capillaries and the muscle tissue. This improves the conditions for nutrition and energy utilization, factors known to be of utmost importance for good endurance. Other important aspects of good endurance are the precompetition nutrition and nutrition during a race, which will be discussed below.

Heat Balance

Because cross-country skiing is often performed in rather cold climates, problems related to cold injuries, breathing problems, and hypothermia might be expected. For the body as a whole, the metabolic heat production during ski racing is usually greater than the heat loss due to convection, conduction, and radiation. Therefore, the skier must sweat to maintain heat balance. During ski races of 15–30 km, the body weight loss, mainly due to sweating, might be 2–3% of body mass. Such dehydration will most likely impair performance in the longer races. Therefore, fluid replacement during races longer than 15–20 km is needed.

Although the heat production during skiing is high, cold injuries to peripheral parts of the body, including fingers, toes, the tip of the nose, and ears, are common during cold weather; high wind velocities, especially during long downhill segments of a course, can be especially dangerous.

Pulmonary ventilation may average 100–150 L/min and increase to more than 200 L/min in some situations. This puts large demands on the airways, because cold air is very dry and must be heated and saturated with water before it reaches the alveoli. Many skiers experience coughing problems after exercise. To avoid local cold injuries and breathing problems, competitions and hard training sessions should be avoided at temperatures below $-20°$ C.

Economy of Movement

It is difficult to establish a value for the mechanical efficiency of cross-country skiing, primarily because external work is affected in a complex manner by factors such as the changing pressure on the skis during each stride, variation in contact area between ski and snow, and variation in the skier's body position. Attempts to calculate mechanical efficiency have resulted in values of about 21% (Niinimaa et al., 1978).

Another way of estimating variability in energy utilization during skiing, i.e., skiing economy, is to compare the oxygen uptakes of different skiers while they ski at given velocities. If the differences among skiers in energy costs for skiing at given velocities are related to ski racing results, it is clear that skiing economy is an important limiting factor in competitive skiing. Åstrand et al. (1963) reported a range of 7% in $\dot{V}O_2 \cdot min^{-1} \cdot kg^{-1}$

during level skiing among members of the Swedish national team, whereas MacDougall et al. (1979) detected even greater differences.

A confounding variable in attempting to produce valid estimates of skiing economy is the method used to compensate for differences in body mass. Traditionally, this is done by dividing the oxygen uptake by body mass. This is likely to underestimate the skill of the light skier because the power needed for skiing increases less than proportionately to body mass (Bergh, 1987; Bergh & Forsberg, 1992b). As yet, it is not possible to suggest a method for equating skiers of different body masses that is valid in all types of terrain.

Given the methodological errors inherent in estimating economy, the real variability in skiing economy among elite skiers is probably less than indicated by the available data. Such potential errors complicate the evaluation of the importance of differences in skiing economy. On one hand, given that differences in $\dot{V}O_2$max among elite competitors are generally small, any real economy differences of 5–10% would seem to be very important for race performances, especially at longer distances. On the other hand, for skiers differing considerably in ability, no significant relationship has been detected between skiing performance and skiing economy measured in a controlled standard manner (MacDougall et al., 1979; Wehlin et al., 1969). Thus, it seems that elite competitors have no distinct advantage as far as skiing economy is concerned. However, in an actual race, the skier uses techniques not included during a test of economy at a controlled, standard, submaximal velocity; thus, the information obtained using standard speeds and movements may not be a valid representation of what occurs during racing conditions. Moreover, the ability to choose the optimal technique for the prevailing conditions during a race may also affect skiing economy. The importance of this quality is presently unknown.

Economy of Different Skiing Techniques

There is good evidence that ski skating is, in general, metabolically more economical than classic skiing. Oxygen uptakes at given velocities are lower during skating than classical skiing (Zupan et al., 1988). Values for heart rate and blood lactate concentration are also lower during ski skating (Hoffman et al., 1990).

There are exceptions to these general trends, including the fact that the classic double poling technique is more economical during level skiing than is ski skating (Hoffman et al., 1990). However, because double poling involves less muscle mass than does ski skating, the strain on the active muscles is higher in double poling. This is consistent with the higher ratings of perceived exertion in the double poling technique.

In general, it is evident that the classic double poling (diagonal) style of skiing is the most costly in terms of metabolic rate and challenge to the cardiorespiratory system. As a result, this technique is now used mostly on uphill terrain. One explanation why ski skating is faster than classic skiing is that velocity changes during the cycle of motion are much smaller during ski skating (Frederick, 1992). Another explanation is that grip wax, which increases frictional drag, is not needed in ski skating. In contrast, skiing velocity is governed by the attainable metabolic power. Skiing styles that require minimal involvement of the legs (such as the skating style) usually cannot elicit maximal oxygen uptake. Hence, an efficient skiing technique may not always be effective if too little power is generated.

Blood Lactate

Another illustration of the high demands on power production in cross-country skiing is the large accumulation of blood lactate during a ski race. For example, in the 1978 World Cup tournaments in Lahti, the average value of blood lactate was 7.8 mM after the men's 15-km race and 8.8 mM after the women's 5-km race, with large interindividual variations. The highest individual values were 13 and 10 mM for men and women, respectively, but lactate concentrations were probably even greater during hilly parts of the course. In longer races, blood lactate levels at the finish are as low as 2–6 mM (Åstrand et al., 1963).

Youth Ski Performance

The importance of developmental maturity for motor fitness and success in skiing was shown in a study by Johansson and Lamberg (1984). They studied young elite skiers in age groups of 11–12 y, 13–14 y, and 15–16 y who participated in a national ski race. Immediately after the race, blood samples were taken for analyses of blood lactate, and both race times and body heights were recorded. The best 10% of the finishers in the 11–12 y and 13–14 y age groups were taller and had higher blood lactate values than did the slower skiers. For the age group 15–16 y, skiing performance was not related to either stature or blood lactate concentration. Thus, differences in maturity, as represented by stature variations, were important factors for the success in the younger, but not in the older age groups. These results are consistent with those reported by Pekkarinen et al. (1989).

One interesting question is whether or not success during the junior years is followed by later success. Over a period of 15 y, there were 22 different winners in the Swedish junior championships. Thirty percent of them became Swedish champions as adults. Among the junior non-winners, only 0.2% won the Swedish championships as adults. Accordingly, winning as a youth is not a very strong predictor of success as an adult; still, young champions are much more likely to succeed as adults than their non-champion counterparts.

NUTRITION FOR CROSS-COUNTRY SKIING

Total Energy Requirements

The energy cost of cross-country skiing is high, e.g., 4–5 MJ for a 15-km race and 13–15 MJ for a 50-km race. During the preparation phase of training, which often includes two daily training sessions, the estimated total energy cost is about 20–25 MJ/d; during training camps, it may be 4–8 MJ higher. To provide adequate energy intake for such a high demand, skiers typically eat three main meals plus small meals after each training session. A carbohydrate-rich meal consumed just before bedtime facilitates restoration of the glycogen stores in muscle and liver.

Quality of the Meal

The glycogen concentration in exercised arm and leg muscles is low or essentially empty in many muscle cells at the end of a ski race or a long training session (Tesch et al., 1978). Thus, a meal rich in carbohydrates is an essential part of an elite cross-country skier's diet. The post-training meal is particularly important because glycogen resynthesis and accumulation in the muscles seems to be faster just after the exercise (Coyle, 1991; Ivy et al., 1988). Unfortunately, most skiers are not hungry immediately after a race.

Of interest to the hard training cross-country skier is that Zawadzki et al. (1992) showed that the post-exercise muscle glycogen concentration can be enhanced above that achieved with a carbohydrate meal when a carbohydrate-protein meat is eaten in place of the carbohydrate. This effect seems to be the result of the interaction of carbohydrate and protein on stimulating insulin secretion.

Racing and prolonged hard training sessions may damage the muscle cells, as indicated by a leakage of proteins and other molecules from Type I fibers (Takala et al., 1989). This may explain why the rate of glycogen resynthesis may sometimes be reduced after exhaustive exercise, especially exercise that extensively involves eccentric muscle actions (Doyle et al., 1993; Widrick et al., 1992). Therefore, it might not always be possible to fully replenish glycogen stores within 24–48 h after hard races and training sessions.

Rehydration and Carbohydrate Replenishment During Skiing

During races, skiers sweat profusely, even in a cold environment. Body mass loss for long ski races may be in the range of 2–4% of initial body mass (Holm et al., 1976). It is a well-known fact that such dehydration can impair physical performance and that rehydration is of great importance for counteracting the negative influence of dehydration. However, rehydration is not the only important factor. During prolonged exercise, as in cross-country skiing, carbohydrate intake will also enhance performance (for references see Coyle & Coggan, 1984; Lamb & Brodowicz, 1986; Maughan, 1991). The mechanism underlying the beneficial effect of carbohydrate feedings on performance is not certain, but it is most likely that the glucose uptake from the blood may contribute considerably to aerobic energy production.

Skiers typically consume 100–200 mL of a 5–10% carbohydrate drink every 10–15 min in races lasting 1 h or longer; the overall rate of carbohydrate intake is roughly equivalent to the minimum of 40–60 g/h suggested by Coyle (1991).

Many athletes in endurance events experience symptoms of central nervous system fatigue (aversion and mental tiredness) during competition and training. It has been suggested that these symptoms are caused by a reduction of the concentration of branched-chain amino acids (BCAA) in the blood, which results in an increased uptake of tryptophan into the brain (Newsholme et al., 1992); tryptophan is converted into 5-hydroxytryptamine (5-HT) in the brain, and 5-HT is associated with sleep onset and depression of mood states. Consistent with the hypothesis that exercise-induced increases in brain 5-HT might adversely affect performance is a report by Bailey et al. (1992) that increased 5-HT concentration in the brains of rats impaired physical performance. Blomstrand et al. (1991) showed in a double-blind study on 196 runners that the group that ran between 180–210 min and ingested BCAA during a marathon race performed 3% better than did the control group. However, there were no significant effects on faster runners.

Vitamins and Minerals

It is common knowledge that vitamin and mineral deficiencies impair general health and human functions and that in most developed countries vitamin deficiencies are rare. Cross-country skiers have high energy intake levels, and because nutrient intakes generally follow energy intakes even when athletes consume no supplements (Blixt, 1965), there is general agreement that skiers consume sufficient nutrients without vitamin or mineral supplements. However, van der Beek (1991) has presented indications that vitamin status may be marginal in athletes engaged in prolonged training programs. This may be caused by a redistribution of vitamin pools in the body consequent to some adaptation to long-term training, rather than by inadequate vitamin intake or increased vitamin requirement. A combination of low bodily stores of thiamin, riboflavin, vitamin B-6, and vitamin C could potentially impair physical performance in an unknown way (van der Beek et al., 1992). It is too early to know whether or not this justifies the recommendation to supplement cross-country skiers engaged in intensive training with these vitamins.

FACTORS PREDICTING PERFORMANCE

There are three main ways to identify factors important to the performance of a given sport:

- to assume that extraordinary characteristics, e.g, a high $\dot{V}O_2$max or great arm strength, of elite competitors are required to achieve success in the sport
- to determine during training or competition the requirements for $\dot{V}O_2$ and other variables that are assumed to be important for performance
- to correlate various types of data obtained in athletes at rest and during exercise with their competitive performance

We have used all three approaches to demonstrate that $\dot{V}O_2$max has a profound influence on competitive skiing performance. In contrast, and contrary to prevailing opinion, there is little information to support the hypothesis that skiing economy is critical to skiing success. Finally, the evidence is quite clear that muscle strength has little bearing on ski racing performance.

In running long distances such as the marathon, performance has been predicted rather accurately from $\dot{V}O_2$max and running economy (Sjödin & Svedenhag, 1985). In skiing, however, it is more difficult to make accurate predictions from such data (Bergh & Forsberg, 1992a). In skiing, factors such as waxing and snow conditions cause excessive variability in the energy costs of movement. As indicated previously, a valid method for determining skiing economy has yet to be determined.

World class skiers have higher values for $\dot{V}O_2$max than do medium class and less successful skiers (Ingjer, 1991), and elite junior skiers exhibit lower $\dot{V}O_2$max values than do elite adult skiers. Although these data illustrate that maximal aerobic power is a dominant factor for success in cross-country skiing, they do not necessarily mean that $\dot{V}O_2$max is a good predictor of the outcome of a race. Thus, the correlation between $\dot{V}O_2$max and race performance may vary considerably from one race to another (Bergh & Forsberg, 1992a), probably as a result of variations in other factors that contribute to performance.

TRAINING

Important characteristics of cross-country skiing, some of which have been previously discussed, include the following:

- energy requirements are met mostly by aerobic metabolism
- oxygen uptake can be taxed maximally, but only with certain techniques of skiing

- the techniques of skiing must be learned
- glycogen stores may be emptied in the longer events
- only an extremely well-conditioned individual can endure the training required to achieve an elite quality of performance

As a consequence of these characteristics, the training should include practices that provide a considerable challenge to the cardiovascular system, activate all muscles used during competitive skiing, improve skiing techniques, and last for hours. Moreover, the amount of training should be increased gradually during the course of each year and from one year to the next; otherwise, there is a considerable risk of overtraining and overuse injuries.

Running and roller-skiing can elicit approximately the same oxygen uptake (Bergh, 1982). In individuals trained for cross-country skiing, either ski-walking (walking up a steep hill using poles to simulate skiing) or cross-country skiing produces a slightly greater oxygen uptake than does running (Hermansen, 1973; Strömme et al., 1977). Roller-skiing has an advantage over running for training the upper body. Training of the arm and trunk muscles is important because these muscles are used in ski poling, which contributes significantly to performance in the classic skiing style. Moreover, individuals who can attain relatively high $\dot{V}O_2$ values during upper body exercise can attain greater $\dot{V}O_2max$ values during combined arm and leg exercise when compared to those with less upper body aerobic capacity (Bergh et al., 1976).

One possible disadvantage of roller-skiing is that the skier can roll quite fast without a high metabolic demand; therefore, the cardiovascular system may not be challenged sufficiently unless the skier makes a compensatory increase in speed. However, skiers typically do not substantially increase their speeds when roller-skiing either on flat or on uphill terrain (Forsberg & Karlsson, 1987). This may suggest that skiers who use mostly roller-skiing in their off-snow training should either use roller-skis with a resistance corresponding to that of snow skiing or roller-ski at faster speeds. The intensity must be such that blood lactate concentrations are elevated over resting values by at least a few mmol/L for most of the training session.

Elite skiers rarely use free weights or resistance training machines to improve muscle strength. However, repeated double poling on roller-skis at maximal speed for 10–30 s is used as strength training, but only for 3–5% of the training time during summer and early fall.

Skiing technique should be learned by snow skiing, because electromyographic recordings show that other activities, e.g., roller-skiing and ski-walking, do not elicit the same patterns of motor unit recruitment that are observed during snow skiing (Petterson et al., 1977). In general, it is preferable to concentrate on technique with youngsters because they learn more easily than adults.

MEDICAL CONSIDERATIONS

Orthopedic Injuries

Orthopedic injuries are fairly uncommon in cross-country skiing. During the summer season, ankle sprains and other injuries from running on roads, paths, and on rough terrain may occur, but these sprains are not specific for cross-country skiing. There is a risk of injuries from falling when roller-skiing; therefore, skiers training on roller-skis should use helmets, knee and elbow braces, gloves, and long clothing that protects legs and arms. Overuse injuries may occur in arms, knees, and the back, but these types of injuries are not specific to skiing and are uncommon in elite skiers.

Internal Medicine Problems

Cross-country skiing puts large demands on the cardiovascular system, but ratings of perceived exertion during skiing are lower at any given power output than during running; the risk for cardiovascular complications in cross-country skiing is similar to that for running (Vuori, 1986). As in all sports, individuals with chronic coronary artery disease (Lehman et al., 1990) or acute diseases should always consult a physician before participating either in races or recreational activity.

Over the years, the biggest problem in elite cross-country skiing has been infections, especially of the upper respiratory tract. Skiers are especially sensitive to these infections because they often train and compete with high pulmonary ventilations in cold, dry climates and are exposed to the viral infections of others in poorly ventilated buildings. Many cross-country skiers report pulmonary problems of an asthmatic type; the use of bronchodilating sprays is very common in skiers.

Immune System. There has been some speculation that prolonged, strenuous physical training and competition might impair the function of the immune system (for references, see Nieman & Nehlsen-Cannarella, 1991). Hours after a prolonged exercise, several immune system variables are depressed (for references, see Heath et al., 1992). Thus, there is the possibility that cross-country skiing may leave participants vulnerable to infections. To address this issue, Berglund and Hemmingsson (1990) studied the incidence of respiratory infections in 53 female and 121 male elite skiers; upper respiratory tract infection was the main reason (75%) given for absence from training or competition in cross-country skiing. There were no differences in the frequency of these infections among hard-training elite skiers, less successful competitive skiers, recreational skiers, and non-athletes. The average time lost was one week in each of these groups. Within each group studied, upper respiratory tract infections were more frequent during the winter, but their incidence was unrelated to the duration or intensity of training.

Anorexia. In all endurance sports, there is a risk that athletes may develop anorexia nervosa. Although most skiers are lean, there is still a real advantage in losing any excess body fat. A skier may be tempted to gain an increase in $\dot{V}O_2max/kg$ body mass through active weight reduction that conceivably could lead to anorectic behavior or to anorexia nervosa. The risk for such a development is greater in female than in male skiers. If an athlete develops anorexia nervosa, $\dot{V}O_2max$ may decrease despite rigorous physical training (Ingjer & Sundgot-Borgen, 1991). It has been estimated that some 15% of elite skiers exhibit anorectic behavior or suffer from anorexia nervosa.

SUGGESTED DIRECTIONS FOR FUTURE RESEARCH

Although research in cross-country skiing has been carried out for many years, many areas of interest should still be investigated. Because most research on cross-country skiing has been conducted on males, more data in all areas of research need to be generated for female skiers.

In both genders, the relative importance of improving anaerobic capacity and/or arm strength needs to be clarified. Furthermore, information about optimal nutrition for skiing is lacking. Studies on different skiing techniques, including metabolic variables as well as biomechanical investigations, are needed to delineate differences in economy among various techniques and among skiers. This is especially true for uphill skiing, in which the relationship between body mass and energy demand has largely been ignored.

SUMMARY

Cross-country skiing, using a variety of techniques, is a dynamic exercise involving a large muscle mass. The energy demand is mainly aerobic, and the cardiovascular system can be taxed maximally during skiing. Therefore, cross-country skiing is an effective mode of endurance training. The elite skier is characterized by an extremely high maximal oxygen uptake, and the skeletal muscles contain predominantly Type I fibers. Body size is typical of the average person of corresponding gender and age. Training is mainly performed by skiing, roller-skiing, and running. The energy demand is very high, and in longer races, the glycogen stores may be emptied. Injuries in cross-country skiing are infrequent, and upper respiratory tract infections are apparently the most common causes of interruptions in training.

BIBLIOGRAPHY

Åstrand, P.O. (1955). New records in human power. *Nature* 176: 922–923.

Åstrand, P.O. (1992). Why exercise? *Med. Sci Sports Exerc.* 24:153–162.

Åstrand, P.O., I. Hallbäck, R. Hedman, and B. Saltin (1963). Blood lactates after prolonged severe exercise. *J. Appl. Physiol.* 18:619–622.

Bailey, S.P., J.M. Davis, and E.N. Ahlborn (1992). Effects of increased brain serotonergic activity on endurance performance in the rat. *Acta Physiol. Scand.* 145:75–76.

Bergh, U. (1982). *Physiology of cross-country ski racing.* Champaign, IL: Human Kinetics Publishers.

Bergh, U. (1987). The influence of body mass in cross-country skiing. *Med. Sci. Sports Exerc.* 19:324–331.

Bergh, U., and A. Forsberg (1992a). Cross-country ski racing. In: R.J. Shephard and P.O. Åstrand (eds.) *Endurance in Sports.* Oxford: Blackwell Scientific Publ., pp. 570–581.

Bergh, U., and A. Forsberg (1992b). Influence of body mass on cross-country ski racing performance. *Med. Sci. Sports Exerc.* 24:1033–1039.

Bergh, U., I.-L. Kanstrup, and B. Ekblom (1976). Maximal oxygen uptake during various combinations of arm and leg work. *J. Appl. Physiol.* 41:191–196.

Berglund, B., and P. Hemmingsson (1990). Infectious disease in elite cross-country skiers: a one-year incidence study. *Clin. Sports Med.* 2:19–23.

Blixt, G. (1965). A study on the relation between total calories and single nutrients in Swedish food. *Acta Soc. Med. Upsala*, 70:117–125.

Blomstrand, E., P. Hassmén, B. Ekblom, and E. Newsholme (1991). Administration of branched-chain amino acids during sustained exercise—effects on performance and on plasma concentration of some amino acids. *Europ. J. Appl. Physiol.* 65:44–149.

Celsing, F., J. Svedenhag, P. Pihlstedt, and B. Ekblom (1987). Effects of anaemia and stepwise-induced polycythemia on maximal aerobic power in individuals with high and low hemoglobin concentrations. *Acta Physiol. Scand.* 129:47–54.

Coyle, E.F. (1991). Carbohydrate feedings: effects on metabolism, performance and recovery. In: F. Brouns et al. (ed.) *Advances In Nutrition and Top Sport.* Basel: Karger, pp. 1–14.

Coyle, E.F., and A.R. Coggan (1984). Effectiveness of carbohydrate feeding in delaying fatigue during prolonged exercise. *Sports Med.* 1:446–458.

Dempsey, J.A., and B.D. Johnson (1992). Demands vs capacity in the healthy pulmonary system. *Schweiz. Z. Sportmed.* 40:55–64.

Doyle, J.A., W.M. Sherman,, and R.L. Strauss (1993). Effects of eccentric and concentric exercise on muscle glycogen replenishment. *J. Appl. Physiol.* 74:1848–1855.

Ekblom, B., and B. Berglund (1991). Effect of erythropoetin administration on maximal aerobic power in man. *Scand. J. Med. Sci. Sports* 1:88–93.

Ekblom, B., and L. Hermansen (1968). Cardiac output in athletes. *J. Appl. Physiol.* 25:619–625.

Ekblom, B., G. Wilson, and P.O. Åstrand (1976). Central circulation during exercise after venesection and reinfusion of red blood cells. *J. Appl. Pysiol.* 40:379–383.

Ekström, H. (1980). Biomechanical research applied to skiing: a developmental study and an investigation of cross-country skiing, alpine skiing and knee ligaments. Linköping studies in science and technology, dissertation no. 53, University of Linköping, Sweden.

Forsberg, A. (1988). Längdskidåkning. In: A. Forsberg and B. Saltin (eds.) Konditionsträning. *Sveriges Riksidrottsförbund*, pp. 246–257.

Forsberg, A., and E. Karlsson (1987). Rullar det för lätt? (Are roller-skis too fast for aerobic training?). *Svensk Skidsport* 7:48–50.

Frederick, E.C. (1992). Mechanical constraints on Nordic ski performance. *Med. Sci. Sports Exerc.* 24:1010–1014.

Frost, P., L. Gabrielsson, and G. Jalderyd (1984). *Kapacitetsanalys av svenska damjuniorer.* (Analysis of racing capacity in Swedish junior female cross-country skiers). Phys. Ed. Thesis Report. 1984:16. Gymnastik- och Idrottshögskolan, Stockholm, Sweden.

Hanson, J. (1973). Maximal exercise performance in members of the US Nordic ski team. *J. Appl. Physiol.* 35:592–595.

Heath, G.W., C.A. Macera, and D.C. Nieman (1992). Exercise and upper respiratory tract infections. Is there a relationship? *Sports Med.* 14:353–365.

Hermansen, L. (1973). Oxygen transport during exercise in human subjects. *Acta Physiol Scand.* (Suppl.) 339.

Hoffman, M.D., P.S. Clifford, P.J. Foley, and A.G. Brice (1990). Physiological responses to different roller skiing techniques, *Med. Sci Sports Exerc.* 22:391–396.

Holm, I., B. Sjödin, J. Nilsson, and A. Forsberg (1976). Muskelfunktionens förändring under vasaloppet (Changes in muscle functions during long distance skiing, the Vasa race). *Svensk Skidsport* 8:27–30.

Ingjer, F. (1991). Maximal oxygen uptake as a predictor of performance in women and men elite cross-country skiers. *Scand. J. Med. Sci. Sports* 1:25–30.

Ingjer, F., and J. Sundgot-Borgen (1991). Influence of body weight reduction on maximal oxygen uptake in female elite athletes. *Scand. J. Med. Sci. Sports* 1:141–146.

Ivy, J.L., A.L. Katz, C.L. Cutter, W.M. Sherman, and E.F. Coyle (1988). Muscle glycogen resynthesis after exercise: effect of time of carbohydrate ingestion. *J. Appl. Physiol.* 64:1480–1485.

Jensen-Urstad, M. (1992). Metabolic and circulatory responses to arm exercise in man. *Opuscula Med.*, Suppl 78 (thesis).

Johansson, G., and E Lamberg (1984). Ungdom på glid. (Youth skiing). Phys. Ed. Thesis Report. 1984. Gymnastik- och Idrottshögskolan, Stockholm, Sweden.

Kanstrup, I.-L. and B. Ekblom. (1984). Blood volume and hemoglobin concentration as determinants of maximal power. *Med. Sci. Sports Exerc.* 16:256–262.

Lamb, D.R., and G.R. Brodowicz (1986). Optimal use of fluids of varying formulations to minimize exercise-induced disturbances in homeostasis. *Sports Med.* 3:247–274.

Lehman, M., G. Huber, and U. Gastman (1990). Heart rates, cardiac arrhythmia, lactate levels and catecholamine excretions in CHD patients during cross-country skiing. *Int. J. Sports Med.* 11:379–382.

MacDougall, J.D., R. Houghson, J.R. Sutton, and J.R. Moroz (1979). The energy cost of cross-country skiing among elite competitors. *Med. Sci. Sports* 11:270–273.

Maughan, R. 1991. Carbohydrate-electrolyte solutions during prolonged exercise. In: D.R. Lamb & M. H. Williams (eds.) *Perspectives in Exercise Science and Sports Medicine, Vol. 4: Ergogenics: Enhancement of Performance in Exercise and Sport*. Indianapolis, IN: Brown & Benchmark, pp. 35–85.

Newsholme, E., E. Blomstrand, and B. Ekblom (1992). Physical and mental fatigue: metabolic mechanisms and importance of plasma amino acids. *Brit. Med. Bull.* 48:477–495.

Nieman, D.C., and S L. Nehlsen-Cannarella (1991). The effects of acute and chronic exercise on immunoglobulins. *Sports Med.* 11:183–201.

Niinimaa, V., M. Dyon, and R.J. Shephard (1978). Performance and efficiency in intercollegiate cross-country skiers. *Med. Sci. Sports* 10:91–93.

Norman, R., G. Caldwell, and P. Komi (1985). Differences in body segment energy utilization between world-class and recreational cross-country skiers. *Int. J. Sports Biochem.* 1:253–262.

Pekkarinen, H.A., A.M. Finne, S.T. Malamäli, and O.O.P. Hanninen (1989). Motor fitness and its relation to body dimensions and growth in young male cross-country skiers and controls. *Scand. J. Sports Sci.* 11:105–111.

Pettersson, L.-G., L. Skogsberg, and U. Zackrisson (1977). Muskelaktivitet under olika träningsformer för längdåkning på skidor. (EMG activity pattern during different training modes for cross-country skiing). Phys. Ed. Thesis, College of Physical Education. Stockholm, Sweden.

Rusko, H. (1976). Physical performance characteristics in Finnish athletes. *Studies in sports, physical education and health no 8*. University of Jyväskylä, Jyväskylä, Finland.

Rusko, H. (1992). Training for cross-country skiing. *Med. Sci. Sports Exerc.* 24:1040–1047.

Saltin, B. (1986). The physiological and biochemical basis of aerobic and anaerobic capacities in man: effects of training and range of adaptation. In: S. Mählum, S. Nilsson, and P. Renström (eds.) *An Update on Sports Medicine. Proceedings from the Second Scandinavian Conference in Sports Medicine*. Oslo: Sofia Moriam, pp. 16–59.

Saltin, B., and P.D. Gollnick (1983). Skeletal muscle adaptability: significance for metabolism and performance. In: L.D. Peachy et al. (eds.) *Handbook of Physiology, section 10: Skeletal Muscle*. Baltimore: Williams and Wilkins, pp. 555–631.

Saltin, B., and L. Hermansen (1966). Esophageal, rectal and muscle temperature during exercise. *J. Appl. Physiol.* 21:1757–1762.

Saltin, B., and P.O. Åstrand (1967). Maximal oxygen uptake in athletes. *J. Appl. Physiol.* 23:353–358.

Secher, N.H., J.P. Clausen, K. Klausen, I. Nore, and J. Trap-Jensen (1977). Central and regional circulatory effects of adding arm exercise to leg exercise. *Acta Physiol. Scand.* 100:288–297.

Secher, N., H. Ruberg-Larsen, R. Binkhorst, and F. Bonde-Pedersen (1974). Maximal oxygen uptake during arm cranking and combined arm plus leg exercise. *J. Appl. Physiol.* 36:515–518.

Sjödin, B., and J. Svedenhag (1985). Applied physiology of marathon running. *Sports Med.* 2:83–99.

Smith, G. A. (1992). Biomechanical analysis of cross-country skiing techniques. *Med. Sci. Sports Exerc.* 24:1015–1022.

Strömme, S.B. , F. Ingjer, and H.D. Meen (1977). Assessment of maximal aerobic power in specifically trained athletes. *J. Appl. Physiol.* 42:833–837.

Takala, T.E., J.I. Vouri, R.J. Rahkila, and E.O. Hakala (1989). Carbonic anhydrase III and collagen markers in serum following cross-country skiing. *Med. Sci. Sports Exerc.* 21:593–597.

Tesch, P., A. Forsberg, and E. Karlsson (1978). Selective muscle glycogen depletion during cross-country skiing. *J. US Ski Coaches Assoc.* 2:12–17.

van der Beek, E.L. (1991). Vitamin supplementation and physical exercise performance. *J. Sport Sci.* 9:77–89.

van der Beek, E.J., W. van Dokkum, J. Schrijver, M. Wedel, A.W.K. Gaillard, A. Weestra, H. vande Weerd, and R.J.J. Hermus (1992). Impact of combined restricted intake of thiamin, riboflavin, vitamin B-6 and vitamin C on functional performance in man. *Am. J. Clin. Nutr.* 48:1351–1362.

Vouri, I. The cardiovascular risks of physical activity. *Acta Med. Scand.*, Suppl. 711:205–214.

Wagner, P.D. (1991). Central and peripheral aspects of oxygen transport and adaptation with exercise. *Sports Med.* 11:133–142.

Wehlin, S., G. Agnevik, B. Sjödin, and B. Saltin (1969). Fysiologiska undersökningar under Engelbrekts-loppet (Physiological studies during the Engelbrekt ski race). *Svensk Idrott* 115-16:1–6.

Widrick, J.J., D.L. Costill, G.K. Mcconell, D.E. Andersson, D.R. Pearson, and J. J. Zachweija (1992). Time course of glycogen accumulation after eccentric exercise. *J. Appl. Physiol.* 72:1999–2004.

Wilmore, J.H. (1983). Body composition in sports and exercise; directions for future research. *Med. Sci. Sports Exerc.* 15:21–31.

Zawadzki, K.M., B.B. Yaspelkis III, and J.L Ivy (1992). Carbohydrate-protein complex increases the rate of muscle glycogen storage after exercise. *J. Appl. Physiol.* 72:1854–1859.

Zupan, M.F., T.A. Shepard, and P.A. Eisenman (1988). Physiological responses to Nordic tracking and skating in elite cross-country skiers (abstract). *Med. Sci. Sports* 20:81.

DISCUSSION

KNUTTGEN: You presented some very interesting data with regard to the oxygen utilization by leg muscles and arm muscles while skiing. In the total race of a particular distance, are there strategies that the racers employ with regard to the relative contribution of legs and arms in the beginning stage, during the middle stage, and while sprinting at the end?

EKBLOM: No, not in the sense that the same plan might work for all courses because there is no "standard" course. The skier uses the technique that is most efficient for the specific portion of the specific course being raced at the time. There can be a change in skiing style after only 5–10 km, or a style can be maintained for several hundred meters. In other words, the skier attempts to optimize arm, leg, and whole body exercise for a specific situation on the specific course. In general, when using the classic skiing style on level terrain, the skier tries to use double poling, which contributes to speed. But this arm activity requires continuous activity of fairly small muscle groups that can become fatigued relatively easily. In a downhill phase, the skier maintains a standing position. There will be a variety of other styles used in uphill phases of the race.

DAVIS: I know you have been working with Eric Newsholme on the central fatigue hypothesis. We have published several papers that suggest rather strongly that elevations in brain serotonin can cause early fatigue during exercise. You refer only to the possibility that raising plasma branched-chain amino acid concentrations might reduce tryptophan uptake into the brain and thereby reduce serotonin synthesis. I believe a better approach is to lower the plasma free-tryptophan concentration with carbohydrate feedings. The increase in plasma free-tryptophan is very large during exercise and can easily be attenuated by carbohydrate feedings. On the other hand, the concentrations of branched-chain amino acids in the plasma change only slightly during exercise. Therefore, the suggestion that athletes should take branched-chain amino acid supplements to reduce central fatigue may not be the best advice, especially because branched-chain amino acids can raise the concentration of ammonia in the blood, and ammonia can also cause early fatigue.

EKBLOM: There may be only a small decline in the concentration of branched-chain amino acids at the start of a race, but the decline may be much greater at the end.

TERJUNG: What are the factors that distinguish the elite skiing performers from those who may eventually become the elite?

EKBLOM: We don't have much data to address this issue very well. However, we know that world class performers in Norway and Sweden have very high values for $\dot{V}O_2$max when expressed in L/min, mL·min^{-1}·kg body mass^{-1}, or mL·min^{-1} × kg body mass$^{2/3}$. The $\dot{V}O_2$max is the best predictor of skiing performance. The number of years of training is also a good predictor of skiing performance. Neither muscle fiber composition nor skiing economy predicts performance very well. Skiers who have high values for $\dot{V}O_2$max as juniors tend to be among the best performers on the national team even 5–10 y later.

TERJUNG: To what extent do you think that technical skill development and proficiency enter into the improvements that are seen between the time when skiers are junior elites and when they later become the senior elite skiers?

EKBLOM: There are certainly small technical improvements that can be made, but it is nearly impossible to tell how well the skier chooses a particular technique over various phases of various courses. Over a series of races, I am convinced that $\dot{V}O_2$max is the most important factor in performance.

GREGG: What is it about cross-country skiing that accounts for the tremendous maximal cardiac outputs achieved by these athletes? There are other sports, e.g., swimming and rowing, that require the use of both upper and lower body masses while training, but neither swimmers nor rowers have the $\dot{V}O_2$max values of cross-country skiers.

EKBLOM: Natural selection may play an important role. Athletes cannot expect to participate in competitive cross-country skiing if they do not start out with $\dot{V}O_2$max values above 65–70 mL/kg. In addition, cross-country skiers train at very high intensities for 700–800 h/y. The standards for training rigor have been increased substantially. This exceptional training load may account for some of the high values for $\dot{V}O_2$max in these skiers. Finally, the combined arm and leg exercises performed at high intensity in an upright posture may enhance maximal cardiac output to a greater extent than the similar exercises of rowers and swimmers in supine or semirecumbent postures.

EICHNER: About a year ago, an article in the journal, *Blood,* reported on a man who had a hematocrit of 68 because he was born in a family supersensitive to erythropoietin. The physicians were worried about the possibility of strokes and heart attacks in this family, but they said the man, now in his fifties, is not only in good health, but has won several gold medals in cross-country skiing. Is it possible that cross-country skiers as a group spend more time at altitude than do swimmers or rowers, which would give skiers greater red cell masses, which could contribute to greater $\dot{V}O_2$max values?

EKBLOM: Nowadays the main issue in training is, How much training at what intensity should be done at what altitude for how many weeks? It is also unknown how long before sea level competition that the athlete should return to sea level. The success of the Norwegian team at the last two international championships has been attributed to their having better athletes who were better trained at high altitude and who had better precompetition preparation. The Norwegian coaches have tried to select the best altitude training scheme for each individual skier. It is safe to say that most international caliber skiers are training almost year-round and spend a lot of time at altitudes of roughly 2,000–2,500 m. However, it is by no means clear that this sojourn at altitude really improves the skiers' $\dot{V}O_2$max values.

GREGG: Why is it that there is such a high correlation between $\dot{V}O_2$max and cross-country skiing performance, when this is not usually true for most other endurance sports?

EKBLOM: I think it is fairly simple. Technique and economy are more important in sports like swimming and rowing than in cross-country skiing, which relies more on raw energy output for a prolonged duration. In other words, the race winner in skiing is going to be the athlete who can produce the most aerobic energy, i.e., the one with the greatest $\dot{V}O_2$max.

HAGERMAN: I should point out that, because rowers do not have to support their body weight, absolute $\dot{V}O_2$ values are more predictive of performance than are values expressed relative to body mass. We find a correlation of about 0.95 between competitive performance and $\dot{V}O_2$ during the last 5 min of an all-out rowing test.

BURKE: I have noticed that cross-country skiers tend to spend more time using the classical style than the skating style, presumably to better maintain their $\dot{V}O_2$ at high levels or to better maintain their cardiovascular conditioning. Why do they seem to like the classical style?

EKBLOM: For most skiers, it is less energetically demanding to maintain a given speed with the classical style than with the skating style. Therefore, it is easier to maintain a high $\dot{V}O_2$ for long periods with the classical style. The skating style is particularly demanding when going uphill; if you lose your speed with the skating style while going uphill, it is much more difficult to regain that speed than it is with the classical style.

KNUTTGEN: How much of a factor in competitive success is the skier's maturity in terms of strategy and reacting appropriately to different conditions? When the elite mature skier and the elite junior skier compete on the same course on five different occasions, the snow texture is different, the temperature is different, and the wind is different. Can it be that the mature skier adjusts better to these changing conditions and, for this reason, has an advantage that contributes to success?

EKBLOM: The mature, experienced skier knows exactly how much he can stress himself without reaching exhaustion too early. The inexperienced skier, for example, can lose 10–20 s during 1 min of an uphill climb because he has pushed himself too far in the earlier stages of the race. The seasoned skier rarely does that.

KNUTTGEN: Is there any evidence that, after the many years of intense aerobic training, the older and more mature elite skier is racing at a higher percentage of his maximal oxygen uptake?

EKBLOM: No one has investigated that idea as far as I know.

KNUTTGEN: You also mentioned that, after many years of training, the respiratory exchange ratio declines at the same relative race speed. Might this greater reliance on fat metabolism help explain how skiers become elite?

EKBLOM: That could be a factor.

BAR-OR: Is there any evidence of co-contraction of agonists and antagonists at any or all terrain profiles during skiing? If this exists, could it be one difference that would separate the more economical skier from the less economical one?

EKBLOM: There are no data available to answer that question.

BAR-OR: You indicated that bronchoconstriction is sometimes a problem in skiers. The high ventilation rates would cause considerable convective cooling of the airway, and the low humidity in the air would result in evaporative cooling. This cooling could play a large role in the bronchoconstriction process. Have skiers tried to use surgical face masks or similar devices to increase the humidification and the temperature of the inspired air?

EKBLOM: Yes, but those available provide excessive resistance to breathing when ventilation rates exceed, for example, 150–200 L/min during uphill skiing. The masks are not efficient enough. Some surveys of cross-country skiers show that more than half of the competitors experience exercise-induced bronchoconstriction. Many of them use $beta_2$ stimulants to counteract bronchoconstriction. I estimate that almost all of the best 10 skiers in the world use these drugs.

HAGERMAN: Our greatest medical problem in rowing is not orthopedic injuries, as one might expect, but serious upper respiratory infections. When the rowers reach national competition levels and the World Championships and Olympic Games, they are living in such close quarters that, if someone develops an infection, it can spread very quickly through the rest of the team. Our worst team performances have occurred when we failed to identify rapidly enough a person with a severe upper respiratory infection, and it spread rapidly to the rest of the team.

BAR-OR: We know that in hot climates people prefer cool beverages during exercise. What is the effect of cold ambient conditions on preferences for a particular temperature of beverages?

EKBLOM: They prefer to drink beverages at temperatures of about 25° C. This seems to allow the skier to consume 150 mL or so of a relatively concentrated carbohydrate drink in a few seconds during a downhill phase of the course. If the drink is too hot or too cold, it cannot be consumed quickly enough to prevent excessive loss of time.

DAVIS: Why do the Scandinavians skiers drink highly concentrated carbohydrate beverages during competition?

EKBLOM: It is very much an individual matter. In addition to a wide variety of sports drinks, there are skiers who drink coffee, soft drinks, and other beverages. In general they tend to use a higher concentration of carbohydrate than do most runners, perhaps because in skiing there is less vertical displacement of the center of gravity with every stride, leading to less gastrointestinal discomfort if the stomach empties slowly.

MURRAY: What can you tell us about the thermoregulatory responses of cross-country skiers? Do they ever experience problems with hyperthermia?

EKBLOM: No. The typical training attire consists primarily of thin "bathing suits." They cool off very quickly in the cool environment. As a matter of fact, there are more problems with frostbite than with hyperthermia.

SPRIET: In ski relays at the World Championships and the Olympics, there are no staggered starts as in the individual events. Thus, two people may be finishing nearly simultaneously in a sprint to the end, as happened in the last Olympics. Would you pick a skier who has demonstrated a good kick in the last several hundred meters to be the anchor of the sprint relay?

EKBLOM: It is obviously important to have a good skier begin the race; if the start is poor, the race will probably be lost. However, as you suggest, most teams generally want to have their best sprinter at the finish.

Index

DATE DUE	
NOV 17 1999	
DEC 15 1999	
JUN 11 2009	